Clinical Presentation of
Ophthalmic
Cases

Clinical Presentation of
Ophthalmic Cases

ML Agarwal MS

Professor Emeritus—Ophthalmology
GR Medical College
Gwalior, MP

Sanjeev Agarwal MS

Professor of Ophthalmology
Regional Institute of Ophthalmology
Gandhi Medical College
Bhopal, MP

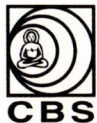

CBS Publishers & Distributors Pvt Ltd

New Delhi • Bengaluru • Chennai • Kochi • Mumbai • Pune
Hyderabad • Kolkata • Nagpur • Patna • Vijayawada

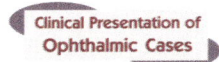

Clinical Presentation of **Ophthalmic Cases**

ISBN: 978-81-239-2293-5

First Edition: 2014

Published by Satish Kumar Jain for
CBS Publishers & Distributors Pvt Ltd
4819/XI Prahlad Street, 24 Ansari Road, Daryaganj, New Delhi 110 002, India.
Ph: 23289259, 23266861, 23266867   Website: www.cbspd.com
Fax: 011-23243014   e-mail: delhi@cbspd.com; cbspubs@airtelmail.in.
Corporate Office: 204 FIE, Industrial Area, Patparganj, Delhi 110 092
Ph: 4934 4934   Fax: 4934 4935   e-mail: publishing@cbspd.com; publicity@cbspd.com

Branches

- **Bengaluru:** Seema House 2975, 17th Cross, K.R. Road,
  Banasankari 2nd Stage, Bengaluru 560 070, Karnataka
  Ph: +91-80-26771678/79   Fax: +91-80-26771680   e-mail: bangalore@cbspd.com
- **Chennai:** 20, West Park Road, Shenoy Nagar, Chennai 600 030, Tamil Nadu
  Ph: +91-44-26260666, 26208620   Fax: +91-44-42032115   e-mail: chennai@cbspd.com
- **Kochi:** 36/14 Kalluvilakam, Lissie Hospital Road, Kochi 682 018, Kerala
  Ph: +91-484-4059061-65   Fax: +91-484-4059065   e-mail: kochi@cbspd.com
- **Mumbai:** 83-C, Dr E Moses Road, Worli, Mumbai-400018, Maharashtra
  Ph: +91-9833017933   e-mail: mumbai@cbspd.com
- **Pune:** Bhuruk Prestige, Sr. No. 52/12/2+1+3/2 Narhe, Haveli
  (Near Katraj-Dehu Road Bypass), Pune 411 041, Maharashtra
  Ph: +91-20-64704058, 64704059, 32392277   Fax: +91-20-24300160   e-mail: pune@cbspd.com

Representatives

- **Hyderabad** 0-9885175004   • **Kolkata** 0-9831437309, 0-9051152362
- **Nagpur**   0-9021734563   • **Patna**   0-9334159340
- **Vijayawada** 0-9000660880

Printed at: R P Printers, Noida

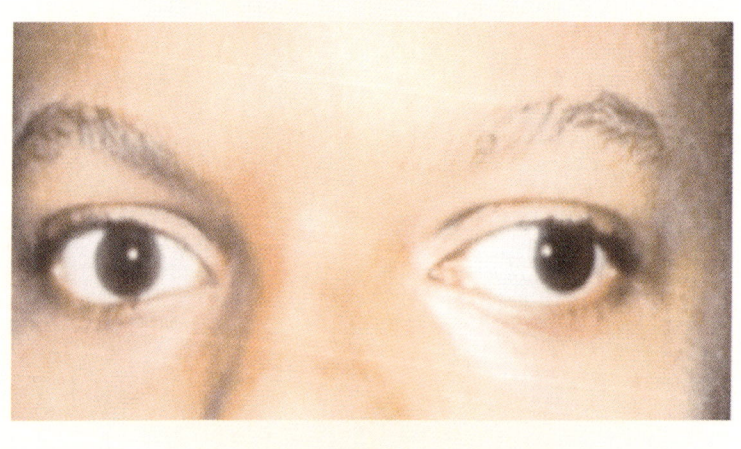

Preface

Medical graduates enter the medical course after scoring very high percentage in pre-medical test by devotional staking their 100% intelligence and diligence foregoing all kinds of extramural activities that are close to their heart to live only one life graced to them and all of us by the creator. All the entrants feel proud to enter the medical fraternity.

Undergraduate and postgraduate medical students are taught theory by lectures and clinical examination of cases by demonstration with case presentation and discussion in out-patient and in-patient department by faculty members on each subject independently.

While all the students do attend the theory classes and practical clinics regularly, yet some students do fail.

This gives rise to the question: Why do the students fail in undergraduate or even postgraduate examinations?

To our mind it is because of the voluminous, strenuous and overburdened course books which cover much more than what they need either at the undergraduate or postgraduate level. All the teachers and faculty members should impart practical knowledge more rather than overburden them and their minds with theoretical and specialized books most of which are merely reference books dealing with all the common and uncommon maladies in detail that are of no use in day-to-day clinical practice even in institutions.

We had felt and still feel that the course books must stick to basic course and faculty should inculcate clinical aptitude to examine the case with patience and care to win confidence and cooperation, and present and discuss the case with faculty and among themselves as required at the undergraduate and postgraduate levels, and later at their clinics or institutions to earn name and fame.

Most of the students do prepare their own notes in concise and point-wise *poetic format* to help them imbibe and reproduce the *prosaic material* to secure high percentage and rank. This book entitled *Clinical Presentation of Ophthalmic Cases* presents the ophthalmic cases in a *poetic format* which will help the student understand, retain and present the maladies easily in theory and practical examinations.

Students can add other clinical features in this book if they feel necessary and as per their own mindset. It shall save their precious time in preparing their own notes in *point-wise poetic composition* that assures them to secure good rank.

ML Agarwal
E-mail: mlapla@rediffmail.com

Sanjeev Agarwal
E-mail: Sanjnino2122@yahoo.com

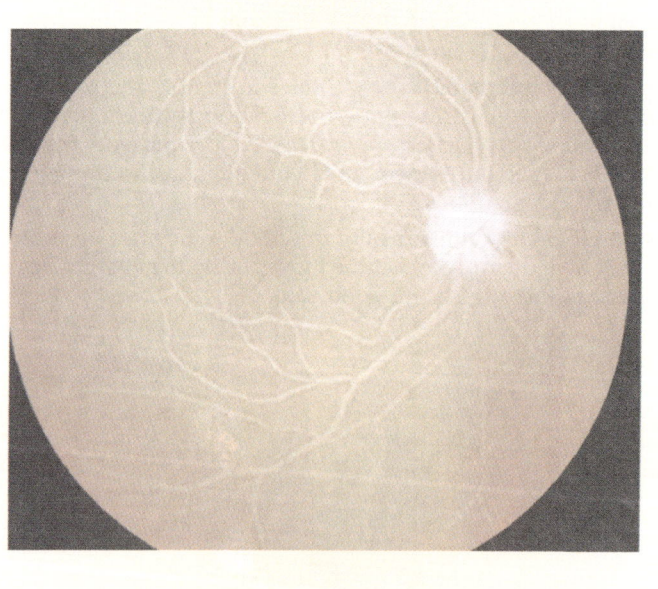

Contents

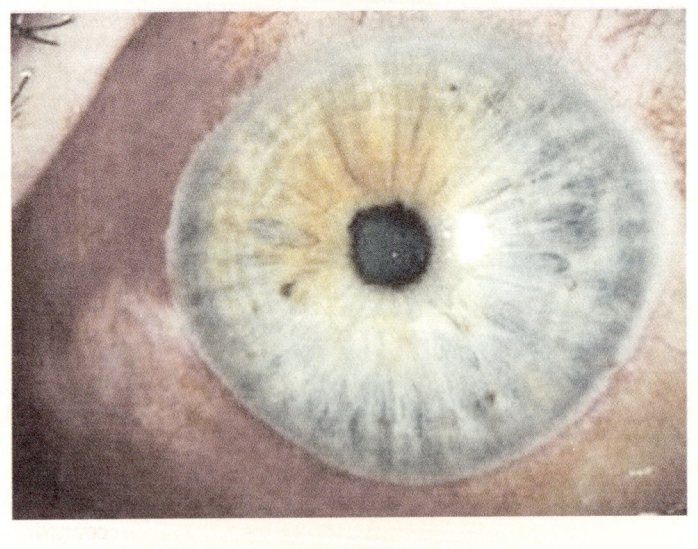

1

Anatomy of Eye

Embryology

- Optic plate • Optic vesicle • Optic cup • Embryonic fissure • Lens • Retina and pigmentary epithelium • Ciliary body, iris and all other structures and • Lids.

Anatomy

- Orbit
- Superior orbital (sphenoidal) fissure
- Inferior orbital (sphenomaxillary) fissure
- Orbital canals
- Orbital spaces
- Orbit and paranasal sinuses
- Lids
- Lacrimal apparatus
- Conjunctiva
- Cornea
- Sclera
- Uveal tract
- Ciliary body
- Choroid
- Anterior chamber
- Posterior chamber
- Lens
- Vitreous
- Retina
- Optic disk
- Macula lutea
- Fovea
- Optic nerve
- Extrinsic ocular muscles
- Arterial supply
- Venous drainage
- Nerve supply of the eye
- Ciliary ganglion

EMBRYOLOGY

- Eye develops from mesoderm and ectoderm.
- Ectoderm is derived from a neural tube, neural ectoderm and from the ectoderm of the surface of the body.
- *Optic plate:* Thickening appears on either side of the neural tube in its anterior part. This optic plate grows towards the surface to form the *optic vesicle.*
- Eyes develop from these two *optic vesicles* and the surface ectoderm and mesoderm in contact with the optic vesicles.
- *Optic vesicles* invaginate from below to form the *optic cups.*
- Line of invagination remains open for sometime as an *embryonic fissure* through which the hyaloid artery enters to provide nutrition to the developing structures. Later the hyaloid artery atrophies and disappears.
- *Surface ectoderm* invaginates and separates to form the *lens.*
- Inner layer of the optic cup forms the *main retina* and the outer layer of the optic cup develops into the *pigmentary epithelium.*
- Neural ectoderm secretes jelly-like structures, the *vitreous* which fills the cavity of the cup.
- Anterior portions of the optic cup and mesoderm surrounding it develop into the *ciliary body and iris.*
- Mesoderm around the optic cup differentiates to form the coats of the eye, orbital

structures, angle of the anterior chamber and main structure of the cornea.

- Surface ectoderm forms the *corneal and conjunctival epithelium*.
- Mesoderm in front of the cornea grows in folds which unite and separate to form the *lids*.

ANATOMY

Orbit

The orbit is a quadrilateral pyramid whose base is formed by the orbital margin and the apex by the optic foramen. Each orbit is formed by the following seven bones (Fig. 1.1):
1. Frontal
2. Ethmoid
3. Lacrimal
4. Palatine
5. Maxilla
6. Zygomatic
7. Sphenoid—greater and lesser wings.

Contents of the Orbit

1. Eyeball
2. Extraocular muscles
3. Lacrimal gland
4. Loose connective tissue
5. Fat, fascia, blood vessels and nerves.

Orbit communicates with the cranial cavity through the following three openings and transmits structures:
  i. Superior orbital fissure
 ii. Inferior orbital fissure
iii. Optic foramen and canal.

Superior Orbital (Sphenoidal) Fissure

The superior orbital fissure (Fig. 1.2) is formed by a gap between the lesser and greater wings of the sphenoid bone. It lies between the roof and the lateral wall of the orbit. It is 22 mm long. It is the largest communication between the orbit and the middle cranial fossa.

It transmits the following ten structures:

1. Lacrimal nerve
2. Frontal nerve
3. Trochlear nerve
4. Superior ophthalmic vein
5. Recurrent lacrimal artery
6. Superior division of oculomotor nerve
7. Nasociliary nerve and sympathetic root of ciliary ganglion

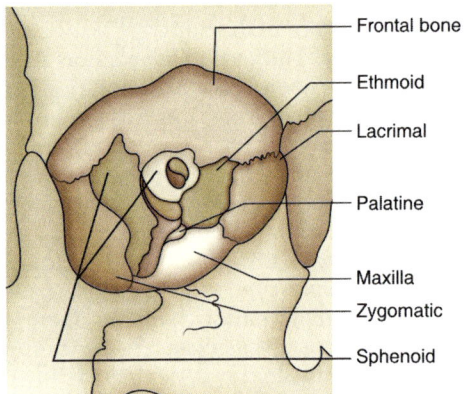

Fig. 1.1: Seven bones of orbit

Frontal bone
Ethmoid
Lacrimal
Palatine
Maxilla
Zygomatic
Sphenoid

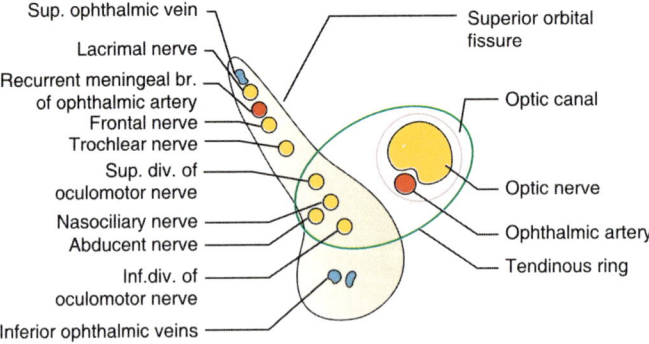

Sup. ophthalmic vein
Lacrimal nerve
Recurrent meningeal br. of ophthalmic artery
Frontal nerve
Trochlear nerve
Sup. div. of oculomotor nerve
Nasociliary nerve
Abducent nerve
Inf. div. of oculomotor nerve
Inferior ophthalmic veins
Superior orbital fissure
Optic canal
Optic nerve
Ophthalmic artery
Tendinous ring

Fig. 1.2: Superior orbital fissure

8. Inferior division of oculomotor nerve
9. Abducent nerve
10. Sometimes the inferior ophthalmic vein.
   The lateral rectus muscle originates from both the margins of the fissure.

Inferior Orbital (Sphenomaxillary) Fissure

It is a gap between the lateral wall and floor of the orbit. Through this fissure, the orbit communicates with the pterygopalatine and infratemporal fossa. It is about 20 mm in length.

It transmits the following four structures:
1. Infraorbital nerve
2. Zygomatic nerve
3. Branches to the orbital periostium from the pterygopalatine ganglion.
4. A communication between the inferior ophthalmic vein and the pterygoid plexus.

Orbital Canals

Anterior ethmoidal canal opens in the anterior cranial fossa near the side of cribriform plate of the ethmoid. It transmits the anterior ethmoidal nerve and artery.

Posterior ethmoidal canal transmits the posterior ethmoidal nerve and artery.

Optic foramen and optic canal transmit the optic nerve with its coverings (dura, arachnoid and pia) and the ophthalmic artery embedded in the dural sheath of the optic nerve. The distance between the two orbital openings of the optic canal is 30 mm. The distance between the two cranial openings of the optic canal is 25 mm.

Orbital Spaces

There are four surgical self-contained spaces in the orbit. The inflammatory process remains confined to its own space for a long time before it spreads to other spaces.
1. Subperiosteal space
2. Peripheral orbital space
3. Central space
4. Tenon's space

Subperiosteal space It lies between the orbital bones and the periorbita. Periorbita is loosely attached to the underlying orbital bones

except at the orbital margin, orbital fissures, foramen and at the lacrimal fossa. The loose attachment permits collection of exudates, blood and pus in this space. The periorbita is very sensitive as it is supplied by the trigeminal nerve. Due to this, there is severe pain, if this space is involved in any inflammatory process.

Peripheral orbital space It lies between the peri-orbita and the extraocular muscles with their facial expansions. The exudates in this space are discharged through the septum orbitale.

Central space It is a closed space between the muscle cone, the intermuscular membrane and the Tenon's capsule. Any lesion in this space leads to proptosis. The common lesion is the optic nerve glioma.

Tenon's space It is a potential space between the Tenon's capsule and the sclera. It is very sensitive. Any inflammatory lesion causes pain especially on the movement of the eyeball.

Orbit and Paranasal Sinuses

The orbit is surrounded by cranial cavity, nasal cavity and three sinuses:
1. Ethmoidal sinus
2. Frontal sinus
3. Maxillary sinus.

   All of these are bad neighbors and are always keen to encroach upon the integrity of orbit by way of infection and extension of tumor.

   Considering all the above anatomical features, any increase in the contents of the orbit by growth or edema is likely to produce proptosis, displacement of globe, diplopia and pain.

Eyelids

Eyelids (Fig. 1.3) are two movable folds in front of the orbit. Lids present:
- Upper and lower *palpebral furrow.*
- *Naso-jugal and malar sulcus* beyond the lower orbital margin.
- Upper eyelid just covers the upper part of the cornea and the lower eyelid is just below the lower margin of the cornea.

- Upper eyelid is much more movable due to especial elevator muscle—*levator palpebrae superioris.*
- Space between the two lids, when the eyes are open, is known as the *palpebral aperture or fissure.*
- Outer angle of the palpebral fissure is known as *outer canthi that are acute and very close to the eyeball.*
- Inner angle of the palpebral fissure is known as *inner canthi* that are rounded and separated from the globe by the *lacus lacrimalis* (tear lake).
- In this area of *lacus lacrimalis*—the tear lake, there is an elevation called as *caruncle* and a semilunar fold known as *plica semilunaris.*
- Margin of each lid is about 2 mm broad and each lid has an anterior and a posterior border.
- Anterior border is rounded with two or three rows of eyelashes.
- Posterior border is sharp and close to the eyeball that helps in drainage of tear fluid and polishing of the corneal surface. The orifices of the meibomian glands open just in front of the posterior border of the lids.
- At the medial end of the lid border, there is a small elevation known as *lacrimal papilla* with *punctum.*
- Shape and the size of the eyes depend on the axis and the width of the *palpebral fissure.* Normally, the axis shows a slope upwards and laterally. The outer canthus is about 2 mm above the inner canthus. Normally, the width of the palpebral fissure is about 15 mm. The eyes having a large width of palpebral fissure appear prominent and seductive. The eyes having a small width of the fissure appear small in size.

Lid consists of the eight structures:

i. Skin
ii. Areolar tissue
iii. Muscles:
- Levator palpebrae superioris
- Orbicularis oculi
- Muller's muscle (palpebral muscle)
iv. Tarsal plate
v. Conjunctiva
vi. Glands
- *Meibomian gland:* Meibomian glands are sebaceous glands situated in the tarsal plate and are about 20 to 25 in each lid. These are arranged vertically in the tarsal plate and their orifices open just in front of the posterior border of the lid. Infection of the meibomian gland manifests as *chalazion.*
- *Zeis gland:* Zeis gland is a sebaceous gland associated with cilia. These are acinous glands like meibomian glands but much smaller in size. Each gland opens into the follicle of a cilium by a short wide duct. They are filled with sebaceous material. The inflammation of zeis gland manifests as *stye.*
vii. Blood vessels:
- Arterial supply is by the medial and lateral branches of ophthalmic and lacrimal arteries.
- Venous drainage is through the ophthalmic vein.
viii. Nerves:
- Seventh cranial nerve supplies *orbicularis oculi.*
- Third cranial nerve supplies *levator palpebrae superioris.*
- Sensory supply is by the first division of the fifth cranial nerve.

Lacrimal Apparatus

Lacrimal apparatus (Fig. 1.4) involves:
- Lacrimal glands
- Accessory lacrimal glands
- Lacrimal drainage system

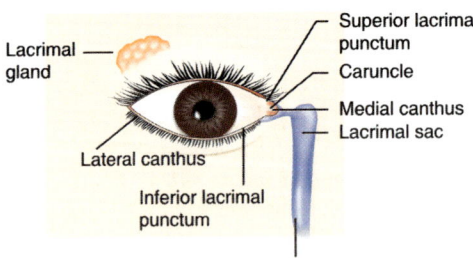

Fig. 1.3: Eyelids

Lacrimal Glands

There are two lobes of the lacrimal gland:

- *Large superior lobe* of the lacrimal gland is lodged in the *lacrimal fossa* which lies in the anterior and outer part of the root of the orbit.
- *Small inferior lobe* of the lacrimal gland lies just above the outer part of the upper fornix of the conjunctiva.

Lacrimal gland secretes lacrimal or tear fluid: The ducts from both the lobes empty the tear fluid into the lateral part of the superior conjunctival fornix.

The gland derives its vascular supply from the lacrimal artery.

The nerve supply is from three sources, namely (i) the lacrimal nerve, (ii) the great superficial petrosal nerve, and (iii) the sympathetic nerve.

Accessory Lacrimal Glands

There are four accessory glands:

i. Krause's glands
ii. Wolfring's glands
iii. Infraorbital glands
iv. Glands in the caruncle and plica semilunaris.

Lacrimal Drainage System

The lacrimal drainage system consists of the following structures.

i. Lacrimal punctum
ii. Lacrimal canaliculi
iii. Lacrimal sac
iv. Nasolacrimal duct

1. Lacrimal Punctum

- Lacrimal punctum is situated on the lacrimal papilla.
- Each punctum appears as a small opening which may be round or oval in shape.
- Upper punctum is about 6 mm and lower punctum is about 6.5 mm from the inner canthus.
- Normally, the punctum is not visible unless the lid is slightly everted.

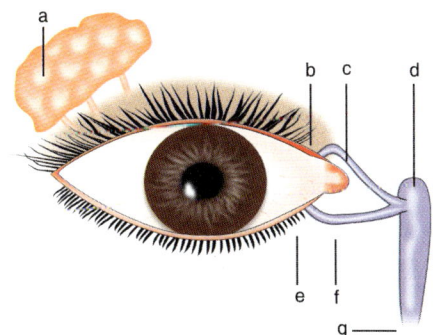

Fig. 1.4: Lacrimal apparatus (a: lacrimal gland; b, e: punctum; c, f: canaliculi; d: sac; g: nasolacrimal duct)

- With each blink, the punctum glides in the lacus lacrimalis and the lacrimal fluid is sucked into the canaliculi.
- Orbicularis oculi muscle plays an important role in this phenomenon of drainage of tear fluid.

2. Lacrimal Canaliculi

- Each lacrimal canaliculus has two parts: *Vertical and horizontal.*
- Vertical part is about 2 mm in length and thereafter it bends at right angle to form the horizontal part which is about 8 mm in length.
- Each canaliculus runs medially piercing the lacrimal sac fascia separately and thereafter unites to open in a small diverticulum of the sac—the *lacrimal sinus of Maier.*
- Internal common punctum opens in the sac at about 2.5 mm from the fundus of the sac.

3. Lacrimal Sac

- Lacrimal sac lies in the lacrimal sac fossa formed by the frontal process of the maxilla and lacrimal bone at the lower part of the medial orbital margin.
- Anterior lacrimal crest on the frontal process of the maxilla forms the anterior boundary of the lacrimal sac fossa.
- Posterior lacrimal crest of the lacrimal bone forms the posterior boundary of the lacrimal sac fossa.

- Lacrimal sac fossa is about 14 mm in length and about 6.5 mm in breadth.
- Upper part of the fossa is in relation to the anterior ethmoidal cells.
- Lower part of the fossa is in relation to the middle meatus of the nose, therefore, in the operation of the dacryocystorhinostomy, the ostium is created in the lower part of the lacrimal sac fossa to establish a communication between the lacrimal sac and the nose for artificial drainage of tear fluid in the nose.

4. Nasolacrimal Duct

- Nasolacrimal duct extends from the lacrimal sac fossa to the inferior meatus of the nose.
- Duct is formed by the three bones, namely: (i) maxilla, (ii) lacrimal bone, and (iii) lacrimal process of the inferior turbinate.
- Upper opening is formed by the *hammulus of the lacrimal bone.*
- Lower opening is in the inferior meatus of the nose.
- Average length of the duct is about 12.4 mm and the average breadth is about 4.6 mm.
- Surface anatomy of the nasolacrimal canal is a straight line drawn on face running from the middle of the medial palpebral ligament to the base of ala nasi.
- Most common affection of the nasolacrimal duct is the congenital block in the infants who show watering of the eye since birth.

Conjunctiva

Conjunctiva has three layers:

 i. Conjunctival epithelium
 ii. Adenoid layer or layer of loose connective tissue
iii. Fibrous layer.

Conjunctiva is divided into three parts:

1. Palpebral conjunctiva
2. Bulbar conjunctiva
3. Fornix.

Palpebral Conjunctiva

- Palpebral conjunctiva commences from the anterior margin of the lid to the posterior margin and thereafter lines the tarsus.
- It is firmly attached to the underlying tarsus, therefore, in any inflammation of the conjunctiva, there is swelling of the lids.

Bulbar Conjunctiva

- Bulbar conjunctiva covers the sclera.
- It is loosely attached to the sclera, therefore, any inflammation of the conjunctiva manifests as *chemosis*—the edema of the conjunctiva.

Fornix

The loose fold which unites the palpebral conjunctiva to the bulbar conjunctiva is known as *fornix*. It is loose, therefore, it allows free movement of the eyeball in all the directions.

Transitional zone of the conjunctiva is at two places:
1. From the anterior margin of the lid to the posterior margin and for 2 mm beyond on the tarsus.
2. Near the limbus.

This transitional zone of the conjunctiva has character of both the skin and the conjunctiva, therefore, it is a common site for occurrence of squamous cell carcinoma.

Blood Supply

- Posterior conjunctival vessels from the lids.
- Anterior conjunctival vessels are branches of the posterior ciliary arteries coming from the muscle branches.

Nerve Supply

- Infratrochlear nerve
- Ciliary nerve
- Lacrimal nerve

Cornea

Cornea has five layers:

1. Stratified squamous epithelium.
2. Bowman's membrane (anterior limiting lamina).

3. Substantia propria.
4. Descemet's membrane (posterior limiting lamina).
5. Endothelium:

- Cornea is the anterior part of the outer coat of the eyeball.
- Cornea is transparent and has more curvature than the rest of the eyeball.
- Cornea appears elliptical of about 12 mm in the horizontal meridian and 11 mm in the vertical meridian.
- Radius of curvature of the anterior surface is about 7.8 mm and that of posterior surface is about 6.5 mm in adult males. *These radii are for the central optical zone of the cornea.*
- Cornea is more flat in the periphery. The cornea is 1 mm thick at the periphery and 0.58 mm at the central optical zone.
- Cornea is avascular and gets its nutrition from the air, aqueous humor and diffusion of tissue fluid from the perilimbal capillaries.
- Cornea is very sensitive and supplied by the *first ophthalmic division of fifth cranial nerve.*
- Transparency of the cornea depends on its state of hydration which is controlled by the endothelium. Any change in the state of hydration results in edema of the cornea.
- Transparency of the cornea is also related to the regularity of the stromal components. Any change in the regularity of stromal components gives rise to opacity of the cornea which varies in its density depending on the extent of corneal stroma involved.

Sclera

Sclera forms the posterior five-sixths of the eyeball.

- Sclera is fibrous and protective.
- Its anterior portion is visible and known as *white of the eyeball.*
- It is about 1 mm thick in its posterior part and becomes thin gradually in its anterior part. It is very thin about 0.3 mm at the site of insertion of extraocular muscles.
- The sclera is covered by the Tenon's capsule and conjunctiva with loose areolar tissue in between the two layers.
- All the extra ocular muscles are inserted in the sclera.
- Sclera is almost avascular, therefore, its diseases are chronic in nature.

Lamina Cribrosa

- Optic nerve pierces the sclera at 3 mm to the inner side and just above the posterior pole of the eyeball.
- At this site, the sclera becomes a thin sieve-like membrane known as *lamina cribrosa.* The axons of the ganglion cells of the retina pass through lamina cribrosa in the form of optic nerve.

Posterior apertures in the sclera are situated around the optic nerve and allow the long and short ciliary nerves and vessels to enter the eyeball.

Middle apertures in the sclera are situated 4 mm behind the equator of the eyeball and allow exit to the vorticose veins and some lymphatics. The vorticose veins drain the blood from the choroid.

Anterior apertures in the sclera are situated in the ciliary zone and allow the anterior ciliary vessels to enter the eyeball.

Episcleral tissue: Episcleral tissue is loose connective and elastic tissue covering the sclera.

- It is thin behind the insertion of ocular muscles and thick and vascular in front of the insertion of the ocular muscles.
- There is a capillary network in the anterior zone which is known as *circumciliary congestion.* It is visible in certain diseases of cornea and uveal tissue.

Limbus

- *Cornea is set into the sclera like a* watch-glass *so that the sclera overlaps the cornea all around in the periphery.*

- Junction of these two tissues is known as *limbus*. There is a minute arcade of blood vessels about 1 mm broad at the limbus.
- Cornea gets its nutrition partly from the diffusion of tissue fluid from these peri-limbal capillaries.

Uveal Tract

Iris

- *Iris is a colored circular diaphragm with an aperture in the center of the* pupil.
- Iris divides the space between the posterior surface of the cornea and the anterior surface of the lens into two parts—*anterior and posterior chamber* of the eyeball.
- Pupil regulates the entry of light in the eyeball by virtue of its power to constrict and dilate.
- Color of the iris depends on the pigment in the stromal cells of the iris.

Iris consists of:
- Spongy connective tissue
- Stroma containing branched pigmented cells
- Plain muscle fibers
- Rich supply of vessels and nerves.

Iris is covered anteriorly by the *endothelium* and posteriorly by the double layer of *pigmented epithelium*.

Iris has two plain muscles—the *sphincter and dilator pupillae*.

- *Sphincter pupillae* muscle is a narrow circular band of about 1 mm wide surrounding the pupil and supplied by the oculomotor nerve and causes constriction of the pupil.
- *Dilator pupillae* muscle consists of radial fibers which extend from the ciliary body to the pupillary margin and supplied by the sympathetic nerve fibers and causes dilation of the pupil.

Iris has a *collarette* which demarcates the iris into two portions—the pupillary and ciliary zones which differ in color.

There are pit-like depressions near the collarette and the root of the iris known as *crypts* which allows free flow of aqueous fluid out and in during the act of contraction and dilation of the pupil.

Blood supply Iris is supplied by the *long posterior and anterior ciliary arteries*. The branches of these vessels anastomose freely at the root of the iris to form the *circulus arteriosus iridis major*. The radial branches arise from this and run towards the pupil. Near the pupil, there are arterial and venous anastomoses which form the *circulus vasculosus iridis minor*. The course of these radial branches is sinuous as these become straight, when the pupil constricts and wavy, when the pupil dilates.

Nerve supply Iris is richly supplied by the nerve fibers through the ciliary plexus.

- Sensory nerve fibers are derived from the trigeminal nerve.
- Motor nerve fibers derived from the oculomotor nerve supply the sphincter pupillae muscle.
- Motor fibers derived from the cervical sympathetic chain supply the dilator pupillae muscle.

Ciliary Body

- *Ciliary body forms a ring which is about 5.9 mm on the nasal side and 6.7 mm on the temporal side.*
- Ciliary body starts from the *ora serrata*.
- Easily recognized by its black color in comparison to the choroid which is brown in color.
- Part of the ciliary body just beyond the ora serrata is smooth, therefore, it is known as *pars plana*.
- Region of the ciliary processes is known as *pars plicata*.

Ciliary body has six layers from without inwards:

i. Suprachoroidal lamina
ii. Ciliary muscle
iii. Ciliary processes
iv. Basal lamina and stroma
v. Epithelium
vi. Internal limiting membrane.

Ciliary Processes

Function of the ciliary processes is to secrete the aqueous. In cyclitis, due to fibrosis, the ciliary processes are atrophied, thereby there is no secretion of aqueous which results in soft eyeball, i.e. low intraocular pressure.

Action of Ciliary Muscle

In the act of accommodation, the ciliary muscle slackens the suspensory ligaments of the lens. The slackening of the ligament causes decreased tension on the capsule of the lens, therefore, the lens becomes more convex due to increase in its anterior curvature. The increased curvature of the lens increases the refractive power of the lens, thereby the near objects are seen clearly.

Blood supply Ciliary body receives its blood supply from the following sources:

1. Branches from the circulus iridis major
2. Branches from the long posterior ciliary arteries
3. Branches from the anterior ciliary arteries.

Nerve supply Ciliary body is richly supplied by the following nerve fibers:

- Sensory nerve fibers from the trigeminal nerve
- Motor fibers from the oculomotor and sympathetic nerves.

Choroid

- Choroid is a vascular layer between the sclera and retina and it extends from the ora serrata to the aperture of the optic nerve in the sclera.
- Choroid is loosely attached with the sclera leaving a potential *epichoroidal space* for detachment of choroid.
- Choroid consists mainly of blood vessels and connective tissue containing pigmented cells bounded by the membrane on either side.

It has five layers from without inwards:

1. Lamina suprachoroid (lamina fusca)
2. Layer of large blood vessels (Mailer's layer)
3. Layer of medium size blood vessels (Battler's layer)
4. Choriocapillaries
5. Basal lamina (membrane of Bruch)
   - Choroid is a vascular layer, therefore, it provides nutrition to the retina.
   - Choroid is drained by the vorticose veins.
   - Choroid is supplied with the sensory nerve fibers from the trigeminal nerve and autonomic nerves of vasomotor function.

Anterior Chamber

- Anterior chamber is a space bounded in front by the cornea and behind by a strip of the anterior surface of the ciliary body, iris and lens in the pupillary area.
- Diameter of the anterior chamber varies from 11.3 to 12.4 mm.
- Anterior chamber is about 3 mm deep in the central part and becomes shallow in the periphery.

Anterior chamber is deep in:

- Young age
- Myopes
- Total posterior synechia
- Aphakia

Anterior chamber is shallow in:

- Hypermetropia
- Angle-closure glaucoma.

Its peripheral recess is known as *angle of the anterior chamber.*

Angle of Anterior Chamber

- Peripheral recess of the anterior chamber is known as *angle of the anterior chamber. It is bounded anteriorly by the corneosclera and posteriorly by the root of the iris and ciliary body.*
- In the inner layers of the sclera at this part, there is a venous sinus called the *canal of Schlemm.* The aqueous is drained through this canal. The recess is formed by the *trabecular tissue.*

- Angle can be only visualized by gonioscopy.

Posterior Chamber

- Posterior chamber is a triangular space.
- Apex is formed by the edge of the iris which rests on the lens.
- Base is formed by the ciliary processes.
- Posterior wall is formed by the anterior surface of the lens and anterior zonular fibers.
- Anterior wall is formed by the posterior surface of the iris.

Lens

- Lens is a transparent biconvex lens with a capsule.
- It is situated between the iris and vitreous.
- It has two surfaces, two poles and equator.
- Curvature of the anterior surface is about 10 mm while that of the posterior surface is 6 mm.
- It is suspended by the suspensory ligaments to the ciliary body.
- Lens matter is plastic in nature while the lens capsule is elastic in nature. This property helps the lens to change its curvature in the act of accommodation.
- Anterior capsule of lens is lined by epithelium. There is no epithelium on the posterior capsule.
- Lens derives its nutrition from the aqueous humor.

Vitreous

- Vitreous is a transparent, colorless and avascular gel of semisolid consistency.
- Vitreous fills the posterior two-thirds volume of the eyeball behind the lens.
- Vitreous takes the shape of the eyeball.
- Vitreous has a saucer-shaped depression (*pateliar fossa*) in front for accommodating the crystalline lens. There is a weak adherence of the vitreous with the posterior surface of the lens in a ring form of about 8.9 mm in diameter, known as the *hyaloideocapsular ligament of Wieger*. Within the circle, there is potential space known as *capillary space of Berger*.

- Vitreous is firmly attached anteriorly in a ring of 3 mm width extending from the ora serrata to the pars plana of the ciliary body and posteriorly around the optic disk.
- Hyaloid canal runs through the central region of vitreous.
- Hyaloid artery is lodged in this hyaloid canal (canal of Cloquet) in the fetal life. Some cases may show its remnants in the form of thin thread-like structure hanging free in the vitreous at one or both the ends.

Retina (Fig. 1.5)

- Retina is the innermost layer—a nervous tunic of the eyeball.
- Retina is derived from the optic cup.
- Outer wall of the cup forms the pigment layer of retina which remains attached with the choroid.
- Inner wall of the cup consists essentially of the nuclei and processes of three layers of nervous elements forming synapsis at molecular zones, namely: (i) visual cells, (ii) bipolar cell, and (iii) ganglion cells.

In the detachment, there occurs a cleavage between this and the pigment layer of retina.

The whole retina is usually described as having ten layers from without inward:

1. The pigment epithelium
2. The layer of rods and cones

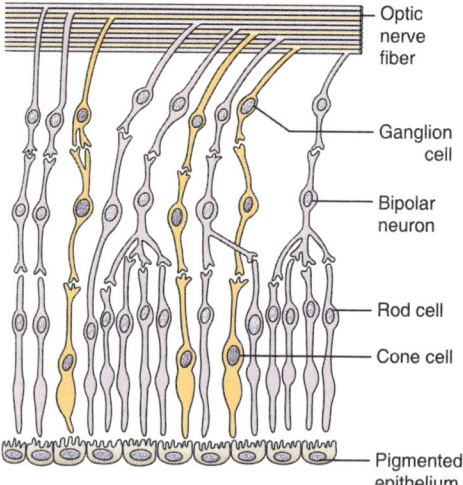

Optic nerve fiber

Ganglion cell

Bipolar neuron

Rod cell

Cone cell

Pigmented epithelium

Fig. 1.5: Structure of retina

3. The external limiting membrane
4. The outer nuclear layer
5. The outer molecular layer
6. The inner nuclear layer
7. The inner molecular layer
8. The ganglion cell layer
9. The nerve fiber layer
10. The internal limiting membrane.

Retina's blood supply is from the *central retinal artery* and *choriocapillaries of the choroid*.

Optic Disk

- Optic disk has only nerve fiber layer, therefore, it does not excite any visual impression so it is known as a *blind spot*.
- Optic disk appears as a nearly circular *disk of 1.5 mm diameter*.
- Optic disk appears pink and the white element is because of *lamina cribrosa and medullated fibers* behind it.
- Depression in the optic disk is called *physiological cup* that varies much in size and form. Its size increases in the *primary open angle glaucoma*.

Macula Lutea

- Macula appears as a dark brown area at the posterior pole of the eye (Fig. 1.6).
- Macula appears browner in color than the surrounding retina due to underlying pigment epithelium and choroid seen through thin retina.
- Macula lies about 3.5 mm lateral to the edge of the disk and just below the middle.
- Macula has numerous ganglion cells arranged in several layers with thick outer molecular layer and there is progressive disappearance of the rods which are replaced by cones.

Fovea

- At fovea, the retina is very thin due to absence of supporting fibers of Muller, ganglion cells, stratum opticum and rods.
- At fovea each cone is connected with one ganglion, thereby it has the best visual acuity.

Optic Nerve

- Optic nerve covered with the pia, arachnoid and dura traverses the optic foramen to enter the orbit and gets attached to the sclera just above and 3 mm internal to the posterior pole of the eye.
- Total length of the nerve is 5 cm the intracranial 1 cm, the optic canal 6 mm, intraorbital 3 cm, intraocular 0.7 mm. *The ophthalmic artery accompanies it in the canal to enter the orbit.*
- In the orbit at optic foramen, the origins of recti muscles surround the optic nerve and the third nasociliary, sympathetic, sixth nerve, ophthalmic artery and vein comes in close relation to it.
- Optic nerve gets the blood supply from the branches of ophthalmic artery, central retinal artery and from short ciliary arteries.
- Optic foramen leads from the middle cranial fossa to the apex of the orbit. It is formed by the two roots of the lesser wing of the sphenoid.

Extrinsic Ocular Muscles (Fig. 1.7)

There are *seven muscles,* namely:
1. Superior rectus muscle
2. Inferior rectus muscle
3. Medial rectus muscle
4. Lateral rectus muscle
5. Superior oblique muscle
6. Inferior oblique muscle
7. Levator palpebrae superioris muscle.

Superior Rectus Muscle

- Arises from the superior part of the common tendinous ring and adjoining dura of optic nerve.
- Inserted into sclera at 7.7 mm from the cornea.
- Main action is *elevation*.
- Subsidiary actions are *intorsion and adduction*.
- Supplied by *third cranial nerve*.

Inferior Rectus Muscle

- Arises from the inferior part of the common tendinous ring.

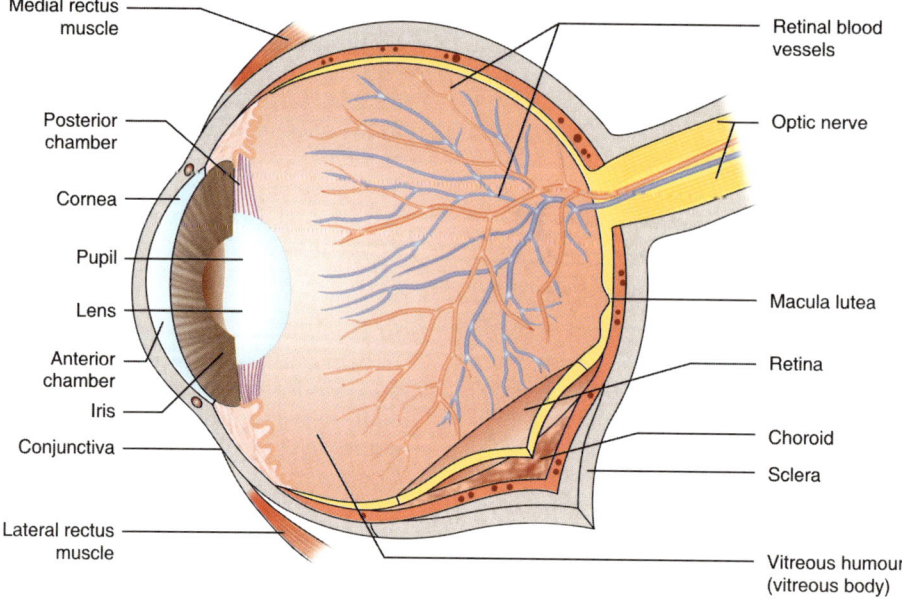

Fig. 1.6: Section of eye

- Inserted into the sclera at 6.5 mm from the cornea.
- Main action is *depressor*.
- Subsidiary actions are *extortion* and *adduction*.
- Supplied by *third cranial nerve*.

Medial Rectus Muscle

- Arises from the medial part of the common tendinous ring.
- Inserted into the sclera at 5.5 mm from the cornea.
- Main action is pure *adduction*.
- Both the medial rectus muscles act together in convergence.
- Supplied by *third cranial nerve*.

Lateral Rectus Muscle

- Arises from the lateral part of the common tendinous ring by two heads which join in a 'V' form.
- Inserted into the sclera at 6.9 mm from the cornea.

- Main action is pure *abduction*.
- Supplied by the *sixth cranial nerve*.

Superior Oblique Muscle

- Arises by a narrow tendon above and medial to the optic foramen.
- Passes forward between the roof and medial wall of the orbit to the *pulley or trochlea* which is situated on the under aspect of the frontal bone a few millimeters behind the orbital margin. The muscle here becomes a rounded tendon of one centimeter before it reaches the pulley. Then the tendon passes through the pulley and bends downwards, backwards and outwards at an angle of 55° passing under the superior rectus muscle and gets attached obliquely in the postero-superior quadrant of the sclera just lateral to the mid-vertical plane.
- Main action is *intorsion*.
- Subsidiary actions are *depression* and *abduction*.
- Supplied by the *fourth cranial nerve*.

Inferior Oblique Muscle

- Arises by a rounded tendon from a small depression on the orbital plate of the superior maxilla a little behind the lower orbital margin and just external to the orifice of the nasolacrimal duct.
- Passes outwards and backwards making an angle of 50° with the visual line between the inferior rectus and floor of the orbit and then under the lateral rectus. Thereafter, it is inserted in the sclera to the back and outer portion of the globe. Its posterior or nasal end is about 5 mm from the optic nerve and thus it lies practically over the macula.
- Main action is *extorsion*.
- Subsidiary actions are *elevation* and *abduction*.
- Supplied by the *third cranial nerve*.

Levator Palpebrae Superioris

- Arises from the under surface of the lesser wing of the sphenoid above and in front of the optic foramen.
- Flat ribbon-like belly passes forward below the roof of the orbit and on the superior rectus muscle. It is inserted in the skin of the upper lid and below the upper palpebral sulcus.
- Main action is to raise the upper lid.
- Supplied by the *third cranial nerve*.

ARTERIAL SUPPLY

Ophthalmic Artery (Fig. 1.8)

- Arises from the internal carotid artery just after leaving the cavernous sinus.

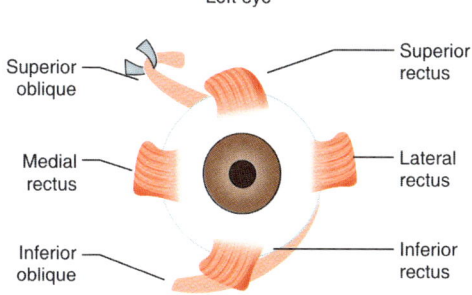

Left eye

Fig. 1.7: Muscles of the eye

- It enters the orbit along the optic nerve within the dura sheath of the nerve.
- In the orbit, it lies in the cone of muscles with ciliary ganglion and the lateral rectus to its outer side and the optic nerve to its medial side.
- It passes forward giving branches and ends by dividing into nasal and frontal branches.

Branches (Fig. 1.8)

1. *The central artery of retina:* It serves to retina.
2. *Posterior long and short ciliary arteries:* The two long posterior ciliary arteries pierce sclera along the side of optic nerve and run between sclera and choroid to supply the ciliary body and then anastomosing with the anterior ciliary arteries to form circulus arteriosus iridis major and supply the iris. The short ciliary arteries come off as 10–20 branches of long posterior ciliary arteries pierce the sclera and enter the choroid.
3. *The lacrimal artery:* It supplies the lacrimal gland, conjunctiva and eyelids.
4. *Recurrent branches:* These arteries run back in the dural sheath of the optic nerve.
5. *The muscular branches:* The lateral branch supplies the lateral rectus, superior rectus,

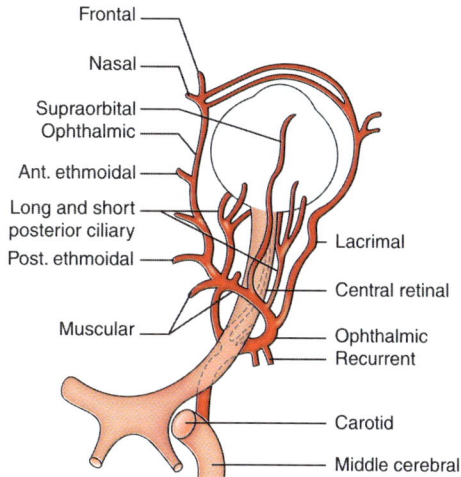

Fig. 1.8: Ophthalmic artery and its branches

levator and superior oblique muscles. The medial branch supplies the inferior rectus, medial rectus and inferior oblique muscle.

6. *The supraorbital artery:* It supplies the upper eyelid, scalp, levator and periorbita.
7. *The posterior ethmoidal artery:* It supplies the mucous membrane of the posterior ethmoidal air cells and upper part of the nose.
8. *The anterior ethmoidal artery:* It supplies the mucous membrane of the front part of nasal cavity, anterior ethmoidal air cells and skin of the nose.
9. *The superior and inferior medial palpebral branches:* These arteries supply the upper and lower lids.
10. *The nasal branch:* It supplies the skin of the root of the nose and lacrimal sac.
11. *The frontal artery:* It supplies the skin, muscles and periosteum of the medial part of the forehead.

Venous Drainage (Fig. 1.9)

Orbit is drained by the *superior and inferior ophthalmic veins.*

These veins communicate with the veins of the face, pterygoid plexus, veins of the nose and cavernous sinus.

Superior Ophthalmic Vein

- It is formed by the union of *angular and supraorbital veins* near the root of the nose.
- It passes into the orbit under the superior rectus to the superior orbital fissure and joined by the inferior ophthalmic vein.
- It leaves the orbit to enter the cavernous sinus.

Inferior Ophthalmic Vein

- It commences as a plexus near the front of the floor of the orbit and runs backwards to join the superior ophthalmic vein.
- It communicates with the pterygoid plexus, anterior facial vein and receives two inferior vorticose veins.

Angular Vein

It is formed by the union of the supraorbital and frontal veins and runs down at the side of nose crossing the nasal end of the medial palpebral ligament some 8 mm from the inner canthus.

Cavernous Sinus

Cavernous sinuses extend on each side of the pituitary body and body of the sphenoid from

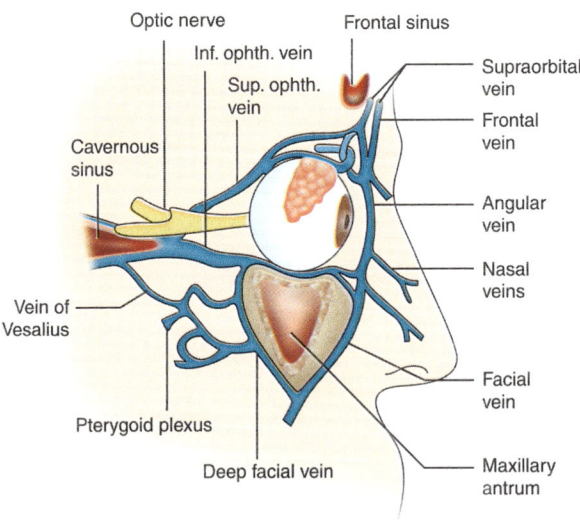

Fig. 1.9: Venous drainage of eyeball

the inner end of the superior orbital fissure to the apex of the petrous part of the temporal bone.

In each sinus, there is internal carotid artery and lateral to it, the sixth nerve.

In the lateral wall of the sinus from above down are the third nerve, fourth nerve and first and second divisions of the fifth cranial nerve.

Nerve Supply of the Eye

- Motor nerve supply is by the oculomotor, trochlear and abducens cranial nerves.
- Sensory supply is by the first division of trigeminal and cranial nerves.
- Sympathetic is derived from the plexus around the internal carotid artery and supplied through the ciliary ganglion.

Oculomotor Nerve

- Oculomotor nerve has two branches.
- Upper branch supplies to *superior rectus muscle* and *levator palpebrae superioris*.
- Lower branch supplies to *medial rectus, inferior rectus, inferior oblique muscle and short branches to the ciliary ganglion*.
- Its paralysis results in ptosis, inability to look upwards, downwards and inwards. The pupil is semidilated and does not react to the light and accommodation.
- The third nerve also supplies to the sphincter pupillae and ciliary muscles.

Trochlear Nerve

It supplies to the superior oblique muscle only.

Its paralysis causes limitation of movements in the downward gaze when the eye is adducted as the superior oblique is only depressor in the adducted position of the eye.

Abducens Nerve

It supplies to the lateral rectus muscle only.

Its paralysis causes convergent squint as the eye becomes unable to move outwards.

Trigeminal Nerve

It is the largest of the cranial nerves.

It has two roots—motor and sensory.

- Motor part supplies six muscles of the mastication.
- Sensory part divides in three branches, namely: Ophthalmic, maxillary and mandibular nerves.

It is the first division or ophthalmic branch of the trigeminal nerve which supplies the whole eye. From the cranial cavity, it runs in the lateral wall of the cavernous sinus and just before it enters the superior orbital fissure, it divides into three branches: (i) lacrimal, (ii) frontal, (iii) nasociliary.

Ciliary Ganglion

It is a small ganglion of about 2 mm situated at the posterior part of the orbit about 1 cm from the optic foramen between the optic nerve and lateral rectus muscle.

It receives three roots—sensory root, motor root and sympathetic root.

- Sensory root comes from the nasociliary. It carries fibers to cornea, iris and ciliary body.
- Motor root comes from the nerve to the inferior oblique muscle. It carries fibers to supply to the sphincter pupillae and ciliary muscle.
- Sympathetic root comes from the plexus around the internal carotid artery. It carries constriction fibers to the blood vessels of the eye and dilator fibers to the pupil.

The ganglion supplies through six to ten short ciliary nerves which enter the eye around the optic nerve.

2

Physiology of Aqueous Humor and Tear Fluid

Aqueous Humor

- Composition of aqueous humor
- Production of aqueous humor
- Drainage of aqueous humor
- Blood–aqueous barrier
- Plasmoid aqueous
- Functions of aqueous humor

Tear Fluid

- Secretion and composition
- Functions of tear fluid
- Basic and reflex secretion of tear fluid
- Tear film
- Tear film break-up time

AQUEOUS HUMOR

Composition of Aqueous Humor

Aqueous humor is a clear watery fluid in the anterior and posterior chambers of the eyeball to maintain clarity of the fluid and vision.

Aqueous humor consists of 99.9% water and 0.1% solids. The solids include protein in traces 5–16 mg%, amino acids, glucose, ascorbic acid, lactic acid, electrolytes, hyaluronic acid, proteolytic enzyme, traces of urea, uric acid, creatinine and oxygen.

Refractive index is 1.33.

Production of Aqueous Humor

Production involves three mechanisms:
1. Ultrafiltration
2. Secretion
3. Diffusion

Ultrafiltration

There is two-way transference of tissue fluid through the capillary walls in the organs of body to supply nutrition and remove metabolites. Permeability of the capillary wall differs in different tissues to suit the need of that particular organ.

Capillaries in the eye are relatively impermeable to colloid molecules so that optical clarity can be maintained for clear and good visual acuity.

Secretion

The ciliary processes secrete about 95% of the total quantity of aqueous humor. The secretory process is conducted by the metabolic activity of the cells of the ciliary epithelium. The exact mechanism of secretion is not clear but a fluid rich in sodium and containing small quantities of ascorbic acid and other substances is secreted into the posterior chamber.

The aqueous humor consists of a dilute solution of all the diffusible constituents of the plasma. The concentration in the aqueous is much less than in the blood. It is rich in sodium. The lactic acid is in higher concentration than in the blood as the lactic acid is an end product of the metabolism of the lens.

Diffusion

It occurs due to osmotic gradient.

Drainage of Aqueous Humor

The intraocular fluid is secreted into the posterior chamber. It flows through the pupil

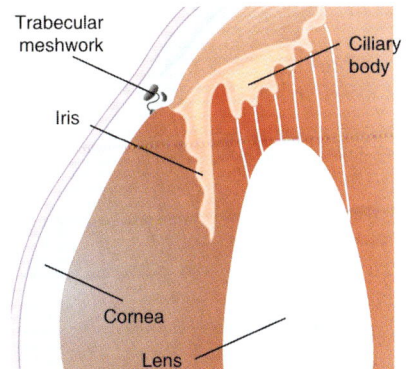

Fig. 2.1: Aqueous drainage through angle of anterior chamber

into the anterior chamber and is drained out by two routes (Fig. 2.1).

Trabecular meshwork outflow It is the main outlet for aqueous from the anterior chamber. There is a free flow of aqueous from trabecular meshwork up to inner walls of Schlemm's canal and then into the episcleral veins. Most of the aqueous about 90% is drained by this route.

Uveoscleral outflow Aqueous passes across the ciliary body into the suprachoroidal space and then drained by the venous circulation in the ciliary body, choroid and sclera. It drains about 10% of aqueous.

Blood–Aqueous Barrier

The system of semipermeable membrane which separates the blood from the ocular cavity is known as *blood–aqueous barrier*.

- *In the posterior segment* of the eyeball the blood–aqueous barrier is formed by the walls of the retinal capillaries, Bruch's membrane and retinal pigment epithelium.
- *In the ciliary region* the blood–aqueous barrier is formed by the two-layered ciliary epithelium.
- *In the iris,* the blood–aqueous barrier is formed by the walls of the capillaries in the iris.

Plasmoid Aqueous

Plasmoid aqueous is an aqueous which is rich in its protein content. Any condition which

results in the dilation of capillaries also increases the permeability of the capillaries, thereby allowing a protein rich fluid to pass through it forming *plasmoid aqueous*.

Increase in the permeability is commonly seen in inflammatory condition of the uveal tract, trauma and lowering of intraocular pressure following paracentesis.

Functions of Aqueous Humor

- It provides nutrition to the non-vascularized tissues of the eye—the cornea and lens.
- It removes the metabolic products of metabolism.
- It maintains the optical clarity of the eye to provide clear and good acuity of vision.
- It helps to regulate the intraocular pressure.

TEAR FLUID

Secretion and Composition

- Tear fluid is a mixture of secretion from lacrimal and accessory lacrimal glands, the goblet cells and the meibomian glands.
- Lacrimal glands—the orbital and the palpebral portion secrete about 95% of aqueous component of the tear fluid.
- Tear fluid is an isotonic fluid that is slightly alkaline and consists of water, potassium, chloride, sodium, urea, glucose, lysozyme, globulins, and albumin.
- Secretion of tear fluid begins only 3 to 4 weeks after birth of a child.

Functions of Tear Fluid

- Keep the cornea as a smooth optical surface.
- Keep corneal and the conjunctival epithelium moist.
- Inhibit the growth of micro-organisms by mechanical action of flushing and by its enzyme the lysozyme.
- Washes away debris and noxious and minute foreign bodies.
- Facilitates movements of lids.
- Flows out through lacrimal drainage system (Fig. 2.2).

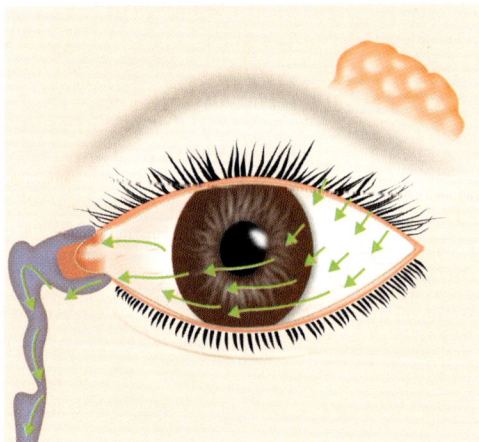

Fig. 2.2: Tear flow

Basic and Reflex Secretion of Tear Fluid

Basic secretion of tears the tear fluid is the resting secretion occurring normally. The reflex secretion of tears is much more and occurs due to stimulus derived from para-sympathetic reflex.

Reflex secretion occurs in both the eyes follo-wing superficial stimulus of one eye. The main and accessory lacrimal glands both respond to reflex stimulus as one unit.

Tear Film (Fig. 2.3)

The pre-corneal tear film has three layers which from posterior to anterior are inner mucin layer, middle aqueous layer and outer lipid layer.

Inner Mucin Layer

*   Mucin is innermost and thinnest layer of the precorneal teal film.
*   Mucin is secreted by the goblet cells in the conjunctiva and also by the crypts of Henle and glands of Manz.
*   Its function is to convert the corneal epithelium from a hydrophobic to a hydrophilic surface. Mucin is a glyco-protein which becomes adsorbed on to the cell membrane of the epithelial cells making them hydrophilic.

Middle Aqueous Layer

The aqueous component is secreted by main and accessory lacrimal glands. Its functions are:
*   Supplies atmospheric oxygen to corneal epithelium.
*   It has antibacterial enzymes; lysozyme, lactoferin and betalysin.
*   Provides a smooth optical surface of cornea.
*   Keeps the eye clean by washing action.

Outer Lipid Layer

The lipid layer is secreted by the meibomian glands. Its functions are:
*   Retards the evaporation of aqueous layer.
*   Increases surface tension so the film is stable.
*   Lubricate the eyelids.

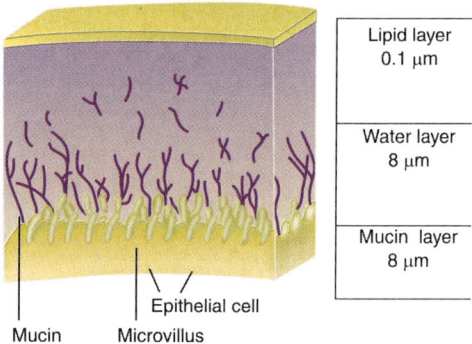

Fig. 2.3: Tear film—three layers

Pathogenesis of Tear Film Break-up

*   Tear film cannot remain stable for a long time.
*   Formation of tear film is a complex process which requires normal blinking reflex, normal lid condition and normal corneal epithelium.
*   With each blink, the mucin is distributed over the corneal epithelium making it hydrophilic and allows the aqueous and lipid layer to spread forming three layers of tear film.

- Evaporation beings immediately and the tear film starts to thin. Some of the superficial lipids will migrate to the tear-epithelial interface usually within a minute creating an area of high interfacial tension over which the tear film becomes unstable, breaks up and forms so called **'dry spots'** (Fig. 2.4).
- With each new blink the surface is recoated and the cycle repeats itself.

Tear Film Break-up Time

The time interval between the blink and appearance of a dry spot in a normal eye is called *'Tear film break-up time'*. This time is usually greater than the time between the two blinks.

- Normal break-up time varies from 15 to 34 seconds.

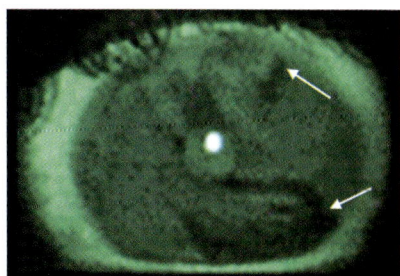

Fig. 2.4: Tear film break-up spots—corneal staining

- Break-up time of less than 10 seconds is taken as abnormal. There is a wide variation of values obtained in the same individual.
- Break-up time of less than 10 seconds obtained on repeat test can be considered positive along with other positive signs of dry eye.

3

Clinical Case History

History Recording Format

- Demographic data
- Present complaints
- History of present complaints
- Past history
- Family history
- Personal history
- Any reports of investigations/treatment

HISTORY RECORDING FORMAT

Recording history is one of the most important clinical norms for students in any clinical study. Once you are apt at it then and then only you shall be able to diagnose the malady by just asking a few leading questions in a short time.

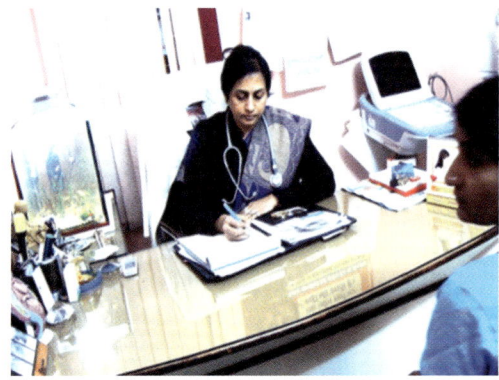

Fig. 3.2: Clinical history notes

Father/Mother's Name

It gives a correct identification as there may be two patients with same name.

Age

Many diseases are related to the age, e.g. presbyopia, arcus senilis, xanthelasma, retinal degeneration, amblyopia exanopsia, arteriosclerosis, and myopia increasing with age.

Sex

Many diseases are related to the sex, e.g. myxedema and migraine; common in female.

Occupation

Occupation plays an important role in occurrence of certain eye disorders. It also helps to advice protective measures, ocular health

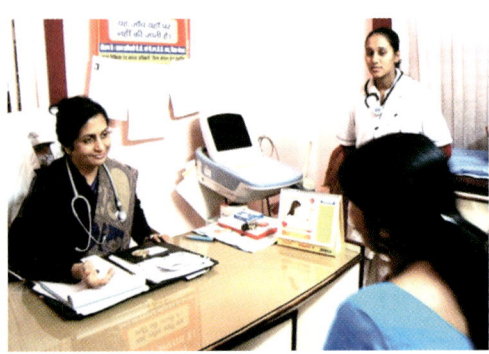

Fig. 3.1: Welcome to patient

Demographic Data

Name

It is recorded for identification.

education and counseling for visual rehabi-litation.

- Industrial worker is prone to mechanical or chemical trauma.
- Grinder, stone cutter or blacksmith often comes with a foreign body which may be superficial or even penetrating.
- Farmer gets vegetative trauma which is likely to be fungal.
- Compositor needs early near vision correction.
- Gardener or table worker is likely to develop glaucoma early.
- Computer vision syndrome in computer professionals.
- Glass blowers are prone to heat cataract.
- Arc welders are prone to photophthal-mitis.

Religion

Some diseases are common in a particular community, e.g. myopia in Jews and Japanese, congenital disorders in Muslims and Parsi community.

Residential Address, e-mail ID and Mobile Number

It is recorded to contact the family members and for follow-up study.

Name of the Next of Kin with his Address

It is recorded to get in touch in case of an emergency especially if the patient has come from out station and is alone as an in-patient.

Present Complaints

Ask about the present complaints and record it in his words.

Most of the complaints from a patient attending out-patient are covered by the following symptoms:

- Dim vision.
- Disturbance in the vision.
- Headache and eye ache.
- Pain in the eye, eyebrow and around the orbit.
- Feeling of burning, tiredness on near work, photophobia and itching, etc.
- Redness of the eyes with watering and discharge.
- Change in the appearance of the orbit, lids and the eyes.

History of Present Complaints

Ask the patient to describe in detail about each symptom felt by him. As most of the patients are unable to describe the details about their own complaints, therefore, it is necessary to ask leading questions about each complaint to elicit a proper and meticulous history.

Dim Vision

Ask the patient about the mode of onset and duration of the dim vision followed by the following leading questions:

- It has affected one or both the eyes.
- Its onset has been gradual or sudden.
- It has affected the distance vision or the near vision.
- Any kind of ocular trauma.
- Watching solar eclipse.
- Systemic use of drugs for a long time.
- Topical steroids for a long time.
- Using hair color dye.
- Recent fever, influenza and sinusitis followed by dim vision.
- Using spectacles.

Disturbance in the Vision

Ask the patient to describe his feeling about the disturbance in his vision. Encourage him to draw a diagram, if possible. The patient is likely to complain of the following problems:

- *Black spot* in front of the eye that moves with the movement of the eyeball—denotes *opacity in the lens.*
- *Floating black spots* of varying hue, shape, size and number which appear to move or float in front of the eyes even though the eyeball is stationary. The patient usually describes these spots as if fly is constantly moving in front of his eyes. Sometimes he may describe these as if small pieces of cotton-wool are moving in front of the eyes. This kind of symptom is disturbing, alarming and annoying to the

patient. *These floating black spots are due to vitreous opacities.*

- *Vision improves in dim* illumination—denotes *nuclear cataract.*
- *Vision improves in bright* illumination—denotes *incipient cataract.*
- *Objects appear wavy, smaller or larger* than their normal sizes—denotes *macular lesion.*
- *Visualizing a curtain* from the side that is shaking and causing gradual loss of peripheral field of vision—denotes *detachment of the retina.*
- *Night blindness*—child feels difficulty in moving about in the dark or dim-illumination. *It is diagnostic for vitamin A deficiency or retinitis pigmentosa.*
- *Photopsia:* Flash of light usually in the upper temporal quadrant—denotes *vitreo-retinal degeneration.*
- *Sudden loss of vision* followed by floaters, red streak and red vision—denotes *vitreous hemorrhage—Eales' disease.*
- *Halos:* Colored rings around the bulb—denotes *incipient cataract or latent primary angle-closure glaucoma.*
- *Diplopia:* See double images of an object. *Unilateral diplopia*—denotes incipient cataract, macular lesion or malingerer. *Bilateral diplopia*—denotes paralysis of extraocular muscle.
- *Polyopia:* See more than two images of an object. *Polyopia is diagnostic for incipient cataract.*
- *Red vision:* Usually after exposure to a strong bright light common in aphakic patient.

Headache

Headache is one of the most common complaints for which patient seeks advice of eye clinician. Ask him about its location, severity, frequency, relation to near work, relation with the time of the day and association with nausea and vomiting.

The following symptoms described by the patient may help to arrive at a diagnosis:
- Headache followed after watching television, movie, or reading and writing can be due to refractive error, astigmatism, heterophoria and presbyopia.
- Tension headache is usually localized in the temporal, frontal, supraorbital or occipital region.
- Tension headache usually affects the patient for all the 24 hours and it has no specific relation to any work. Any kind of emotional disturbance acts as a trigger to it.
- Headache due to migraine manifests usually in association with feeling of nausea. Patient gets relief in a dark, cool and quiet room.

Eye Ache

Eye ache is usually described by the patient with following symptoms:
- Feeling of fatigue all the time without doing any reading or writing work.
- Feeling of pull in the eyes.
- Feeling of tiredness, pressure or pain in the eyes and feels relief on palming the eyes.

The eye is a very sensitive organ. Any disturbance in the normal functioning of the body even of a very mild nature can give rise to all the feelings described above. Apart from excluding an eye problem like refractive error and heterophoria, it is essential to look into his system as a whole. He/she needs comprehensive systemic examination, investigation and counseling for emotional stress, if everything is clinically normal.

Pain in the Eye, Eyebrow and around the Orbit

The pain in the eye, eyebrow and around the orbit is usually due to localized inflammation or referred. The patient shall be able to point out the focus of infection or inflammation or generalized systemic problem.

Feeling of Discomfort in the Eyes

Quite often a patient does feel discomfort in his eyes yet is unable to describe it. The common feelings of discomfort are experienced and expressed as follows:

- Uneasy feeling even after watching a program on the television for only a few minutes. If there is no refractive error then it could be attributed to the brightness of the television picture. Advise him/her to reduce the brightness. It might help him.
- Discomfort in moving out of home in bright daylight. Advise him/her to use umbrella and goggles.
- Falls sleep or feels sleepy even after reading for half an hour. Check for refractive error and heterophoria. Advise him/her to maintain a proper posture, illumination and good ventillation. Advice him/her to sleep continuously for minimum of 7 hours at a stretch.
- Feeling of dryness of the eyes.
- Feeling of wet eyes.
- Feeling of grittiness in the eyes.
- Itching of the eyes.
- Feeling of burning sensation in the eyes as if the whole eyeball is hot like a burning coal.
- Desire to rub the eyes again and again even after reading for short time. Advise him/her to wash the face and to avoid direct blast of fan.

Redness of the Eyes with Watering and Discharge

The redness of the eyes with watering and discharge is common. The location of the redness and the type of discharge helps to arrive at a diagnosis.

The following description shall be helpful:
- Redness of the bulbar and the palpebral conjunctiva occurs most commonly in the conjunctivitis.
- Redness of the lower bulbar conjunctiva and lower fornix favors an allergic or irritative factor.
- Redness localized in the palpebral area is diagnostic for angular conjunctivitis.
- Redness around the limbus indicates a lesion in the cornea, uveal tract and glaucoma.
- Localized redness along with a nodule is seen in scleritis, episcleritis and phlyctenular conjunctivitis.

- Redness of the eye or eyes is always associated with watering of the eyes and discharge.
- Sticky and ropy discharge is diagnostic for vernal conjunctivitis (spring catarrh).
- Discharge may be mucus, mucopus or purulent depending on the virulence of the organism affecting the conjunctiva.
- Formation of a crust at the lid margin is diagnostic for squamous blepharitis.

Change in the Appearance of the Orbit, Lids and the Eyes

Any change in the appearance of the orbit, lids and the eyes is easily noticed by the patient and his/her friends and relatives. The patient seeks advice early for cosmetic embarrassment. Usually, the patient is able to describe the symptoms well and in detail. Ask about the duration and mode of onset.

The following changes are commonly seen:
- *Swelling* all around the orbit or in any part of it.
- *Constant twitching* of the lid or muscles of the face usually on one side.
- *Ptosis*: Lid may appear drooping affecting one lid or both the lids.
- *Lagophthalmos:* One eye remains open even on forced closure of the lid. It is due to facial paralysis.
- *Retraction of the lids:* Eyes appear prominent and bulging in Graves' disease and high myopia.
- *Proptosis:* Eyes may bulge forward.
- *Squint:* Eye may deviate inward or outward.
- *Ecchymosis*: Skin around the eyes and lids appears black due to subcutaneous hemorrhage.
- *Allergic dermatitis*: Skin of the lids near the lid margin appears dark and dry with intense desire to itch with nail of little finger.
- *Blepharitis:* Lid margin may show crust formation.
- *Chalazion:* Single or multiple nodules in the lid.
- *Nodule* at the limbus or in the sclera.

- *Xanthelasma:* Symmetrical yellow spots on the lids at the inner angle of the orbit.
- *Bitot's spot:* White foamy patch in the conjunctiva due to xerosis of the conjunctiva.
- *Pterygium:* Triangular patch in the conjunctiva encroaching on cornea.
- *Dacryocystitis:* Swelling in the lacrimal sac region.

Past History

- The past history of any chronic ailment plays an important role in the diagnosis and prognosis of a case.
- If there is no past history mentioned by the patient even then ask leading questions about tuberculosis, diabetes, hypertension and any kind of other illness he/she may remember and about any surgical intervention undergone.

Family History

There are many diseases which are familial in character. The patient is ignorant about them. Ask a few leading questions as mentioned below.

- Any member of the family suffered from tuberculosis any time.
- Any history of diabetes, hypertension, epilepsy, convulsions, night blindness, retinal detachment, glaucoma, or any congenital abnormality of the skull or long bones.
- Any history of using myopic glasses by any member of the family either from paternal or maternal side.

Personal History

The personal habits and addictions play an important role. Ask him/her in private and after taking in confidence.

The following queries shall be helpful:

- Addiction to alcohol, tobacco or cannabis.
- Addiction to any drugs.
- Used contraceptive pills to prevent pregnancy.
- History of miscarriage or abortion.
- Discharge from the genital organs.
- Boils or infection around the genital organs.
- Pets in the family, e.g. dog, cat, parrot and rabbit.
- History of unprotected sex.

Any Reports of Investigations/Treatment

Ask about reports of past or present investigation, previous record of eye examination and treatment undergone either surgical or medical.

4

Clinical Ocular Examination

General Examination of a Case

- Preliminary inspection

Clinical Examination of the Case

- Orbit
- Eyeball
- Palpebral aperture
- Lids
- Lacrimal sac
- Conjunctiva
- Cornea
- Sclera
- Anterior chamber
- Pupil
- Iris
- Lens
- Vitreous
- Fundus

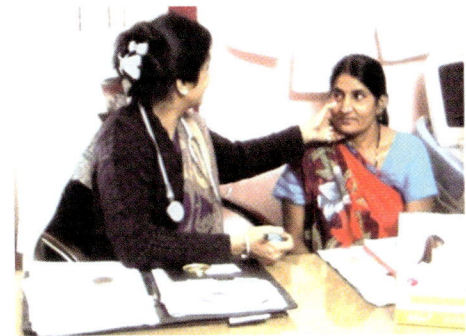

Fig. 4.1: General examination

GENERAL EXAMINATION OF A CASE

The general examination of a case (Fig. 4.1) is conducted by preliminary inspection.

It begins with entrance of the patient in the clinic and the clinician asks him to come and sit down on chair while facing the patient sitting on his revolving stool.

Preliminary Inspection

Patient as a Whole

- Watch his/her gait and expression of his/her face as he/she enters the clinic.
- Assess his/her age.
- Assess his/her built thin, average or obese.

Head

- Look for any abnormality of skull, e.g. oxycephaly.
- Look for the position, i.e. any head tilt or face turn.

Face

- Look for any asymmetry of face.
- Look for facial paralysis.
- Any changes in the skin of the face.
- Any change in the appearance of the orbit, lids and eyes.
- Look for malar and nasojugal sulcus.

Eyebrows

- Elevation of eyebrow due to action of frontalis muscle usually seen in a case of ptosis.
- Loss of hair usually on the outer aspect of the eyebrow, e.g. leprosy and myxedema.

Palpebral Aperture

- Normal on both the sides
- Narrow in one eye, e.g. unilateral ptosis
- Narrow in both eyes, e.g. bilateral ptosis
- Wide on one or both sides, e.g. Graves' disease due to lid retraction.

Lids

- Drooping of lid on one or both the sides
- Retraction of lid on one or both the sides
- Lagophthalmos.

Orbit

- Any deformity
- Any swelling in any part, e.g. dermoid, lipoma
- Any discharging sinus, e.g. tubercular osteomyelitis.

Eyeball

- Small eyeball—microphthalmus
- Shrunken eyeball—atrophic or phthisis bulbi
- Large eyeball—buphthalmos
- Bulging of eyeball—thyrotoxicosis
- Prominent eyeball—high myopia
- Deviated eyeball—squint
- Oscillation of eye—nystagmus
- Limbus—congestion, nodule, patch, pigmentation, scar or growth.

CLINICAL EXAMINATION OF THE CASE

In this era, the clinical examination of the patient is being conducted by providing a comfortable seat on electronically adjustable ophthalmic chair-cum-table holding; autorefractometer, slit-lamp with applanation tonometer and imaging equipment, gonioscope trial case for subjective verification, direct and indirect ophthalmoscope while consultant sits on revolving and freely mobile adjustable cushioned stool usually with back rest.

Slit-lamp is indispensable for clinical examination of eye (Fig. 4.2).

Clinic provides comfortable and cool environment to both the patient and the consultant with soft background music as relaxant.

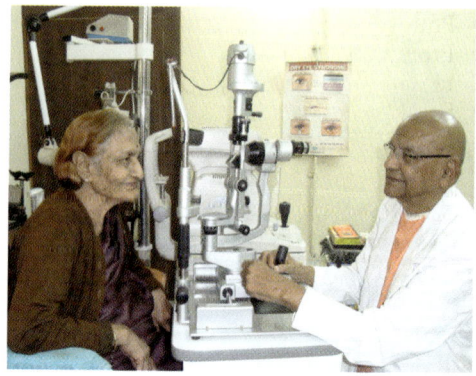

Fig. 4.2: Clinical examination

Orbit

The orbit and its contents are prone to all types of affections: Congenital, inflammatory, vascular, neoplastic, metabolic and trauma.

Inspection

- Any abnormal swelling along the orbital margin
- Any signs of inflammation along the orbital margin
- Any discharging sinus.

Palpation

Palpation of the orbital margin is done with the thumb, index or little finger. Use little finger to feel for any growth which might have grown to reach the orbital margin. The little finger can be easily inserted between the eyeball and the orbital margin. Feel for any tenderness and pulsation.

Ocular Movements

Lesion of the orbit usually causes restriction in the movement of the eyeball. Test the ocular movements carefully in all the direction of gaze.

Eyeball
Inspection

Compare both the eyes and look for the following conditions:

- Proptosis—axial or eccentric
- Enophthalmos

- Phthisis bulbi
- Prominent eyes myopia and natural due to wide palpebral fissure
- Squint
- Nystagmus
- Nodule at the limbus
- Staphyloma.

Palpation

Palpation of the eyeball is done with the palm of the hand.

- Proptosis is *reducible* in thyrotoxic exophthalmos.
- Proptosis is *not reducible* in thyrotropic exophthalmos and growth behind the globe.
- Pulsatile or non-pulsatile.

Ocular Motility

Ocular motility gets affected in many diseases of the eyeball. Test the movements of the eyes in all the direction of gaze and make a note, if there is any restriction of movement of the eye in any direction.

Palpebral Aperture

Palpebral aperture is bounded by the margins of two lids. On closure of the lids, the palpebral aperture becomes a palpebral fissure which is concave upwards in the central portion. With the lids open, the palpebral aperture appears as an ellipse of about 30 mm by 10 mm which is taken as a normal average size. Natural width of palpebral aperture adds to beauty of both the sex.

Inspection

Compare the palpebral aperture of both the eyes.

- Normally the palpebral apertures appear similar in shape and size.
- Palpebral aperture is narrow in one eye or both the eyes in *ptosis and myasthenia gravis.*
- Palpebral aperture is wide in one or both the eyes in *thyroid orbitopathy-thyrotoxicosis* due to lid retraction.

- Palpebral aperture of one eye appears narrow in *facial paralysis* due to lagophthalmos.
- Presences of the horizontal furrows on forehead on raising the eyebrows indicate the *upper motor neuron type of facial paralysis.*
- Absence of the horizontal furrows on forehead on raising the eyebrows indicate the *lower motor neuron type of facial paralysis.*

Lids

Lids play an important role in the cosmetic appearance of a person.

Thus any change in the appearance of the lids, its lashes and margin compels the patient to attend eye clinic.

Inspection
Position of lid

- Look and assess the position of the lid in relation to the cornea.
- In a primary position of the eyes while looking straight, the upper lid just covers the upper part of the cornea and the lower lid remains just below the lower margin of the cornea.

Thickness of the lids

- Normal lid is thin and freely mobile.
- It becomes thick and heavy in *trachoma* due to fibrosis.

Change in appearance Look for any redness, edema, swelling, nodule, growth, roughness, dermatitis, pigmentation, depigmentation, crusts, ulcer and scar mark.

Inspection of lashes

- *Trichiasis:* Misdirection of lashes.
- *Madarosis:* Absence or less number of lashes.
- *Poliosis:* Grey color in old age and Vogt-Koyanagi syndrome.
- *Nits:* At the root of lashes in parasitic infection.
- *Matting:* Due to conjunctival discharge.

Inspection of lid margin

- *Entropion:* In-rolling of lid margin.
- *Ectropion:* Out-rolling of lid margin.

- *Squamous blepharitis:* Crust deposition on lid margin.
- *Ulcerative blepharitis:* Minute ulceration of lid margin.

Palpation

Ask the patient to close the eyes softly. Palpate the lids by the tip of the index finger. The palpation helps to locate any small nodules (chalazion) and any change in the texture of the skin of the lids especially near the lid margin which is the area mostly affected by allergic dermatitis.

Movement

Movement of the lids is controlled by the two muscles:

- Levator palpebrae superioris muscle opens the lid.
- Müller's muscle maintains the open position of the lid.

Test for movement of the lids

- Ask the patient to look at the index finger placed horizontally in front of his/her eyes at about 15 inches and follow the movement of the finger upward and then downwards and observe the movement of the lids. The normal movement of the lids is about 15 mm.
- In a case of ptosis, the movement of the affected lid is restricted.
- Results of surgery are good, if the movement of the affected lid is above 4 mm.

Eversion of the Upper Lid

Ask the patient to look down and instruct him/her to keep looking down during the process of eversion of the lid and slit-lamp examination of the everted lid for; follicles, foreign body, granuloma and scars of healed trachoma.

Technique of eversion of upper lid
Grasp the eyelashes of the upper lid by index finger and thumb of right hand and pull the lid slightly forward and evert it over the supporting thumb of the left hand placed just above the upper margin of the tarsal plate of the lid. The everted lid is kept in this everted position by the left thumb and the examiner uses his right hand to operate slit lamp. After examination, release the lid and ask the patient to look upward and the lid adopts its normal position.

Technique for double eversion of upper lid
Make the patient lie down in a supine position on the examination table. Instill xylocaine 2% as drops in the eyes once. Evert the lid as usual. Grasp this everted lid by a ring forceps from the temporal side and give one turn to the forceps for double eversion. The double eversion is required only to expose the fornix for locating any deep lesion usually a foreign body or any growth.

Lacrimal Sac

Inspection

Look for any swelling, signs of inflammation, scar and fistula.

Regurgitation Test

The regurgitation test should be performed as a routine in every case who attends an eye clinic with epiphora.

Negative test does not rule out dacryocystitis.

Technique
Hold the face of the patient by both the hands supporting the side of the face, keeping the thumbs free for the test. Use the thumb of one hand to slightly pull the lower eyelid exposing the lower punctum and with the thumb of the other hand press at the lacrimal sac area to empty the contents of the sac. There shall be either no regurgitation or regurgitation of mucus or mucopurulent discharge from the lower punctum under observation.

- Positive test is diagnostic of chronic dacryocystitis.
- Negative test does not rule out the lacrimal sac disease.

Syringing of the Lacrimal Sac

Syringing of the lacrimal sac is mandatory in any case who attends eye clinic with symptom of unilateral epiphora or repeated unilateral conjunctivitis with negative regurgitation test.

Technique

Instill xylocaine 2% as drops in the eye once. Use a 2 cc syringe fitted with a curved lacrimal cannula. Fill it with antibiotic eye drop solution. If the patient is a child or an infant then immobilize him/her. The assistant holds the head of the child along with his/her hands kept along the side of his/her head. The other assistant is asked to stretch the legs of the child and keep a firm and soft pressure on the knees. This immobilizes the child without causing any harm to him/her. The surgeon exposes the lower punctum of the eye by pulling the lower lid with the help of his/her thumb. With the other hand, he/she dilates the punctum by the punctum dilator and thereafter inserts the lacrimal cannula in the dilated punctum and canaliculi. Once the surgeon is sure of the proper insertion of the cannula the fluid in the syringe is pushed slowly.

- Fluid passes down the nose and throat, if the passage is patent.
- Fluid regurgitates through the upper punctum or even the same punctum if the passage is blocked.

Dacryocystography

Dacryocystography gives information about the size and shape of the lacrimal sac and also the site of the block in the lacrimal passage. This information helps the ophthalmologist to plan the surgery.

Technique For dacryocystography—a radiopaque dye is injected in the lacrimal sac with the same method as for syringing the lacrimal sac. The X-ray is taken with forehead-nose position. The radiopaque dye outlines the canaliculi, sac and nasolacrimal duct. If the X-ray shows a big dilated sac, then the case is fit for performing dacryocystorhinostomy.

Conjunctiva

The conjunctiva has three parts:
- Bulbar conjunctiva
- Palpebral conjunctiva
- Fornix.

To examine the conjunctiva, follow the pattern mentioned below:

- *Lower bulbar, palpebral and fornix:* It can be easily examined by asking the patient to look upward and by pulling the lower lid downward.
- *Upper bulbar conjunctiva:* It can be examined by asking the patient to look downward and pulling the upper lid upward.
- *Upper palpebral conjunctiva and fornix:* The upper palpebral conjunctiva can be examined by eversion of the upper lid and the upper fornix can be examined by double eversion of the upper lid.
- *Bulbar conjunctiva in the palpebral aperture:* It can be examined by asking the patient to look straight in the primary position of gaze.
- *Plica semilunaris and caruncle:* Ask the patient to look outward.

Inspection

- Congestion—generalized or localized.
- Conjunctival congestion. ⎤
- Circumciliary congestion. ⎦ Table 4.1
- Congestion in the palpebral aperture.
- Nodule at the limbus with or without congestion—*pinguecula.*
- Chemosis—edema of conjunctiva.
- Discharge—watery, mucus, mucopus, purulent and ropy.
- Petechial hemorrhage.
- Subconjunctival hemorrhage.
- Follicles or papillae on the palpebral conjunctiva.
- Membrane on the palpebral conjunctiva.
- Scarring of the palpebral conjunctiva.
- Xerosis.
- Dry and lusterlessness.
- Bitot's spots.
- Pigmentation.
- Triangular growth encroaching on the cornea *pterygium.*
- Polygonal flat nodules on the palpebral conjunctiva.
- Gelatinous thickening with brownish color at limbus all around or involving a sector only *vernal conjunctivitis.*
- Foreign body.
- Concretion.

Table 4.1: Differences between conjunctival and circumciliary congestion

Conjunctival congestion	Circumciliary congestion
1. Intense at the fornix	Intense around limbus
2. Conjunctivitis	Uveitis and acute glaucoma
3. No pain	Intense pain with photophobia
4. Mucopurulent discharge	Only watering of the eyes
5. Congestion is of bright red color	Congestion is of pink color
6. Superficial vessels	Deep vessels

Note: This difference is most marked in the early phase of the disease. Later the congestion becomes generalized.

Cornea

Inspection by Slit-lamp

- *Diameter of the cornea:*
  - *Normal size* of the cornea is 12 mm in the horizontal and 11 mm in the vertical meridian.
  - Small diameter in *microcornea*
  - Large diameter in *buphthalmos or mega-locornea*

Curvature of the cornea is markedly increased in *keratoconus.*

- Irregularity in the corneal surface can be diagnosed by *Placido's disk.*
- Opacity on the cornea can be *nebular, macular or leukomatous.*
- *Adherent leukoma* is a condition wherein there is incarceration of iris in the corneal scar usually following perforation of the cornea.
- *Staphyloma* is a condition in which the corneal scar is incarcerated with the iris tissue which bulges forward.
- *Keratopathy:* Band-shape degeneration of cornea.
- *Nodule or nodules:* Phlycten which may be single or multiple.
- *Tumor:* Dermoid at the limbus
- *Filamentary keratitis:* One end of the filament is attached to the cornea while the other end is freely mobile.
- *An abrasion of the cornea* can be easily diagnosed by the use of fluorescein staining of the cornea.
- *Vascularization of cornea:* Vascularization can be superficial or deep diagnosed by slit-lamp.

- *Keratic precipitates* on back of cornea diagnosed by slit-lamp.

Corneal Staining with Fluorescein

Instill a drop of fluorescein solution or touch the wetted strip of fluorescein in the lower fornix. Ask the patient to keep the eye closed for one minute and then examine the cornea by slit-lamp with cobalt filter.

Staining of the cornea appears bright green in color and it is better appreciated under a cobalt filter.

The corneal staining helps to detect the following lesions:

- Minute abrasions
- Multiple erosions
- Superficial punctate keratitis
- Corneal ulcer

Corneal Sensitivity Test

Touch the cornea with a wisp of moist cotton wool and compare it with the opposite normal eye.

Zone of very sensitive cornea is a small area of 5 mm in the center of cornea.

Corneal sensitivity decreases with:

- Age with malnourishment
- Wearing contact lens
- Herpes simplex.

Placido's Keratoscopic Disk

The Placido's disk has black and white circles painted alternately with a central hole to observe. The surgeon holds the disk in his hand and looks through the central hole in it. The image of the Placido's disk is reflected on the patient's cornea due to light placed just on the side and slightly behind at the level of his/her ear.

- If the cornea of the patient is smooth and regular, then the reflected image of rings on the cornea of the patient appears smooth and regular.
- If there is irregularity due to facet or a minute nebular opacity, then the reflected image of the rings on the cornea appears broken or irregular in that sector.

Specular Microscopy of Corneal Endothelium

The surgeon can observe large number of corneal endothelial cells and can study their morphology and photograph also. The magnification is at 200. The average endothelial cell count is 2800 cells per square millimeter.

Significant decrease in the cell count with age and after cataract operation.

Cell loss with cataract operation is from 0 to 8% with intracapsular extraction.

Cell loss with intraocular lens implant is from 24 to 62%.

It is very essential to conduct the cell count before using donor cornea for grafting. Cells do not regenerate.

Keratometry (Ophthalmometry)

The keratometry helps to assess the corneal curvature accurately and with ease. It is useful in prescription of contact lens and for IOLs implant.

Pachometry

Pachometer is used to measure the thickness of the cornea.

Central corneal thickness varies between 0.49 and 0.56 mm.

Reading above 0.6 mm suggests an endothelial affection.

1. *Optical pachometry* uses the image splitting device in the Haag-Streit slit-lamp.
2. *Ultrasonic pachometry* is useful in cases of radial keratotomy.

Pachometry is useful in the following conditions:

- Corneal decompensation
- Keratoconus
- Corneal ulcers
- Corneal transplant
- Radial keratotomy.

Sclera

Inspection

- *Flat or a raised nodule with localized congestion.*
- Ectasia of the sclera around the limbus or in any sector of the limbus.
- Flat grey-colored areas are diagnostic for healed scars of scleritis.
- Pigmentation at the point of entry of anterior ciliary vessels is common and normal.
- Blue sclera in infants is normal.

Palpation

If there is a raised or a flat nodule in the sclera, then ask the patient to close the eyes and thereafter gently press the area of nodule.

Feeling of tenderness is a positive sign for scleritis/episcleritis.

Anterior Chamber

- *Shallow* in glaucoma and in the intumescent stage of cataract.
- *Deep* in iridocyclitis with total posterior synechia.
- *Funnel-shaped,* i.e. deep in center and shallow in periphery in iridocyclitis with ring synechia.
- *Unequal,* i.e. shallow in some part and deep in other part in subluxation of the lens.
- *Absent* in detachment of choroid and leak following intraocular surgery.

Contents of the Anterior Chamber

- Cells and aqueous flare *in iridocyclitis.*
- *Hypopyon* in iridocyclitis and hypopyon ulcer.
- *Hyphema* following trauma.
- *Lens matter* following trauma.

Pupil

Normal pupil is centrally placed, circular, optically clear and varies in its size from 3 to 4 mm and reacts briskly to the light reflex and near reflex.

Size of Pupil

- Pupils are small in size in infants and old age.
- Pupil is small in size with use of miotics.
- Pupil is large in size with use of mydriatic.
- Pupil is constricted in uveitis.

Shape of the Pupil Margin

Irregularity in the shape of the pupil is due to synechia.

Pupillary Aperture

Any exudate in the pupillary area indicates uveitis.

Reaction of Pupil

Abnormal pupillary reaction indicates involvement of the optic nerve, macula or retina.

Reflex from the Pupil

- *Red reflex* from a pupil is normal.
- *Grey reflex* from the pupil in refractive error, early cataract, glaucoma and myopia.
- *White reflex* from the pupil in detachment of the retina, cyclitic membrane, retrolental fibroplasia and retinoblastoma.
- *No reflex* in massive vitreous hemorrhage.

Iris

- Pattern of the iris.
- Color of the iris.
- Atrophic patches.
- Iridectomy hole
- Iridodialysis, i.e. torn iris in the periphery.
- Tremulousness of the iris is seen in the subluxation and aphakia.
- Synechia which may be—anterior, posterior, ring, total posterior and peripheral anterior synechia.
- Congenital coloboma of iris.
- New vessels on the iris, e.g. rubeosis iridis.
- Persistent pupillary membrane.

Lens

The normal lens is optically clear and transparent. Dilate the pupil to examine the lens in detail. Examine the lens by slit-lamp and ophthalmoscope to get complete information about any change in it or its capsule.

Look for the following signs:
- Opacity in the lens or its capsule appears black against the red background.
- Wedge-shape spokes of opacity with clear area in between are seen in the incipient stage of cataract formation.
- Opacities in the posterior capsule are seen in cases of retinitis pigmentosa and choroiditis.
- Multiple blue dot cataract.
- Pigments left over the lens may be due to broken synechia or due to persistent pupillary membrane.

Vitreous

Vitreous is a clear, avascular, gelatinous gel filling the space bound by the lens, retina and optic disc.

Slit-lamp and ophthalmoscope help to examine vitreous.
- Look for any opacity constant in the field of vision or floating.
- Cells, flare, bands, membrane, new vessels, empty spaces.
- Liquid or gel.

Fundus

Examine by ophthalmoscope or slit-lamp with three or four mirror contact lenses.
- *Optic disk*: Look for changes in its color, margins, physiological cup, vessels, hemorrhage and edema.
- *Macula*: Look for edema, pigmentation, hemorrhage, hard exudates, lamellar hole, macular hole, cherry red spot, degeneration and scarring.
- *Retinal blood vessels*: Look for narrowing, tortuosity, sheathing, crossing defects and pulsation.
- *General background:* Superficial or deep hemorrhages, micro-aneurysms, hard and soft exudates, pigmentation, drusens, neovascularization, bands, fibrous membranes, tumor, detachment, etc.

5

Clinical Ocular Investigations

Visual Acuity

- Visual acuity for distance vision
- Visual acuity for near vision

Refractometry

- Computerized autorefractometer

Ophthalmoscopy

- Indirect binocular ophthalmoscopy
- Direct ophthalmoscopy

Slit-lamp Biomicroscopy

- Cornea
- Lens
- Vitreous
- Fundus with Hruby lens
- Fundus with posterior fundus contact lens
- Fundus and angle of anterior chamber with three-mirror contact lens

Gonioscopy

- Three-mirror contact lens, four-mirror contact lens

Tonometry

- Digital tonometry
- Schiotz indentation tonometry
- Applanation tonometry

Color Vision

- Polychromatic plates of Ishihara

Angiography

- Fundus fluorescein angiography

Exophthalmometry

Ultrasonography

- A-scan (time amplitude)
- B-scan (intensity modulation)
- Electroretinography (ERG)
- Dark adaptative (adaptometry)
- Electro-oculography (EOG)
- Visually evoked response (VER)
- Optical coherence tomography

Computerized chair, auto-refractometer, slit-lamp and many new automated electronic gadgets have totally replaced the traditional unventilated, humid and environmentally boring dark room procedures.

Now ophthalmologist conducts ocular investigations in a well ventilated, air condition, interiorly decorated clinic (Fig. 5.1) and soft background music with young intelligent, soft and beautiful hands to assist.

VISUAL ACUITY

Visual Acuity for Distant Vision (Fig. 5.2)

The visual acuity for distant central vision is universely tested by *Snellen test type*. These are constructed upon the standard that the average minimum visual angle is one minute. The test type consists of a series of letters arranged in lines, each line diminishing in respect to the size of letters from above to downwards. The breadth of the lines of each letter is composed in such a way that the edges of each letter subtend an angle of one minute

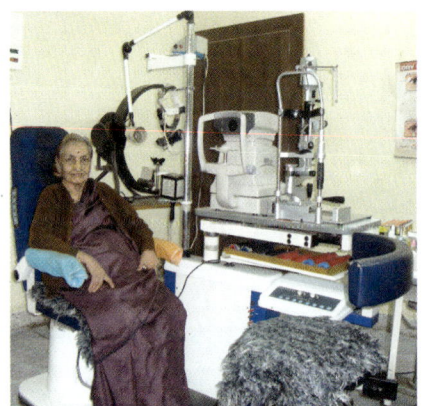

Fig. 5.1: Ophthalmic clinic

at the nodal point of the eye at a particular distance. Each letter is of such a shape that it can be placed in a square the sides of which are five times the breadth of the lines of letter. Due to this, the whole letter subtends an angle of five minute at the nodal point of the eye, if it is 60 meters from the eye. The letters in the subsequent lines subtend an angle of five minute, if they are at 36, 24, 18, 12, 9 and 6 meters from the eye.

For recording the visual acuity, it is not possible to keep the letters at the desired distance. For practical purpose the patient is kept at a fixed distance of 6 meters from the Snellen test type. At the distance of 6 meters, the rays coming from the letters of Snellen test type are considered parallel and the eye is at rest with no accommodation. A person with normal visual acuity should be able to read all the letters from the top 60 meter line to the bottom 6 meters line.

To record the visual acuity, make the patient sit in a comfortable testing automated chair facing the Snellen distant test type drum. Put a trial frame and ask the patient to read slowly and loudly from the top letter to the bottom line. Test each eye separately by putting an occluder in the trial frame left eye first and thereafter the right eye. Make a note of the visual acuity recorded according to the value which corresponds to the line the patient is able to read correctly. The convention for recording is 6/60, 6/36, 6/24, 6/18, 6/12, 6/9, and 6/6 in which the numerator is the

distance of the test type from the patient which is constant always at 6 meters and the denominator is the distance in meters marked along the line up to which a patient is able to read on the Snellen test type. The normal visual acuity of 6/6 means that the patient is able to read from a distance of 6 meters the letters which are supposed to be read at a distance of 6 meters. The visual acuity of 6/18 means that the patient is able to read from the distance of 6 meter the letters which are supposed to be read from the distance of 18 meter. Thus, the distant vision is recorded as V-6/18. The normal vision is V-6/6.

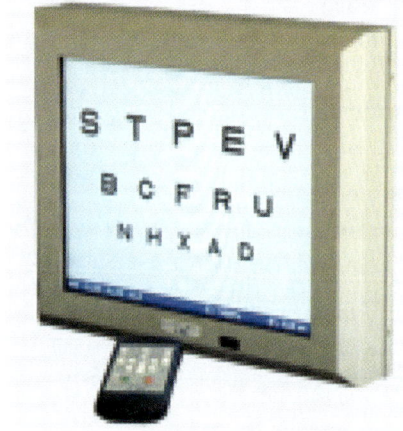

Fig. 5.2: Automated visual acuity unit for distance vision

If the patient is unable to read the top letter, i.e. his/her visual acuity is less than 6/60 then ask patient to get up and walk slowly towards the test type and stop soon, when he is able to read the top letter. If this distance is 3 meters then his/her visual acuity is recorded as V-3/60 thus the numerator, i.e. 3-meter is the distance at which the patient is able to read the top letter and the 60 meters shall be the denominator.

If the patient is unable to see the top letter even from a close distance of about one meter, then ask him/her to count the extended fingers of the ophthalmologist's hand held up in level with his eyes. The visual acuity is recorded as V-fingers at one meter.

If the patient is unable to count the fingers also then ask him/her to observe the movements of the extended hand of the ophthalmologist. If he/she can see the movements of the hand then the visual acuity is recorded as V-hand movements.

If the patient is unable to see even the hand movements then throw the torch light on the patient's eye and ask him/her whether he/she can perceive the torch light or not. If the patient is able to perceive the light, then the visual acuity is recorded as V-PL (perception of light, present). If the patient is unable to perceive the light, then the visual acuity is recorded as V-no PL (patient denies perception of light).

If the patient is able to perceive the light, then the torch light should be shown to him from four cardinal directions—up, down, right and left; and make a note about the direction in which he can perceive the light and the direction from which he is unable to perceive the light. The visual acuity is recorded as V-PL and PR from all directions (projection of light from all direction), or V-PL from the direction from which he/she can perceive the light.

Visual Acuity for Near Vision (Fig. 5.3)

For recording the visual acuity for near vision, the cards with modern Times Roman type in various sizes from 5 pt to 48 pt is used. These have been standardized by the faculty of ophthalmologists and numbered from N 5 to N 48 corresponding to modern Times Roman type in various sizes from 5 pt to 48 pt as N5, N6, N8, N10, N12, N14, N18, N24, N36 and N48. A person with normal distant vision is able to read the near vision test type up to N5 without any difficulty up to the age of 40 years. After this age, the near point recedes away from the comfortable near point and he/she needs near glasses.

The patient is given the near vision test type card and asked to keep it at a distance at which he/she is normally used to read and work. The paragraph up to which he/she is able to read clearly and comfortably is noted with the size marked over it. The near vision is recorded as N12. if he/she is able to read this paragraph clearly or as N14 if patient is able to read this paragraph clearly. For correction of near vision, assess the near point with distant correction. According to the requirement of the patient, the near vision is corrected. The near vision correction closer than 28 cm is not well tolerated.

REFRACTOMETRY

Computerized Autorefractometer (Fig. 5.4)

- Refractometry is an objective method of assessing errors of refraction by the use of refractometers.
- Presently, computerized autorefractometers are popular and in demand.
- It is a quick method of assessing refractive errors in term of sphere, cylinder with axis and interpupillary distance.

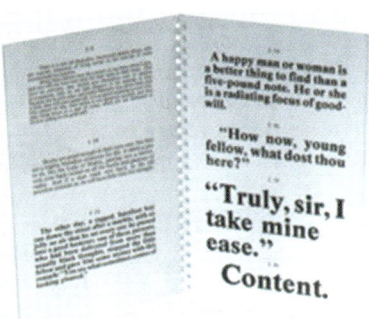

Fig. 5.3: Near vision chart

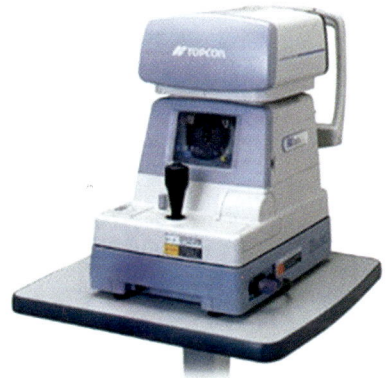

Fig. 5.4: Computerized autorefractometer

- It is handy, accurate and fast procedure for clinics, eye out-patient clinics and for mass screening, research work and epidemiological study.

OPHTHALMOSCOPY

Indirect Binocular Ophthalmoscopy (Fig. 5.5)

Principle

- Eye is made highly myopic irrespective of its refraction by placing a convex lens in front of the eye so that a real and inverted image of the fundus is formed between the observer and the convex lens.
- *Image is magnified:* The amount of magnification depends upon the refraction of the eye, the power of the convex lens, and the distance at which the convex lens is kept from the eye.
- *In emmetropia:* If the power of the lens used is plus 13 dioptre and the lens is placed at its focal distance from the anterior focal point of the eye then the image is magnified to five times and reflexes are at their minimum allowing a clear view of the fundus.
- *In myopia:* The image forms close to the lens than in the emmetropia.
- *In hypermetropia:* The image forms further away than in a case of emmetropia.
- A convex lens weaker than 13 dioptre gives more magnification but less bright image of the fundus.

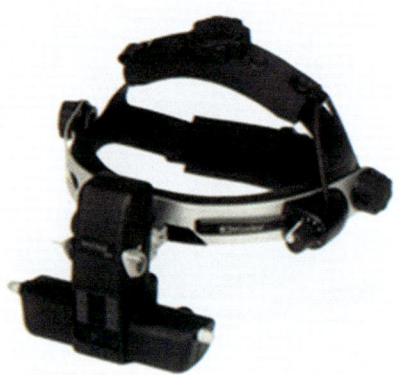

Fig. 5.5: Binocular indirect ophthalmoscope

- A convex lens stronger than 13 dioptre gives less magnification but brighter image of the fundus.
- Most of the eye surgeons use strong convex lens usually of 20 dioptre.

Technique

The pupil must be fully dilated with a cycloplegic. The eye surgeon adjusts the head band, the light and the pupillary distance as per his need. The patient is made to lie down supine on an examination coach about two feet in height. The surgeon stands on the head side and directs the light of the ophthalmoscope on the patient's right eye and the convex lens held between the index finger and thumb is placed near the eye. Thereafter, it is gradually moved away from the eye until the image of the fundus is seen clearly occupying the whole lens.

It is essential to remember that the plane surface of the convex lens is placed towards the eye.

Light reflexes can be dodged by slightly tilting the lens.

Periphery of the fundus can be examined by scleral depression.

Advantages

- Stereoscopic view
- Large field
- Bright image
- Magnification can be varied
- Extreme periphery of the retina can be seen by scleral depression.

Disadvantages

- *As the image formed is real and inverted, therefore, there is a problem of orientation of fundus lesions unless one gets used to it.*
- Magnification is only 5 times while in the direct ophthalmoscopy it is 15 times.

Direct Ophthalmoscopy

Direct ophthalmoscopy is for fundus and media examination. While conducting direct ophthalmoscopy, it is presumed that the observer is emmetropic and has learned the art to relax his accommodation.

Direct ophthalmoscopy is most popular, convenient technique for fundus and media examination. It is conducted by a self-luminous direct ophthalmoscope (Fig. 5.6). The direct ophthalmoscope has handle and head in which there is a disk of lenses ranging from plus 30 to minus 30, a control disk and a sight-hole.

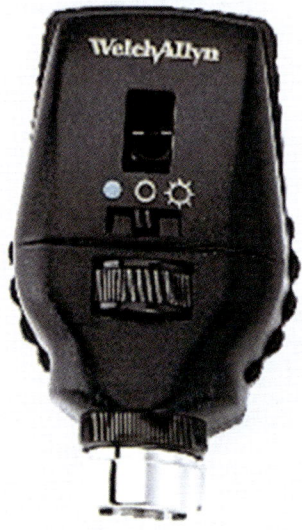

Fig. 5.6: Direct ophthalmoscope

Principle

- The observer receives the emergent rays from the fundus of the patient directly.
- If the patient is an emmetrope, then the emergent rays are parallel and brought to focus on the retina of the observer directly and he will be able to see the fundus clearly.
- If either of the two, the patient or the observer is ametropic or accommodates during examination then the observer shall have to change the lenses in the ophthalmoscope to bring the retina in focus.
- The image formed is virtual erect and magnified to about 15 times.
- Magnification of the image of fundus is somewhat less in hypermetropia and more in myopia.

- Area of fundus observed varies with the distance of the ophthalmoscope from the eye and also on the refractive state of the patient's eye.
- Area of fundus observed increases as the eye is approached closer.
- Area of fundus observed is greater in hypermetropia and lesser in myopia than in emmetropia.
- Ophthalmologist views large area with less magnification in a hypermetropia and a small area but more magnification in myopia.

Technique

- Dilated pupil allows better view of the fundus, therefore, it is better to dilate the pupil by mydriatic eye drops.
- Make the patient sit comfortably in a chair and ask him/her to look at a distance or a spot light in the Snellen test type drum.
- For examination of the fundus of the right eye, stand on the right side of the patient. Hold the ophthalmoscope in the right hand and examine him/her by your right eye and vice versa for the left eye.
- Viewing through the sight-hole of the ophthalmoscope and the light focused on the patient's eye, approach the patient with the light beam on the pupil until you see a red glow and soon the details of the fundus.
- Bring the fundus in focus by changing the lens in the ophthalmoscope by rotating the lens disk.
- Clear image of the fundus is visible, if both—the patient and the observer are emmetropic, do not accommodate and the anterior focal points are coinciding.

Advantages

- Direct ophthalmoscope is handy, portable and self-luminous.
- Image is erect and magnified 15 times, so better orientation.
- Opacities in the vitreous and lens can be viewed by changing convex lenses from 0 to plus 20 dioptre and slightly withdrawing from the eye. The opacities

appear as black spots against the red background of red glow.

- Ophthalmologist can thoroughly explore the eye from the fundus to the surface of the cornea.
- Detached retina can be seen by putting up convex lenses and slightly withdrawing from the eye.
- Refractive state of the eye can be assessed, when the degree of ametropia is high.
- Difference in the level of the lesion can be measured. *It is helpful in glaucomatous cupping and papilledema.* The base of the cupped disk will be relatively myopic to the edge of the disk and similarly the top of the swollen disk in papilledema will be relatively hypermetropic to the edge of the disk. Therefore, in a case of cupped disk, concave lens is required to focus vessels at the bottom while convex lens is required to focus the vessels on the top of the swollen disk. Difference of three dioptre is equivalent to approximately one mm difference of level at the fundus.
- *To get the correct reading, it is essential that the correcting lens in the ophthalmoscope is at the anterior focus of the emmetropic eye and accommodation of the observer and the patient is fully relaxed.*

Disadvantages

- Periphery of the fundus cannot be examined even with full dilation of the pupil.
- Uniocular view and not the stereoscopic view.

SLIT-LAMP BIOMICROSCOPY

The slit-lamp is the most useful instrument for the examination of the eyeball as a whole specially the cornea, iris, angle of anterior chamber, lens, vitreous and retina.

Slit-lamp stereoscopic microscope basically consists of an illuminating system and a movable binocular microscope. The light beam can be adjusted to vary the width, height and angle of incidence. The microscope and the light beam can be aligned or redirected to view the lesion from a different angle. The most common and popular slit-lamp Haag-

Streit model 900 (Fig. 5.7) is in focus at about 95 mm in front of the objective lens of the microscope or 280 mm (11 inches) from the examiner's eyes. The cornea, iris, lens and vitreous can be examined by the slit-lamp directly. For the examination of the angle of the anterior chamber and the retina, one needs a three/four mirror contact lens of *Goldmann.* With this lens in place on the cornea, one can examine the posterior pole and the periphery of the fundus and the angle of the anterior chamber.

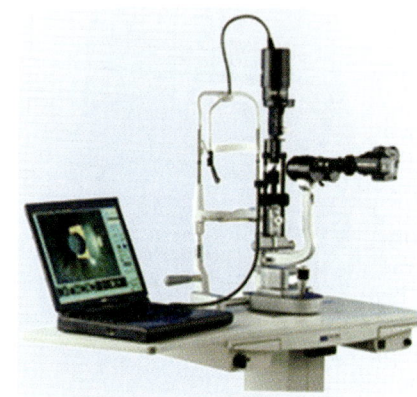

Fig. 5.7: Slit-lamp—Haag-Streit with imaging unit

Cornea

There are 6 techniques for examination of the cornea:

1. Diffuse illumination
2. Sclerotic scatter
3. Direct focal illumination
4. Retroillumination
5. Specular reflection
6. Indirect illumination.

Diffuse Illumination

Use a wide beam and keep it out of focus and view the whole cornea from one side to the other. It is like an examination with a torch.

Sclerotic Scatter

Direct a narrow beam at the temporal limbus and focus the microscope centrally on the cornea. In this technique, the light from the temporal limbus is transmitted within the cornea by the total internal reflection and exits at the opposite nasal limbus. In a normal cornea, no light is seen. Any stromal or epithelial opacities get illuminated. This technique is useful to diagnose any lesion of the stroma or epithelium of cornea.

Direct Focal Illuminaiton

Focus the slit-beam and microscope at coincident points. This technique provides direct view of the structure under observation. By altering the direction of beam and making it narrow, it helps to locate the position of the opacity and the depth of the lesion. This is the most common method of examination of cornea by a slit-lamp.

Retroillumination

The cornea is illuminated by the light reflected from the fundus and the iris. Focus the light beam behind the cornea and the microscope on the cornea. By this technique, any change in the epithelium, stroma and the endothelium can be observed especially small stromal opacities and keratic precipitates.

Specular Reflection

The cornea is observed adjacent to the beam. By altering the angle of the beam, a point is reached at which the reflection of the posterior corneal surface allows visualization of mosaic pattern of the endothelial cell, endothelial changes and folds in the Descemet's membrane. Similarly, by altering the angle of beam, the reflection of the anterior corneal surface allows visualization of the precorneal tear film.

Indirect Illumination

Direct the beam of the light at the corneal opacity and observe with the microscope. The changes in the adjacent area like new vessels stand out prominently in the scattered light.

Lens

Slit-lamp is the best appliance for examination of lens from various angles and magnifications as required. It is essential to dilate the pupil fully with a cycloplegic to examine the lens thoroughly and preferably with low illumination in the room.

- *Diffuse illumination* is helpful in the survey of the anterior and posterior surfaces of the lens and large opacities in the lens.
- *Retroillumination* is used for viewing the anterior capsular changes.
- *Direct focal illumination* is useful for viewing the zones of discontinuity. The zones appear as bright stripes in the parallelepiped because they are formed by abrupt changes in the refractive index and occur between different layers of the lens. The zones are concentric to one another and are as follows; capsule, line of disjunction, adult nucleus, infantile nucleus and fetal nucleus which contains the anterior and posterior Y-sutures.
- *With specular reflection,* the opacities, elevations or depressions of the anterior lens capsule may appear as dark spots.

Vitreous

Set the slit-lamp to the brightest beam and adjust the beam to a narrow slit. Bring the beam from a very wide possible angle. This will create black background against which the delicate fibrillar elements and posterior vitreous face are visible. With the silt beam aimed vertically, the general shape of the posterior vitreous face can be examined. The posterior vitreous face is visible only when the vitreous is detached. The fluid vitreous takes longer time to settle down while the healthy gel merely quivers a little.

Fundus with Hruby Lens

The Hruby lens has a planoconcave surface attached to the slit-lamp. The dioptric power of the lens is –58.6 D so that the image of the fundus is brought to focus at the distal focal point of the lens which lies in the anterior segment of the eye. It provides a small field with low magnification and fundus is visible only up to equator. The concave surface of the Hruby lens is towards the patient.

Fundus with Posterior Fundus Contact Lens

The posterior fundus contact lens is a modified Koeppe lens. The image formed is erect, virtual and situated in the anterior vitreous cavity. It allows view of the posterior fundus only.

Fundus and Angle of Anterior Chamber with Three-mirror Contact Lens

Three mirrors in the Goldmann three-mirror contact lens (Fig. 5.8) are placed in the cone; each mirror with a different angle of inclination. Two mirrors are rectangular and one mirror is semicircular in shape.

- Central part of the lens allows examination of the posterior fundus.
- Long rectangular mirror allows examination of the peripheral part of the fundus.
- Small rectangular mirror allows examination of the extreme periphery of the fundus even up to ora serrata.
- Semicircular mirror is used to examine the angle of the anterior chamber.

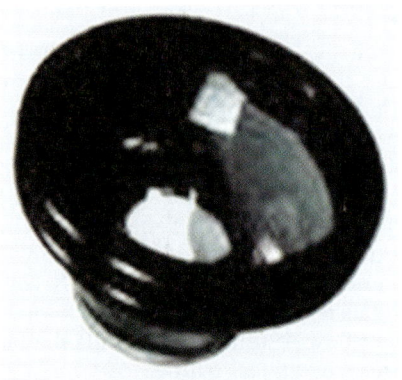

Fig. 5.8: Goldmann three-mirror contact lens

For the complete examination of the peripheral fundus and the whole angle of anterior chamber, the mirror should be rotated along with the beam of the slit-lamp.

GONIOSCOPY

- Semicircular mirror is used for visualizing angle of anterior chamber and it needs complete rotation to visualize the angle.

- Four-mirror gonioscope (Fig. 5.9) allows complete anterior chamber angle viewing with minimal lens rotation.

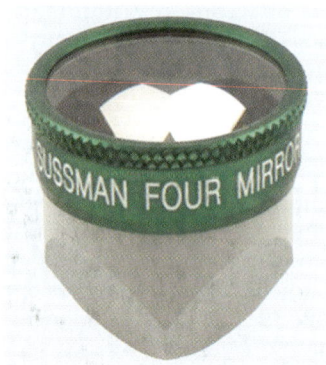

Fig. 5.9: Four-mirror goniolens

Technique

Anesthetize the cornea by instillation of lignocaine hydrochloride 2% as topical drops once. Make the patient sit in front of a slit-lamp and adjust the instrument and the patient in a comfortable position. Explain him/her to get his/her cooperation. Pour methyl cellulose drops in the cup of the lens and insert it between the lids to fit properly on the cornea. Holding the lens by fingers of one hand to adjust the light beam of slit-lamp light on the semicircular mirror of the lens. With slight adjustment of the lens and the beam, the angle becomes visible. By rotating the lens and accordingly the beam of light, one can examine the whole angle.

Interpretation

- *In wide angle:* All the structures of the angle are seen. The narrow beam of the light deflects at the transition between the anterior wall of the angle and the recess and again deflects at the transition between the ciliary body and the root of the iris. *In wide angle, the anterior surface of the ciliary body forms the recess of the angle.*
- *In close angle:* Only the Schwalbe's line (glistening white line) and anterior part of the trabecular band are visible. The crowding of the iris in periphery conceals

the lower part of the trabecula, ciliary body and root of the iris. There is a deflection of the beam of light. *This parallactic displacement of light beam indicates that some part of the angle is open.*

- *In close angle during attack or after:* The periphery of the iris appears to be adherent at the anterior wall of the angle. *In a completely closed angle, there is no parallactic displacement of beam.* The beam appears to meet at a point. The periphery of the iris is bulging forward making the chamber very shallow.

TONOMETRY

Digital Tonometry

It is done in the same manner as testing for fluctuation in nodule or cyst in other parts of the body. Ask the patient to close both the eyes and look down. Perform digital fluctuation first in normal eye and then compare it with the affected eye. Place the bulb of two index fingers a short distance from one another above the upper border of superior tarsal plate and perform fluctuation test softly. Repeat the test 2–3 times in both the eyes and compare. Hard feeling or no fluctuation indicates raised intraocular pressure.

It is easy and handy method for out-patient screening for glaucoma.

Schiotz Indentation Tonometry

The Schiotz tonometer (Fig. 5.10) is most popular tonometer used for measuring the intraocular pressure because of its simplicity, reliability, low price, relative accuracy, portability, easy to use, and used without slit-lamp.

- *Indentation tonometry is based on the principle of indentation of the eye by the plunger of the Schiotz tonometer.*
- Amount of indentation is measured on a scale. The reading of the scale is converted into millimeters of mercury (mm Hg) by referring to the chart available with the tonometer.
- Scleral rigidity plays an important factor in the measurement of intraocular pressure. A person with low scleral rigidity

shows false low reading on tonometry, whereas patient with high scleral rigidity shows false high reading on tonometry, when compared with applanation tonometry.

- Abnormal scleral rigidity can be detected by Schiotz tonometer by taking two readings with two different weighs. If the two readings are the same, then the scleral rigidity is normal. Difference in the reading indicates scleral rigidity.

Technique

- Make the patient lie down on the examination table. Instill a drop of lignocaine hydrochloride 2%. Explain the patient about the technique and ask for his/her cooperation in looking straight up at a spot light on the ceiling or one finger placed directly in his line of gaze and not to squeeze the lids.
- It is customary to start with 5.5 g weight.
- Apply the tonometer properly and softly on the cornea to get the correct reading of pressure.
- Separate the lids by fingers of one hand and apply tonometer plunger on the cornea by the other hand. Place the plunger centrally on the cornea and make note of the reading on the scale.
- If the scale reading is four or less, then take another reading with 7.5 g weight.
- If the intraocular pressure is 20–25 mm Hg or more, consistently for three readings in

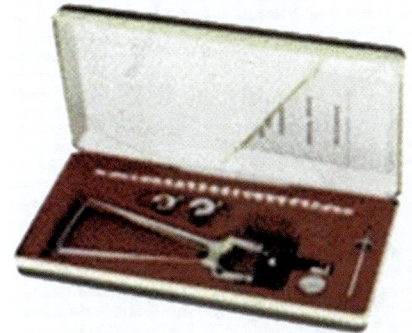

Fig. 5.10: Schiotz tonometer

day and for three days then label the patient as a case of glaucoma.

- *Note the reading on the scale of tonometer only when the lever of the tonometer shows pulsation. The lever shows pulsation, if tonometer is placed centrally and softly. The lever shows pulsation as the intraocular pressure varies with the cardiac pulse pressure.*
- The normal reading varies from 12–22 mm Hg.

Sources of Error

- *Scleral rigidity:* The scleral rigidity is low in high myopia, dysthyroid exophthalmos and following glaucoma surgery.
- *Improper calibration of tonometer:* Test the tonometer each time by placing it on the testing plate to confirm its calibration. The lever must move freely and show proper calibration.
- *Improper application:* The tonometer must be placed centrally on the cornea. Even slight misplacement can give a false reading. Take reading, when the lever shows pulsation.
- *Uncooperative patient:* Patient is uncooperative because of apprehension and improper local anesthesia. Squeezing of the lids causes rise in the pressure. Take reading, when the patient is relaxed or has relaxed his/her lids. Take care not to separate the lids by force against his/her squeeze as it raises the pressure.

Precautions

- Sterilize the tonometer at least once a day. It can be easily sterilized by formalin vaporizer. A non-sterile tonometer can spread infection from one patient to another.
- Clean the foot plate with moist cotton swab before using it on each patient.
- Improper application of tonometer can cause minute abrasions on the cornea.
- Perform tonometry carefully with full cooperation from the patient.

Applanation Tonometry

The principle of applanation tonometry is based *on 'imbert-fick law'* which states that the pressure inside a sphere (P) is equal to the force (W) required to flatten its surface divided by the arc of flattening (A).

$$\text{That is; } P = W/A$$

Scleral rigidity plays no role in applanation tonometry.

Applanation tonometer (Fig. 5.11) consists of a double prism that has a diameter of 3.06 mm mounted on slit-lamp.

It is essential to handle the applanation tonometer gently to get the correct reading at correct time with semicircles in correct position.

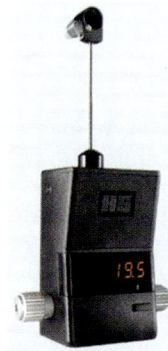

Fig. 5.11: Applanation tonometer

Technique

- Make the patient sit on stool in front of slit-lamp.
- Instill lignocaine hydrochloride 2%
- Stain the tear film by fluorescein strip.
- Adjust the tonometer and view. The cornea and biprisms are illuminated with cobalt blue light from the slit-lamp. When the prism touches the apex of the cornea, then the observer can see two fluorescent semicircles. These semicircles represent the stained tear film touching the upper and lower halves of the prism. Adjust the applanation force against cornea until the inner edges of two semicircles just touch. These semicircles never stay still but are constantly pulsating with cardiac pulse.
- Take the reading at midpoint. Note the reading on the dial of the tonometer and multiply by ten to get the intraocular pressure in mm Hg.

COLOR VISION

- *Color sense* provides us an ability to differentiate the colors as excited by the light of different wavelengths.
- *Cones* appreciate colors only in the light of good intensity.
- *Objects appear grey with different hue* in low illumination or dark-adapted eye.
- *Trichromatic color:* Three pigments in the cones which absorb different wavelengths of light corresponding to three *primary colors—red, green and blue.*
- *Test for color vision* is essential for recruits in the military services, railway services, air and road transport services.

- *No disability*: As such no one is ever disabled due to being a color deficient or color blind and leads a normal life like any normal human being.

Polychromatic Plates of Ishihara (Fig. 5.12)

These plates are made up of dots of the primary colors printed on the background of similar dots in a confusion of colors. The dots of primary colors are set in a pattern of bold numerical or a wavy line. A person with normal color vision can read the numbers or trace the wavy line correctly but the person having total color blindness or color deficiency reads the numerical or trace the line wrongly or cannot read or trace at all.

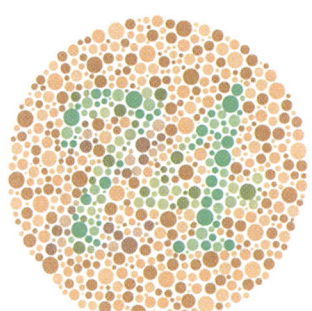
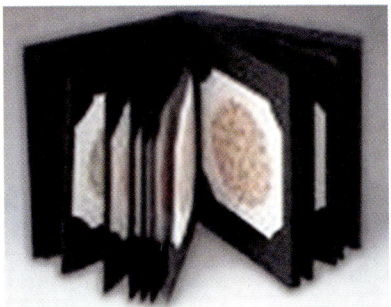

Fig. 5.12: Polychromatic plates of Ishihara

Technique

The patient is asked to hold the book of Ishihara chart and read out the numerical number or trace the wavy line and a note is made of the outcome. The result of each plate is given and accordingly the surgeon can find out whether the patient is a color deficient or color blind.

It is necessary that the illumination should not be less than 50 feet candle for correct assessment.

ANGIOGRAPHY

Fundus Fluorescein Angiography

Fundus fluorescein angiography is one of the important diagnostic techniques to assess ocular pathophysiological mechanism. The fluorescence can be observed directly by slit-lamp or ophthalmoscope, and can also be photographed for the permanent record.

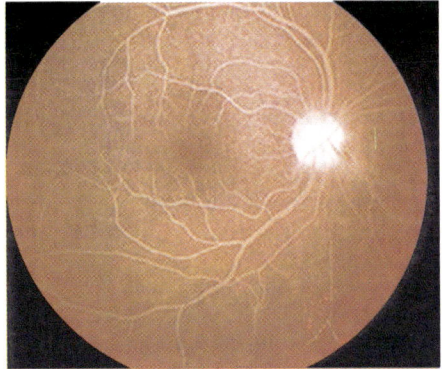

Fig. 5.13: Normal fluorescein angiogram

Normal angiogram (Fig. 5.13) consists of overlapping phases; *pre-arterial phase, arterial phase, arteriovenous phase, venous phase.*

Fluorescein angiography of the anterior segment is gaining importance as a valuable diagnostic aid and providing information about late complications which otherwise may be missed by slit-lamp.

Technique

Fluorescein is an alkali dye of the sodium fluorescein. Its low molecular weight and high solubility in water allow rapid diffusion.

- For angiography, 5 cc of 10% solution of sodium fluorescein is injected intravenously in the cubital vein very fast preferably through the wide bore needle.
- Injection is given after the patient has been adjusted for slit-lamp viewing and photography.
- Fluorescein can cause nausea and vomiting. It can also cause urticaria and allergic reaction.
- All patients have slight yellow skin discoloration for about 12–24 hours after fluorescein injection.
- Fluorescein is mainly excreted in urine with a small amount in bile.

Interpretations

Hyperfluorescence is an increased fluorescence as compared to normal. It is seen in vascular tumors, neovascularization, and in conditions where the pigment epithelium is defective.

Hypofluorescence is decreased fluorescence as compared to normal.

It is seen in conditions such as retinal vascular occlusion, atrophy of choriocapillaries, hemorrhages, abnormal tissue proliferation and increased pigmentation.

Retrofluorescence occurs when nonfluorescent structures come in the way of fluorescent background.

Fluorescein leakage and pooling The fluorescein crosses the physiological barrier of the retinal vessels or pigment epithelial cells and spreads into spaces between the cells or between tissue layers. It is seen in cases of macular degeneration, central serous retinopathy.

Fluorescein staining It occurs due to attachment of the dye to the tissue, thereby causing fluorescence. It can be seen in drusen.

EXOPHTHALMOMETRY

Periodic reading of exophthalmometry is essential to assess the forward projection of the eyeball and for the follow-up to assess the prognosis of exophthalmos and proptosis.

The normal range of the reading of exophthalmometry is 12–20 mm indicating the anterior distance of the cornea from the lateral orbital margin.

Any reading above 20 mm is pathognomonic, therefore, the patient should be further investigated and kept under the observation. *Technique of exophthalmometry by Hertel's exophthalmometer* (Fig. 5.14) *:* Make the patient stand close to the wall of the clinic and ask him to look into the examiner's eyes. Fix the concave part of the exophthalmometer against the lateral orbital margins adjusting it to fit properly and make a note of the bar reading on the exophthalmometer.

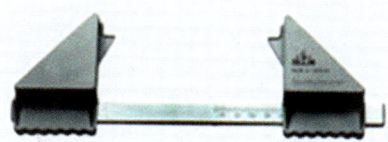

Fig. 5.14: Hertel's exophthalmometer

It is essential to fix the instrument, at the same bar reading for follow-up recording.

After fixing the instrument the examiner shall observe an image of the cornea of the right eye in the mirror of the appliance. The mirror is adjusted to line up the cornea with the scale and note the reading.

During this process, the patient is asked to look with his right eye in the observer's left eye.

Repeat the process by asking the patient to look with his/her left eye in the observer's right eye.

A typical reading is noted as follows:

With a bar reading of 98 mm, the right eye 18 mm and left eye 20 mm. Difference of more than 2 mm is seen with suspicion and patient should be kept under observation for follow-up.

IMAGING TECHNIQUES

Ultrasonography

Ultrasonography was initially used by military but later on it was used in the industry also. The diagnostic ophthalmic ultrasound was first reported in 1956 by Mundt and Hughes. Now, we have ultrasound A-scan and B-scan. All the diagnostic ophthalmic ultrasounds are based upon pulse echo technique. The ultrasonic energy is beamed into the ocular and orbital tissues. The returning signals are detected, amplified, and converted into display forms for interpretation. The processed signals are displayed on the cathode ray tubes in one of two modes: A-scan or B-scan.

A-scan (Time Amplitude)

In A-scan (Fig. 5.15), the horizontal dimension of the display screen is proportional to time and calibrated for distance measurement. *Vertical deflections from this line depict the position of an echo while the height of the vertical deflection is proportional to echo intensity.* Use of A-scan unit allows detection of any intraocular lesion which is elevated more than 0.75 mm from the sclera.

B-scan (Intensity Modulation)

In B-scan (Fig. 5.16), the horizontal dimension of the display screen is still related to time and distance. *The echoes are represented as intensity-modulated dots.* The strong echoes are white and weaker echoes are shades of grey depending on their strength. In B-scan ultrasonography, both the *water bath and contact* methods are available.

Water bath technique allows visualization of the anterior segment of the globe.

Contact technique: The probe is held directly against the closed lids with methyl cellulose as coupling agent and the anterior segment cannot be visualized with this.

Clinical Application

Ultrasonography helps to evaluate the condition of fundus, when the ocular media is opaque. It can help to detect, localize, measure, differentiate and follow-up a lesion in the eye or orbit.

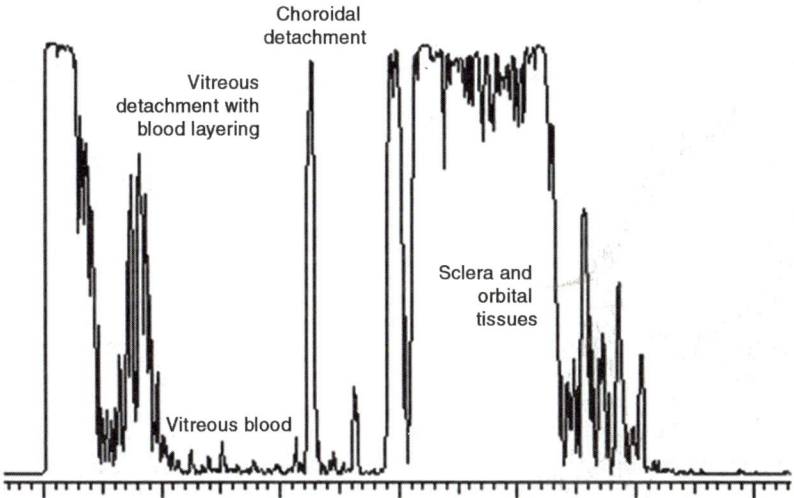

Fig. 5.15: A-scan ultrasound

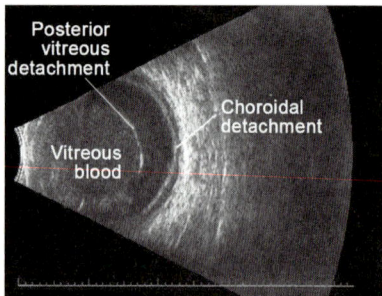

Fig. 5.16: B-scan ultrasound

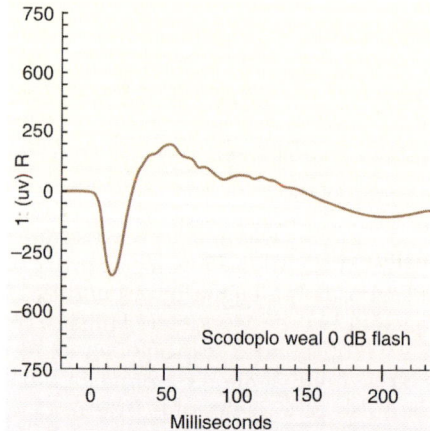

Fig. 5.17: Normal electroretinogram (ERG)

It is only by combining the reports from A-scan and B-scan that a reliable diagnosis can be made.

Useful in:

- Biometric studies using A-scan to calculate power of IOLs to be implanted.
- Vitreous opacities
- Senile vitreous degeneration
- Vitreous hemorrhage
- Retinal detachment
- Intraocular tumors
- Intraocular foreign bodies
- Orbital foreign bodies
- Orbital mass lesions
- Exophthalmos.

Electroretinography (ERG)

The electroretinogram (Fig. 5.17) is the record of an action potential produced by the retina, when it is stimulated by flash of light.

Recording

Active electrode embedded in a contact lens is placed on the cornea. Reference electrode is placed on patient's forehead. The potential between the two electrodes is then amplified and the response is displayed on a pen recorder. The electroretinogram can be obtained both in the light adapted (photopic) and dark adapted (scotopic) states. The usual response is biphasic.

- *a-wave*: It is the initial negative deflection.
- *b-wave*: It is the large positive deflection. The amplitude of the b-wave increases with dark adaptation and in the intensity of the light stimulus.

- *c-wave:* It is also positive wave.
- Eectroretinogram shows the function of the first two neurons of the retina.
- Electroretinogram does not help in the diagnosis of the function of the ganglion cells and optic nerve.
- Electroretinogram is *flat or extinguished* in retinitis pigmentosa, central retinal artery occlusion, total detachment of the retina, and in the case of advanced siderosis.
- Electroretinogram shows *subnormal response* in the condition of advanced retinopathy wherein large areas of retina has become atrophic or ischemic.
- Electroretinogram shows *negative response* in cases with gross disturbances of the retinal circulation.

Dark Adaptation (Adaptometry)

The test is clinically useful in the cases who complain of night blindness due to disorder of the retina as in a case of retinitis pigmentosa.

Electrooculography (EOG)

The electrooculogram measures the standing action potential which exists between the cornea which is electrically positive and the back of the eye which is electrically negative. It is based on the activity of the retinal pigment epithelium and the photoreceptors. This means that an eye blinded by any lesion proximal to photoreceptors will show a normal electrooculogram. An advanced disease of the retinal pigment epithelium shows a significant electrooculogram response. This test is supplementary to electroretinogram.

Visually Evoked Response (VER)

Visually evoked response is an electrical signal generated by the visual cortex in response to light stimulus of the retina. As most of the visual cortex represents the macula, therefore, this test is essentially a method of testing the macular function. This is the only test which can assess the function of the visual path beyond the retinal ganglion cells. Thus, an abnormal visually evoked response with a normal electroretinogram and electrooculogram shows lesions of visual pathway beyond ganglion cells to the visual cortex.

Visually evoked response is nothing but electroencephalography (EEG) recorded at the occipital lobe.

Uses of VER

- *To diagnose a lesion in the optic nerve-demyelination*
- Determination of visual acuity in infants
- Detection of a malingerer
- Evaluation of macular lesions.

Optical Coherence Tomography

Optical coherence tomography is non-invasive diagnostic method. It performs a cross-sectional imaging of retina and optic nerve with a resolution of 5–10 micron.

There are two types of machines—Time domain and spectral OCT. Spectral OCT is faster with better resolution (3–5 micron).

It is an invaluable non-invasive technique to study retinal changes in maculopathies especially in age-related macular degeneration when used along with fundus fluorescein angiography.

Optical coherence tomography has found wide applications in neuro-ophthalmology. All the neuro-ophthalmic diseases of afferent visual system involve damage to retinal nerve fiber layer which coalesces to form the optic nerve. Therefore, OCT becomes valuable diagnostic tool for the multiple sclerosis, parachiasmal lesions, Alzheimer's disease and tumors compressing anterior visual pathways.

It is very useful in cases with:
- Vitreomacular traction
- Epiretinal membrane
- Macular hole
- Vascular blocks
- Diabetic maculopathy
- Age-related macular degeneration
- Central serous retinopathy
- Any lesion in retina or optic disc especially macula.

6

Optical System of Eye

Optical System

- Optical system of normal eye
- Optical system of hypermetropic eye
- Optical system of myopic eye
- Optical system of aphakic eye

OPTICAL SYSTEM

Optical System of Normal Eye
(Schematic and Reduced Eye)

Optical system of an eye comprises four refractive media, namely: Cornea, lens, aqueous humor and vitreous.

Center of curvature of the cornea and the lens are on the same straight line, *the optic axis* of the system.

Refractive medium in front of this optical system is the *air*.

Refractive power of cornea is about 43 dioptre as the optical medium in front of cornea is air and the optical medium behind the cornea is the aqueous humor both having different refractive indices, thereby more refraction at the cornea. Refractive power of the lens is about 15 dioptre which is much less than the cornea due to optical medium of nearly equal refractive index on both sides. Thus, the total dioptric power of the *schematic eye* forming a homocentric complex lens system is plus 58 dioptre. *The object of this optically complex system of refraction is to shorten the focal distance of the system so that a small eye can perform a good function.*

Reduced Eye

From the optical point of view, the entire system of the eye can be regarded as one lens with its:

- *Principal point* is 1.5 mm behind the anterior surface of cornea.
- *Nodal point* lies in the posterior part of the crystalline lens at 7.2 mm behind the anterior surface of cornea.
- As the rays enter and leave the eye through media of varying refractive indices, therefore, the anterior and posterior focal point and length are different.
- *Anterior focal point or length* is 15.7 mm in front of the anterior surface of cornea.
- *Posterior focal point or length* is 24.4 mm behind the anterior surface of cornea.

Posterior focal distance in a normal emmetropic eye is exactly at the place of retina in a normal eye. The parallel rays of light coming from infinity form a focus at 24 mm behind the cornea, i.e. on the retina. Thus, it is deduced that the normal eye is so constituted that the distant objects form the image upon the retina.

Axis and Angle of the Eye (Fig. 6.1)

Optical axis is the line-AR passing through the center of cornea-(P), center of lens-(N) and meets the retina-(R) on the nasal side of fovea.

Visual axis is the line of joining the fixation point-(O), nodal point-(N) and the fovea-(F) on the retina. *Visual axis* meets the retina at the *fovea centralis*—the best spot for distant acuity of vision. Here, just as in a convex lens, the image formed on the retina is inverted. This inverted image is reinverted psychologically in the brain.

Fixation axis: It is a line-OC joining the fixation point-(O) and center of rotation-(C) at the center of eye.

Angle alpha: It is the angle-ONA formed by optical axis and visual axis at nodal point.

Angle gamma: It is the angle-OCA formed by optical axis and fixation axis at the center of eyeball.

Angle kappa: It is the angle-OPA formed by visual axis and pupillary line represented by the center of cornea-(P). Clinically, the positive angle kappa manifests as pseudoexotropia and negative angle kappa manifests as pseudoesotropia.

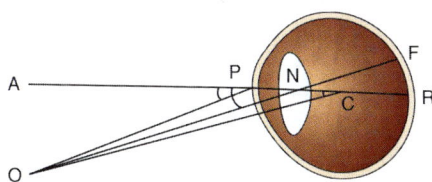

Fig. 6.1: Optical axis and angles of eye

- Optical axis-AR
- Visual axis-OF
- Fixation axis-OC
- Angle alpha-ONA—between optical axis-AR and visual axis-OF, at nodal point-N
- Angle kappa-OPA—between optical axis-AR and pupillary line-OP, at center of cornea.
- Angle gamma-OCA—between optical axis-AR and fixation axis-OC at center of eyeball.

Optical System of Hypermetropic Eye

In hypermetropia, the eyeball is short, thereby the retina is placed forward than its normal position at 24 mm behind the cornea. Therefore, in a hypermetropic eye, the parallel rays

coming from a distant object come to focus behind the retina.

Far point in hypermetropic eye is *virtual, i.e. behind the eyeball.* That is why, a hypermetrope cannot visualize neither distant nor near objects clearly with his/her eyes at rest since the far point is virtual and it is not possible to place an object at that point.

A young hypermetrope, i.e. a young person with low degree of hypermetropia can alter his refractive power by virtue of his accommodation and thereby can manage to see distant as well as near objects clearly. Continuous use of accommodation causes eye ache or headache.

Hypermetropia is treated by providing requisite amount of convergence to the rays before they enter the eye by convex lens. The convex lens provides convergence and brings the rays to focus on the retina (Fig. 6.2).

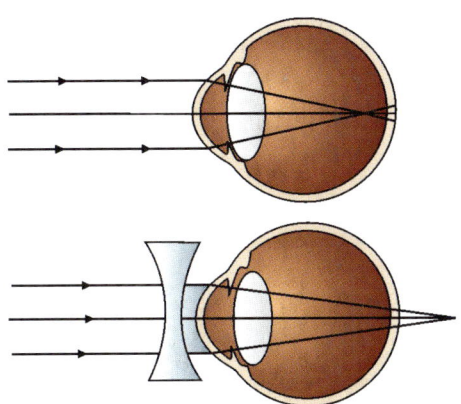

Fig. 6.2: Convex lens brings rays to focus on retina

Optical System of Myopic Eye

In myopic, the eyeball is longer than normal, thereby the retina is placed far backward than its normal position. In myopia, the parallel rays coming from a distant object come to focus before reaching the retina, i.e. the focus is formed in front of retina.

Far point in myopic eye is *real, i.e.* in front of the eyeball.

Myope cannot see distant objects clearly but can see the near objects clearly with his/her eyes at rest, i.e. even without use of accommodation.

Myope cannot alter his/her refractive power by virtue of his/her accommodation. He/she can see objects at a distance better, if he/she screws up his/her eyes making a narrow slit to see through.

Myopia is treated by providing requisite amount of divergence to the rays before they enter the eye by concave lens. The concave lens provides divergence and brings the rays to focus on retina (Fig. 6.3).

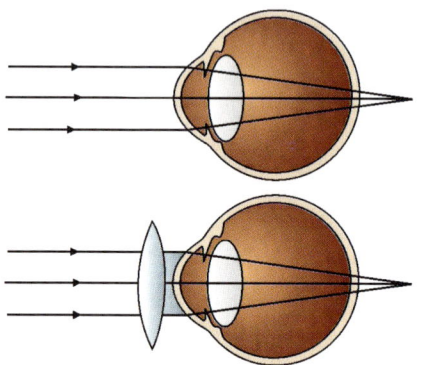

Fig. 6.3: Concave lens brings the rays to focus on the retina

The optician aims at placing the optical center of spectacle lens 13–15 mm from the cornea. It is to be noted that if the convex lens is placed away from the anterior focal distance of the eye, then its power increases. Similarly, if the concave lens is placed away from the anterior focal distance of the eye, then its power decreases.

In other words, if convex lens is to be kept away from the anterior focal distance of the eye, then it should be slightly weaker in its power. Similarly, if concave lens is to be kept away from the anterior focal distance of the eye, then it should be slightly stronger in its power.

The distance of the spectacle lens from the anterior focal point of the eye has an effect on the *size of image*. If the spectacle lens is more than 15 mm from the cornea, then the retinal image in hypermetropia is larger and the retinal image in myopia is smaller than the emmetropic image. The increase in the size of the retinal image is advantageous in a

hypermetrope but diminution in the size of retinal image is a disadvantage in myopia.

Thus in myopes, the spectacle lens should be slightly close to the eye and in hypermetropes the spectacle lens should be slightly away from the eye to give an advantage to the patient for good and clear vision without any eye ache or headache.

In myopia, the parallel rays come to focus in front of the retina, therefore, the image formed by divergent rays on the retina is a blurred image. In myopia only divergent rays come to focus on the retina, therefore, the object must be brought close to the eye (closer than 6 meters) so that it emits divergent rays which form a focus on the retina.

Far point in myopic is the farthest point at which objects can be seen clearly.

In emmetropic, it is at infinity.

In myopic, it is at a finite distance away from the eye.

This distance of far point from the eye gives us the degree of myopia. If the far point is 2 m away, then there is myopia of 0.5 dioptre. If the far point is 1 m away, then there is 2 dioptre of myopia as the dioptric power is reciprocal to the focal distance.

In myopia, the *far point* is at finite distance from the eye, i.e. within 6 m of distance. The *near point* is very close to the eye, therefore, a myopic can read from a very close distance.

The range of accommodation is also very small and so the amplitude of accommodation is also less. For example, a myopic patient can see clearly at 50 cm thus he/she has myopia of 2 dioptre. His/her near point is 10 cm. At this point of 10 cm, the refractive power shall be 10 dioptre. Thus, his/her range of accommodation shall be 40 cm, and his/her amplitude of accommodation shall be 8 dioptre.

Conclusive dictums:

- The far point is at finite distance, i.e. within 6 meters from the eye.
- The near point is very close to the eye.
- The range of accommodation is small.
- The amplitude of accommodation is less.
- The distant objects are not seen clearly.
- The near objects are seen clearly even without any effort of accommodation.

- The image formed by myopic eye is larger than the image formed by an emmetropic eye.
- There is an apparent convergent squint due to a large negative angle alpha.
- The myopia can be corrected by prescription of suitable concave lens for providing necessary divergence to the rays coming from distance so that they form a focus on the retina.

Optical System of Aphakic Eye

- The optical system consists of cornea separated by two media of different refractive indices; the air in front and aqueous and vitreous behind.
- *Anterior focal point* is at 23.2 mm and *posterior focal point* is at 31 mm from the cornea in aphakic eye as compared to *anterior focal point* at 15 mm and *posterior focal point* at 24 mm for the normal eye.

7

Maladies of Refractive Error

REFRACTIVE ERRORS

Emmetropia

Emmetropia is a condition in which the incipient parallel rays of light coming from infinity (distance of more than 6 m) come to focus on the light sensitive layer of retina (Fig. 7.1) when the eye is at rest.

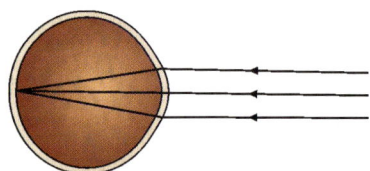

Fig. 7.1: Emmetropic eye—rays are focused at retina

In an emmetropic eye, the axial length and curvature of the cornea may vary a little, therefore, one concludes that emmetropia is a result of integration of all the factors mentioned above, i.e. one factor compensating for the other. Most of the infants are born as hypermetrope. Most of them reach to emmetropia and those who fail remain hypermetropic and those who overshoot become myopic.

A minor degree of low ametropia should be considered as a biological variant and not regarded as pathological.

Ametropia

Ametropia is a condition in which the incipient parallel rays of light from infinity (distance of more than 6 m) do not come to focus upon the light sensitive layer of the retina, when the eye is at rest.

It can be due to the following factors:

1. Axial Ametropia

Axial ametropia is due to abnormal length of the eyeball.

An eyeball longer than normal results in *myopia* and eyeball shorter than normal results in *hypermetropia*.

2. Curvature Ametropia

Curvature ametropia is due to abnormal curvature of cornea and the lens.

Increased curvature results in *myopia* and decreased curvature results in *hypermetropia*.

3. Index Ametropia

Index ametropia is due to change in the refractive index of the lens.

- High refractive index of the lens nucleus results in *myopia*. It is commonly seen with sclerosis of lens nucleus in aged people.

- High refractive index of cortex of the lens results in *hypermetropia.* It is commonly seen in aged people in early stage of maturation of cataract.

4. Position of Lens

The forward displacement of the lens than its normal position results in *hypermetropia.* It is seen after subluxation or in a congenital anomaly of the lens.

5. Absence of Lens

In the absence of lens as seen in aphakia or dislocation of the lens, the error is *hypermetropia.*

Myopia

Patient presents with prominent eyeballs with complain of short sight, i.e. unable to see distant objects clearly though he/she can perform near work for hours without any eye strain.

Myopia is a dioptric condition of the eye in which with accommodation at rest the incipient parallel rays from infinity come to focus anterior to the light sensitive layer of the retina (Fig. 7.2).

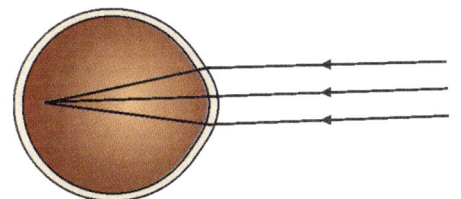

Fig. 7.2: Myopic eye-rays come to focus in front of retina

1. Congenital Myopia

It is rare. The patient is born with an abnormal long eyeball. The fundus examination may show lack of pigmentation with choroidal vessels and crescent near the optic disk. The error is usually about 10 dioptre. It is usually bilateral. It is non-progressive. Both the eyes show convergence and nystagmoid movements. Congenital myopia may be associated with congenital anomalies. Early treatment is desirable.

2. Simple Myopia

Simple myopia results as a variant in frequency curve of axial length. These cases do not progress after adolescence and the refractive error is usually within 5–6 dioptre. It may show an increase in the physical state of debility. There are no degenerative changes in the fundus. The corrected visual acuity is near to normal.

3. Pathological Axial Myopia

Pathological axial myopia is degenerative and progressive. The myopia appears in childhood that increases rapidly and steadily up to the age of 25 years or more. The error may be around 15–25 dioptre. Pathological myopia is strongly hereditary common in females and has a racial tendency also being common in Jews and Japanese.

Etiology

1. It is considered as a disturbance of growth superimposed by degenerative phenomenon which is beyond the normal biological variations of growth.
2. Heredity and general growth factors play important role.
3. Endocrine and nutritional factors play as incidental factors.
4. Debility and chronic illness may increase the tendency.
5. Environmental factors like excessive near work, poor illumination, bad posture have been thought to play a part.

Pathogenesis

Probably, the abnormally long eyeball is not due to stretching of the sclera but it is due to primary degeneration of the coats of the eyeball including the posterior half of the sclera. The increase in the length of the eyeball affects the posterior pole of the eye and the anterior half is normal. In very high degree of myopia, the sclera may bulge out at the posterior pole to manifest as *posterior staphyloma.*

Symptoms

- *Low or indistinct vision for distance:* Patient complains of poor distant vision. A low degree of myopic may not come for eye check-up for a long time until his vision has reduced considerably to the extent of about 6/60 or less. This is due to the fact that he/she can continue his/her near work without any eye problem.

- *Discomfort after near work:* Patient complains of discomfort after near work. This discomfort is due to imbalance between the use of accommodation and convergence. Myope does not use the accommodation for near work but uses his/her convergence to see near objects thus there is an imbalance between the two which results in discomfort after near work.
- *Floaters before the eyes:* Patient complains of seeing black spots floating before the eyes.

    Floaters are due to vitreous degeneration.

    Vitreous becomes fluid and the particles float in this fluid vitreous which appears as black spots floating before the eyes.
- *Flashes of light:* Patient complains of occasional flash of light. It is due to irritation of the retina caused by the fluid vitreous coming in contact with degenerative thin retina in the periphery on movement of the eyes.

    Patient with complaint of constant flashes of light even with slightest movement of the eye must be thoroughly investigated for detachment of the retina.

    High myope is prone to detachment of retina due to degenerative changes in the retina and the vitreous.

Signs

- *Prominent eyeball:* In a case of unilateral high myopia, it may give an appearance of unilateral proptosis. If there is myopia affecting both the eyes, then it may appear as bilateral proptosis. Low vision and refraction shall help to differentiate it from other causes of proptosis.
- *Deep anterior chamber with dilated sluggish pupil:* Anterior chamber is deep as the eyeball as a whole is elongated. Pupil is comparatively more dilated with sluggish

reaction as the patient does not use accommodation thus there is less constriction of pupil for near work.

- *Apparent convergent squint:* Apparent convergent squint appears due to large negative angle alpha.
- *Real divergent squint:* Cover test reveals a real divergent squint. Eye with more refractive error is likely to diverge out due to poor visual acuity and no use of accommodation.
- *Refraction:* Autorefractor shows myopia.
- *Ophthalmoscopy:* In a pathological myopia, there are always changes in the fundus.

Large optic disk Optic disk appears larger than in an emmetropic eye. It is due to the fact that the image formed in myopia is larger than the normal.

Myopic crescent
- *Temporal crescent* is due to separation of the retina and choroid from the temporal margin of the optic disk leaving the sclera to shine through.
- *Annular crescent* appears in high myopia due to separation all round the disk.
- *Supertraction crescent* appears due to overriding of the retina on the nasal side of the disk resulting in blurred appearance.

Chorioretinal myopic degeneration The chorioretinal myopic degeneration affects mostly the central fundus but the changes also occur in the periphery. The pigment layer of the retina loses much of its pigment, therefore, the fundus is tigroid and choroidal vessels are seen. There are numerous patches of chorioretinal atrophy, i.e. white areas surrounded by pigmentary changes. Atrophic patches give rise to scotomas.

Posterior staphyloma It is seen as a crescentic shadow two to three disk diameters away on the temporal side. It is concentric with the optic disk. There is kinking of vessels as seen in cupping of the disk.

Foster-Fuchs' fleck A myope may occasionally present with a sudden loss of vision. On ophthalmoscopy, there is a dark circular area at the macula. It is probably caused by sub-retinal neovascularization and choroidal hemorrhage.

Posterior vitreous detachment (PVD) Detachment of the vitreous may occur at the posterior pole. On ophthalmoscopy there is reflex streak seen on its posterior face in front of the retina.

Vitreous floaters Numerous vitreous floaters are seen floating freely in the liquefied vitreous due to degeneration of vitreous.

- *Field charting:* On charting the central and peripheral fields, there shall be scotoma corresponding to the chorioretinal atrophic lesions. There is enlarged blind spot due to myopic crescent.
- *Electroretinography:* Electroretinogram may be subnormal due to chorioretinal atrophy.

Complications

1. Vitreous degeneration
2. Detachment of retina
3. Complicated cataract
4. Foster-Fuchs' fleck
5. Vitreous hemorrhage.

Prognosis

The prognosis is good in simple myopia. The patient can lead a good normal life except that he/she has to wear glasses. The prognosis in pathological myopia depends upon the degree of myopia. A patient with high myopia should choose profession that leads to sedentary life style to avoid complications associated with pathological myopia due to exertive lifestyle.

Management

1. **Optical procedures:** Treatment of myopia is to prescribe concave lenses to correct the myopic refraction.
   - *Spectacle concave lens:* Resilens offer safety over glass lens. Myopes are more likely to be involved in injury and many eyes are lost due to shattering of glasses, causing rupture of globe.
   - *Contact lens:* Contact lens gives an improvement in the appearance, visual acuity and field of vision.

- *Low vision aids:* Telescopic lens is helpful for the distance vision. A high myope gets adjusted to read at his far point comfortably.

2. **Refractive surgical procedures**
   - *Radial keratotomy (RK):* This procedure involves deep radial incisions in the peripheral part of the cornea leaving the central 4 mm optical zone. On healing, these incisions flatten the central cornea, thereby reducing its refractive power. It gives good correction in low to moderate myopia of 2 to 6 D.
   - *Photorefractive keratectomy (PRK):* In this technique, central optical zone of anterior corneal stroma is photo-ablated using eximer laser to cause flattening of the central cornea. It gives good correction for 2 to 6 D of myopia.
   - *Laser in situ keratomileusis (LASIK):* In this technique, a flap of 130–160 micron thickness of anterior corneal tissue is raised. Then the midstromal corneal tissue is ablated directly with an ***excimer laser beam*** to flatten the cornea. This is the most considered choice of treatment for myopia of up to 12 D.
     - *Aphakic intraocular lens implant, if myopia is more than 12 D.*
     - *Phakic intraocular lens implant.*
     - *Intercorneal ring implantation*
     - *Orthokeratology*

Myopia Hygiene

- *Proper posture:* Advise myopic not to read with a stooping position. Patient should be advised to keep his/her back straight while reading or writing. For this, the height of the table and chair should be adjusted to give the patient proper posture and height to maintain proper distance from the books. Proper posture will help avoid congestion of the eye due to stooping and proper distance shall help avoid extra effort on the accommodation and convergence.
- *Correction of refraction:* The patient must get himself/herself examined every

6 months to correct his/her refraction so that there is no strain on the eyes and proper balance is maintained

- *Nutrition:* Pay proper attention for intake of animal protein and vitamins. The intake of food should be properly timed to provide a child with calories all the day.
- *Early treatment for any febrile or systemic illness:* Any febrile or debilitating illness can cause increase in myopia. It is advisable to take an early treatment to check progress of myopia.
- *Illumination and ventilation:* The study room should be properly illuminated. The light should not fall directly on the book or the eyes. The room should have proper ventilation for flow of fresh air.
- *Avoid hard and jerky exercise or games:* A patient with myopia of 10 D or above must be advised to avoid hard exercises and games which involve jerks and fast movements. It is advisable to get interested in indoor games.
- *Marriage counseling:* Two high myopes should avoid marriage. As it is a hereditary disease. The offsprings are likely to have myopia.

Hypermetropia

An adult mother presents her healthy child with complain of eye strain and headache even after near work for a short period. Child plays well and can watch television for hours without any complain of any kind. Child comes home with eye strain and does not like to finish his/her home work.

Hypermetropia *is a dioptric condition of the eye in which with accommodation at rest, the incipient parallel rays from infinity come to focus posterior to the light sensitive layer of the retina (Fig. 7.3).*

Etiopathogenesis

Axial hypermetropia The majority of cases of hypermetropia is axial, i.e. there is a shortening of the anteroposterior axis of the eyeball.

A decrease of 1 mm in the anteroposterior axis produces hypermetropia of 3 dioptre.

Hypermetropia is considered as a stage in normal development. At birth, practically all eyes are hypermetropic of about 2 to 3 dioptre. By the time the person is above adolescence age, he/she should be an emmetrope. Most of the cases reach to emmetropia. Those who do not become emmetropic, remain as low hypermetropes and those who overshoot become myopic. Normally, the hypermetropia does not exceed 6 dioptre, i.e. the shortening of the eyeball rarely exceeds 2 mm.

Curvature hypermetropia The curvature hypermetropia is commonly seen in cases of cornea plana. A decrease of 1 mm in the curvature of cornea produces a hypermetropia of 6 dioptre.

Index hypermetropia Index hypermetropia occurs due to change in the refractive index of the cortex of the lens. A high refractive index of the cortex of the lens results in hypermetropic refraction commonly seen in old age.

Optical Condition in Hypermetropia

In hypermetropia, the parallel rays from infinity come to focus behind the retina. The image formed at the retina is blurred and indistinct. The far point is behind the eyeball; therefore, a hypermetrope cannot see distant objects clearly unless the converging power of the optical system of the eyeball is increased. It can be increased by two ways: (i) by use of accommodation, and (ii) by prescription of convex lens. A low hypermetrope can see distant objects clearly by use of his/her accommodation. A high hypermetrope needs help of convex lens for distance to spare his/her accommodation for near work.

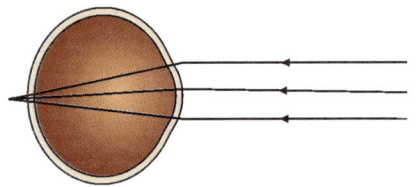

Fig. 7.3: Hypermetropic eye—rays are focused behind retina

Hypermetropia and its Components

Total hypermetropia is the total amount of refractive error that is estimated after complete cycloplegia with atropine.

Total hypermetropia consists of latent and manifest hypermetropias.

Latent hypermetropia Latent hypermetropia of about 1 dioptre is normally corrected physiologically by the normal tone of the ciliary muscle.

Manifest hypermetropia Manifest hypermetropia cannot be corrected by the normal tone of the ciliary muscle. It is further divided into two types:

- *Facultative hypermetropia* is the hypermetropia which is overcome by the patient due to his effort of accommodation.
- *Absolute hypermetropia* is the hypermetropia which cannot be overcome by the patient even with his/her effort of accommodation.

The abovementioned different components of hypermetropia can be determined clinically as follows.

Make the patient sit in a chair and ask him/her to look at the distant test type. Put a trial frame and then place convex lenses as follows to determine the different types of hypermetropia. The patient is unable to see a distant test type clearly. Place convex lenses of gradually increasing strength in the trial frame until patient can just see clearly. At this point he is able to see with the help of the convex lens and his/her accommodation. The amount of the hypermetropia corrected by convex lens is the absolute hypermetropia. So it can be concluded that the *absolute hypermetropia* can be measured by the weakest convex lens with which maximum visual acuity can be obtained. Now, gradually add stronger convex lenses until the patient can see clearly. In this process, we have been replacing the converging power of accommodation by the convex lenses. So, this hypermetropia corrected by further addition of convex lenses is the facultative hypermetropia which was normally corrected by the effort of accommodation. Thus, it can be concluded that the *facultative hypermetropia*

is measured by the difference between the strongest and weakest convex lenses with which maximum visual acuity is obtained.

The strongest convex lens is the measure of the *manifest* hypermetropia.

Now instill cycloplegic, atropine and after complete paralysis of ciliary muscle, again add the convex lenses to get the maximum visual acuity. Thus, the *total hypermetropia* is measured by the strongest convex lens with which the maximum visual acuity is obtained.

The difference between the strongest convex lens before and after use of atropine gives the measure of *latent hypermetropia*. The difference is of about 1 dioptre.

Symptoms

- *Eye strain with headache:* The patient usually complains of eye strain after close work even for a short period. The eye strain may manifest as eye ache, burning of the eyes, dry feeling in the eyes, more blinking and lacrimation. A hypermetrope uses more accommodation in comparison to the convergence, therefore, there is an imbalance between the two and it results in eye strain. These symptoms manifest in cases with high hypermetropia even after short period of near work.
- *Early presbyopia*: Presbyopia sets early as patient is using a part of accommodation for seeing the distant objects clearly.
- *Apparent divergent squint:* It is due to large positive angle alpha.

Signs

- *Eyeball:* The eyeball is small in all the directions. The cornea is small but the lens is of normal size, therefore, the anterior chamber is shallow. Eye is predisposed to develop primary closed-angle glaucoma.
- *Ophthalmoscopy:* The optic disk is small and red with blurred margin; the vessels are full, tortuous with abnormal branching.

The fundus simulates optic neuritis—pseudopapillitis. There is a grey areola around the disk. There is a peculiar sheen—a reflex effect known as *shot-silk retina*.

- *Real convergent squint:* It is due to excessive use of accommodation, therefore, excessive use of convergence.

Management

1. **Optical procedures:** Treatment of hypermetropia is to prescribe convex lenses to correct the hypermetropic refraction.

   If there is no symptom, no treatment is required. A young low hypermetrope can correct his/her distant and near vision by virtue of his/her accommodation. There is no need of prescribing convex lenses as there is no complaint of eye strain or headache.

   It is better to under-correct rather than over-correct.

2. **Refractive surgical procedures**
   - *Holmium laser thermoplasty*
   - *Hyperopic PRK with excimer laser*
   - *Hyperopic LASIK*
   - *Conductive LASIK*

Refractive surgery in hypermetropia is neither effective nor reliable as for myopia.

Astigmatism

Patient presents with complain of mild eye strain, asthenopia or running of letters in each other soon after involving in near work especially reading and writing and computer application. Though the patient has 6/5 visual acuity yet he/she does miss one or two words while reading the Snellen's chart usually in his/her first attempt. An alert ophthalmologist should clinch the diagnosis and prescribe lowest cylinder acceptable.

Astigmatism is a dioptric condition of the refraction wherein a point of focus of light cannot be formed upon the retina.

Etiopathogenesis

The astigmatism can occur due to an error of curvature, centering or refractive index.

Curvature astigmatism It is the most common type of astigmatism observed. It is due to a change in the curvature of cornea. It is usually a congenital anomaly. The most common error in the curvature is one wherein the vertical curvature is greater than the horizontal curvature of the cornea. It is accepted as physiological and is probably due to constant pressure of lids.

An acquired astigmatism is due to a change in the curvature of cornea. It can occur due to congenital deformity, e.g. conical cornea, trauma and operative scar at limbus, etc.

Decentering of lens A decentered lens may cause astigmatism. It is seen as a congenital anomaly or follows subluxation of the lens.

Refractive index astigmatism It is seen as a physiological change in the lens during maturation of cataract. It is due to sectorial alteration in the refractive index of lens during formation of spoke-like lens opacities in the periphery of lens. The patient complains of polyopia.

Optical Condition

In astigmatism, instead of a single focal point, there are two focal lines separated from each other by a *focal interval* of *Sturm*. The bundle of rays formed by the two surfaces is known as *Sturm's conoid.* The length of this focal interval is the measure of the degree of the astigmatism and the correction of the astigmatism is accomplished by reducing these two foci into one. This is achieved by prescription of cylindrical lenses.

In Figure 7.4, V to V is the vertical meridian of the cornea which is more curved and the rays passing through this meridian are brought to focus at B. The H to H is the horizontal meridian of the cornea which is normal in curvature so rays are brought to focus at the retina F. Thus, there are two foci, one at B and another at F. The distance between the foci B and F is the *focal interval of Sturm*. The whole bundle of rays so formed is known as *Sturm's conoid*. It is difficult to represent this conoid on a plane surface, but we can see the sections of bundle of rays at different distance from the refracting surface the cornea.

Types of Astigmatism

1. Regular astigmatism:
   - Astigmatism with rule
   - Astigmatism against the rule

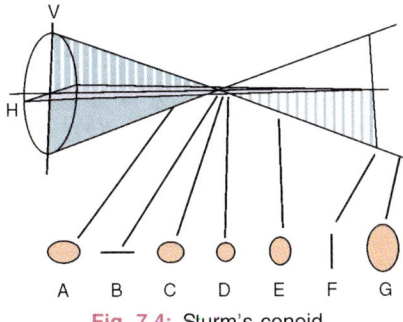

Fig. 7.4: Sturm's conoid

- Simple hypermetropic astigmatism
- Simple myopic astigmatism
- Compound hypermetropic astigmatism
- Compound myopic astigmatism
- Mixed astigmatism
- Oblique astigmatism
- Bioblique astigmatism.

2. Irregular astigmatism

Regular Astigmatism

Normally, the vertical curvature of the cornea is slightly more curved than the horizontal curvature of the cornea. It has been accepted as physiological.

- *Astigmatism with-the-rule:* It refers to a condition in which the vertical curvature is more than the horizontal curvature of cornea.
- *Astigmatism against-the-rule:* It refers to a condition in which the horizontal curvature is more curved than the vertical curvature of the cornea.
- *Simple hypermetropic astigmatism:* It is a dioptric condition of the refraction in which one axis of the cornea is emmetropic and the other axis is hypermetropic, i.e. one focus forms on the retina and the other focus behind the retina.
- *Simple myopic astigmatism:* It is a dioptric condition of the refraction in which one axis of the cornea is emmetropic and the other axis is myopic, i.e. one focus forms on the retina and the other focus in front of the retina.
- *Compound hypermetropic astigmatism:* It is a dioptric condition of the refraction in

which both the vertical and the horizontal axes of the cornea are hypermetropic with varied curvatures, therefore, both the foci form behind the retina but at different levels.

- *Compound myopic astigmatism:* It is a dioptric condition of the refraction in which both the vertical and the horizontal axes of the cornea are myopic with varied curvatures, therefore, both the foci form in front of the retina but at different levels.
- *Mixed astigmatism:* It is a dioptric condition of the refraction in which one axis of the cornea is myopic and the other axis is hypermetropic, i.e. one focus forms in front of the retina and the other focus forms behind the retina.
- *Oblique astigmatism:* It is a type of regular astigmatism wherein the two principal meridians are not the vertical and horizontal yet these are at right angles to each other.
- *Bioblique astigmatism:* It is a type of regular astigmatism wherein two principal meridians are not at right angle to each other.

All types of regular astigmatism can be resolved by spherocylindrical combination.

Irregular Astigmatism

It is seen in corneal nebular opacity, facet, incipient cataract, conical cornea and lenticonus. Most commonly the surface of cornea is irregular so the rays are also refracted irregularly without any symmetry and different groups of rays form foci in various positions. Patient complains of defective vision, distortion of objects and polyopia. Irregular astigmatism due to corneal affection can be easily diagnosed and assessed by Placido's disc and photokeratoscopy.

- It cannot be resolved by any combination of spherocylindrical lenses.
- It can only be improved to an extent by contact lens which replaces the anterior irregular surface of cornea for refraction to certain extent.
- Phototherapeutic keratectomy is helpful in cases with superficial corneal scars.

Symptoms

The only symptom is that of *eye strain or asthenopia*. It is more pronounced in a low degree of astigmatism than in the high degree of astigmatism. The patient may complain of a feeling that the letters in the book appears to be *running in each other*. One feels fatigued after reading even for a short time. All these symptoms are due to patients endeavor to accommodate so as to produce a circle of least diffusion upon the retina.

Signs

Autorefractor reveals different power in two meridians.

A thorough examination of the eye should be done to exclude any change in the surface of cornea and in the shape and position of the lens. A slit-lamp examination is helpful to locate a small and faint corneal nebular opacity or a facet.

Investigations

- Autorefractometry
- Keratometry
- Astigmatic fan test

Management

1. **Optical procedures**
   - If there are no symptoms, the patient requires no treatment at all.
   - If there are symptoms of eye strain or asthenopia, then the patient needs correction of his astigmatic error, however, small the error may be.
   - A correction by cylindrical lenses or combination of spherocylindrical lenses is the treatment of choice.
   - Contact lens can be prescribed in selected cases.
2. **Refractive surgical procedures**
   - Astigmatic keratotomy
   - Photo-astigmatic refractive keratotomy
   - LASIK

Anisometropia

Isometropia is a dioptric condition of refraction wherein the refraction in two eyes is equal in its degree or kind.

Anisometropia is a dioptric condition of the refraction wherein the refraction of the two eyes is unequal in its degree or kind.

Anisometropia is found in every possible variety, i.e. one eye is emmetropic and the other eye may be hypermetropic, myopic or astigmatic. Both the eyes may be ametropic varying in degree or in its kind, i.e. one eye may be low myopic and the other eye may be of high myopic or one eye may be hypermetropic and the other eye may be myopic.

Vision in Anisometropia

The vision is usually affected in cases with anisometropia.

Binocular vision is a rule in low degree of anisometropia usually below 3 dioptre.

Alternating vision is seen, when one eye is low hypermetropic and the other eye is myopic. In this case, the low hypermetropic eye is used for distant vision and the myopic eye is used for near vision. Such a patient feels very comfortable as he/she has not to use accommodation, therefore, no symptoms.

Uniocular vision is seen, when one eye is low ametropic and the other is having a very high refractive error. In such cases, the eye with low refractive error is used for all the work and the other eye is completely excluded from the vision at an early stage in life. The defective eye which is being not used tends to become *amblyopic*. This eye in due course of time manifests as *divergent squint*. This type of *amblyopia ex anopsia* is a preventable condition by correcting the refractive error at an early stage of life before amblyopia and divergence set in.

Treatment

1. **Optical procedure**
   - Only treatment is early and full correction of refractive error.
   - Patient should be advised to use glasses constantly.
   - In a high degree of refractive error, the more ametropic eye may be undercorrected for a few weeks so as to give enough time for the eyes to adjust to

the new images formed by the use of lenses. Gradually, correct the ametropic eye to its full correction.

Anisometropia is extremely common in small degree and especially with an astigmatic error and is well tolerated without any symptom.

2. **Refractive surgical procedure:** Refractive corneal surgery can be performed for unilateral high myopia and astigmatism.

Aniseikonia

Aniseikonia is a condition wherein the images projected to the visual cortex from two retinae are abnormally unequal in size and/or shape. Aniseikonia up to 5% is well tolerated by the patient.

Etiopathogenesis

1. *Optical aniseikonia*: It is due to inherent or acquired high degree of anisometropia.
2. *Retinal aniseikonia*: It usually occurs due to retinal edema at fovea.
3. *Cortical aniseikonia:* It is due to asymmetrical simultaneous perception in spite of equal size of images formed on retina.

Symptoms and Signs

Patient complains of asthenopia, diplopia and problems in depth perception.

Management

Optical aniseikonia can be managed by aniseikonic spectacle glasses, contact lenses or intraocular lens.

Retinal aniseikonia can only be treated by treating the causative factor.

Aphakia

Aphakia is a condition of the eye in which the lens is absent from the pupillary area.

In other words, the aphakia is a condition of the eye in which there is absence of lens either due to surgery or dislocation by the trauma.

Aphakia results in high degree of hypermetropia.

Optical Condition

1. There is hypermetropia of about 10 dioptre.

2. There is astigmatism against the rule as the corneal section is in the upper part that makes the corneal flattening in the vertical meridian. The astigmatism amounts to about 2 to 3 dioptre which diminishes gradually in due course of time.
3. There is a complete loss of accommodation as the lens has been removed or dislocated.
4. The retinal image is about a quarter larger than the emmetropic retinal image. This large image is a visual problem for aphakic patient as everything appears big to him/her. This enlarged image also causes diplopia, if the opposite eye has a normal vision. The diplopia is due to disparity of the retinal images of two eyes; the normal and aphakic eyes.

Optical System of Aphakic Eye

- The optical system consists of cornea separated by two media of different refractive indices; the air in front and aqueous and vitreous behind.
- *Anterior focal point* is at 23.2 mm and *posterior focal point* is at 31 mm from the cornea in aphakic eye as compared with *anterior focal point* at 15 mm and *posterior focal point* at 24 mm for the normal eye.

Diagnosis

- History of operation or trauma with scar mark at limbus
- Deep anterior chamber
- Jet black pupil
- Iridodonesis or tremulousness of the iris
- Absence of 3rd and 4th Purkinje's images.

Symptoms

- *Defective vision* due to high hypermetropia and loss of accommodation.
- *Glare from the bright light* is due to absence of lens. Help him by prescribing sun glasses and avoid bright light.
- *Enlarged image* is due to absence of lens and aphakic glasses. Prescribe contact lens. If the opposite eye is normal, then let him/her use normal eye and does not correct the aphakic eye.

- *Distortion of objects* is due to prismatic effect of the periphery of thick convex lens of high power. There is *Jack-in-the-box phenomenon or Roving ring scotoma* effect. Prescribe contact lens.
- *Disorientation* is due to prismatic effect of thick convex lens and also due to astigmatism associated with aphakia. It causes problem of physical co-ordination and movement.
- *Red vision* is due to entry of infrared rays into the eyes due to absence of lens. Ask him/her to avoid bright light.
  Pin cushion effect is due to spherical aberration.

In this era, IOLs implant eradicates all types and kind of defective vision due to thick aphakic lens.

Signs

- *Limbal scar*
- *Deep anterior chamber*
- *Iridodonesis*
- *Jet black pupil*
- *Purkinje's test shows only two images.*

Management

- Spectacles give rise to many visual problems.
- Contact lens helps to eliminate or reduce visual problems.
- Intraocular lens implant is the first choice in every case unless absolutely contraindicated. **Pseudophakia** is a condition wherein aphakia has been corrected by intraocular lens implant—IOLs.

8

Maladies of Accommodation

Accommodation

- Mechanism of accommodation
- Range of accommodation
- Amplitude of accommodation
- Availability of accommodation
- Acts associated with accommodation

Anomalies of Accommodation

- Insufficiency of accommodation
- Cycloplegia or paralysis of accommodation
- Spasm of accommodation

Presbyopia

- Correction of presbyopia
- Management of presbyopia

ACCOMMODATION

Accommodation is a phenomenon in which there is an increase in the refractive power of the lens due to increase in the curvature of the lens in the act of accommodation.

In a person with normal vision, the eye is so constituted that the parallel rays coming from distance, i.e. beyond 6 m are brought to focus on the retina with eye at rest. The near object emits divergent rays and obviously these rays cannot form a focus on the retina. These divergent rays are converged to form a focus on the retina in the act of accommodation.

Mechanism of Accommodation

To understand the mechanism of accommodation, it is essential to keep the following facts in mind:

- Lens has a considerable degree of plasticity, i.e. it can mold in any shape. The lens capsule is elastic in nature and is anchored by the suspensory ligaments to the ciliary process.
- Lens capsule is thick in the periphery and thin in the center.
- Radius of curvature of the anterior surface of the lens is 10 mm and that of the posterior surface is 6 mm.
- In accommodation, the posterior surface remains almost same but the anterior surface changes to such an extent that its radius of curvature becomes 6 mm.
- This change in the curvature of the anterior surface of the lens increases the refractive power of the lens, thereby it brings the incident divergent rays from near objects to focus on the retina so that near objects are seen clearly.

In the normal state of the eye the lens capsule and the suspensory ligaments are taut. In the act of accommodation due to contraction of the ciliary muscle, the suspensory ligament is relaxed and the lens capsule becomes slacker or loose. Relieved of the strain the capsule bulges out in the center preferentially at the anterior pole. This causes increase in the curvature of the lens which results in the increase of its refractive power. This increase in the refractive power brings the incipient divergent rays from the near objects to focus on the retina by providing necessary convergence to these rays.

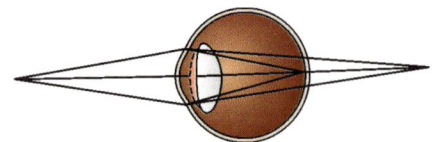

Fig. 8.1: Act of accommodation—rays from near objects are focused on retina for clear vision

That is how an emmetrope is able to see near objects clearly at any desired distance by the act of accommodation (Fig. 8.1).

Control over the ciliary muscle is involuntary and very delicate, i.e. all the objects up to 7 cm close to the eye can be focused clearly in children.

Near Point

The nearest point at which small objects can be seen clearly is called the *near point* or *punctum proximum.* At this point, the accommodation is used at its maximum.

The near point varies with static refraction of the eye and again with the age of the patient.

Far Point

The far point at which an object is visible clearly is called *far point or punctum remotum.* At this point, the accommodation is not used at all.

The far point varies with the static refraction of the eye whether the eye is emmetropic, hypermetropic or myopic eye.

In emmetropia, the far point is at infinity.

In hypermetropia, the far point is *virtual,* i.e. behind the eyeball.

In myopia, the far point is *real* and in front of the eye depending on the degree of myopia.

The accommodation is completely relaxed at the far point (infinity) and it is maximum at the near point.

Range of Accommodation

The distance between the far point and the near point, i.e. the distance over which the accommodation is effective is known as the *range of accommodation.*

Amplitude of Accommodation

The difference in the refractivity of the eye at the far point and the near point is known as the *amplitude of accommodation.*

Availability of Accommodation

Emmetrope or a low hypermetrope with the use of accommodation is able to see distant as well as near objects clearly though a low hypermetrope shall have to use accommodation for all the range.

High hypermetrope may see distant objects clearly by using his/her accommodation but needs aid of glasses to see near object clearly.

Myope has far point close to the eye thus he/she needs the aid of myopic glasses for distant vision but is able to see near objects clearly without use of any accommodation.

Acts Associated with Accommodation

Three synkinetic acts associated with accommodation:

1. Convergence by internal rectus muscles is essential to receive the incipient divergent rays from the near objects.
2. Pupillary contraction by sphincter pupillary muscle is essential to prevent entry of more light from near objects and also helps to diminish the optical aberrations.
3. Act of accommodation by the ciliary muscle is essential for near work.

All three muscles; internal rectus, sphincter pupillary and ciliary are supplied by the third cranial nerve.

ANOMALIES OF ACCOMMODATION

Insufficiency of Accommodation

Insufficiency of accommodation denotes that the range of accommodation is below the lower limit of the normal for the patient's age.

It is commonly seen in following:
- Weakness of the ciliary muscle due to anemia and debility.
- Advancing age due to sclerosis of the lens.
- With primary open angle glaucoma.

Treatment should be done by treating the cause and by prescribing suitable glasses for near work.

Cycloplegia or Paralysis of Accommodation

Cycloplegia is usually seen:
- Following use of cycloplegic drug.
- Contusional injury.
- Paralysis of third nerve.

It is often unilateral.

Bilateral paralysis of accommodation is seen in syphilis, diabetes, alcoholism and meningeal diseases.

Pupil is well dilated in cycloplegia.

Treat the cause.

Spasm of Accommodation

Spasm of accommodation is found in young people and particularly in myope.

Spontaneous spasm of accommodation can occur in cases with some kind of refractive error and who have been subjected to near work in an unfavorable environment, i.e. a bad posture, poor illumination, mental anxiety, emotional and intellectual stress.

Spasm of accommodation can be produced by use of myotic. Treat by correcting any refractive error, use of topical atropine and counseling.

PRESBYOPIA

Patient presents with headache or eye ache following reading, writing or any kind of near work even after short period.

Presbyopia is an anomaly of accommodation and not the error of refraction.

Presbyopia is a condition in which the near point of the emmetropic eye has receded far away so that it is beyond the comfortable reading or near working distance.

In an emmetropic at the age of about 10 years, the *near point* is about 7 cm from the eye having an accommodative power of about 14 dioptre.

The control over ciliary muscle is involuntary and very delicate and that is why all the distances from the infinity to near point of 7 cm can be accurately focused in childhood.

The near point varies with the age of the patient as the lens becomes less elastic with the advancing age. It has been seen that the lens is a mass of epithelial cells, the central part of lens being the oldest. With the age, this central part of lens becomes sclerosed forming a relatively hard nucleus. The hard nucleus is less plastic than the soft cortex of younger years, therefore, it responds less and less to the change in the tension of lens capsule in the act of accommodation with advancing age.

Thus it can be concluded that the near point gradually recedes away from the eye throughout the life. The near point at the age of 40 years is about 25 cm, the distance at which most of the people are used to read, write and do all their near work. At the age of 40 years with a near point at 25 cm, the accommodative power left with the patient is 4 dioptre. With further advance in age or his/her profession demanding the near point closer than 25 cm shall put him/her at a disadvantage. It is at this age and his/her demand for a near point closer than 25 cm, a normal emmetrope needs correction for his/her near vision.

The near point also varies with the static refraction of the eye whether hypermetrope or myope.

Myopic patient does not use his/her accommodation as his/her near point is very close to the eye, i.e. patient can read and write at a close distance for long hours even in advancing age without any eye ache or headache.

Hypermetropic patient uses a part of his/her accommodation to see distant objects clearly, therefore the near point recedes at an early age. Due to this, either patient needs distant correction or near correction at an early age.

Correction of Presbyopia

For presbyopic correction, the most popular test type employed are numbered from N5 to N48. The test type for near vision corresponds to modern Times Roman type in various sizes from 5 to 48 pt.

The patient is asked to hold the text type chart in his/her hand at a distance at which patient is used to work or would like to work or read and write. Now add the convex lenses in the trial frame so that the letters size N5 becomes distinct to patient at his/her near point as per his/her requirement.

It is better to under-correct than over-correct for near vision. The overcorrection causes problem with patient's convergence and also the range of amplitude becomes limited. Usual practice is to correct patient's near vision at 25 cm. It is well tolerated as it provides a wide range of amplitude and less convergence.

In case of myopia or hypermetropia the near correction should be added to patient's distance correction. Again it is better to under-correct him/her.

Management of Presbyopia

In this era, the management of presbyopia is a challenge to ophthalmologists. The aim of presbyopic management is to maintain the distant vision and restore the progressively changing near vision. There is growing number of presbyopic patients. Therefore, ophthalmologists cannot afford to ignore this malady. The perfect treatment for presbyopia is the need of this era more than ever before. Many modalities for presbyopic treatment are available and under evolution. Today, one needs to choose the modality wisely for each individual patient.

Presently, following lens-based modalities are available.

1. Monovision
2. Multifocal IOLs
3. Accommodating IOLs
4. Presbyopic LASIK
5. Intracorneal inlays

Monovision

In monovision, one eye is corrected for distance vision and the other eye is corrected for near vision to compensate for the loss of accommodative capacity. This modality works through intraocular blur suppression that is automatic or unconscious ability of the patient to suppress the blurred image from one eye; the eye corrected for distance vision so that it does not interfere with the focusing near image from the other eye; the eye corrected for near vision.

The patient has to learn this art consciously to adapt to contact lens monovision for distance. This modality of monovision affects binocular visual acuity, stereopsis and contrast sensitivity. The opinion varies about which vision is to be corrected first; distance or near vision. The entire outcome depends on the accurate calculation of IOL power, whether for near or for distance vision.

Multifocal IOLs

The multifocal IOLs have near and distance foci simultaneously in a single optic. These IOLs affect contrast sensitivity and produce glare and halos. These IOLs need neuroadaptation. Some cases do show improvement in vision after months of surgery—not explained by optics and can be explained only on the ability for neuroadaptation by the patient. Multifocal IOLs are options open to patients who desire to ward off the use of glasses.

Accommodating IOLs

Accommodating IOLs are being evolved to achieve active ciliary muscle-derived accommodation by 'Optic shift' principles. Accommodating IOLs are the best treatment for presbyopia. Such IOLs shall be free from reduced contrast sensitivity, glare and halos offered by multifocal IOLs.

- *Synchrony IOL:* It is a dual-optic, silicon, single-piece, foldable, accommodating IOL and features a high plus powered front optic with minus-powered rear optic depending on the target. The front and rear optic power is individualized. Ultrasound biomicroscopy studies have demonstrated that the lens does move forward, when the patient accommodates.
- *Crystalens:* It is a modified plate-haptic, 5 mm optic, silicon accommodating intraocular lens designed to flex anteriorly in response to ciliary muscle contraction in the act of accommodation.
- *Fluid vision*: A fluid-filled flexible membrane that bulges with accommodation known as fluid vision.

- *Liquid lens:* A sandwich of flexible material that bulges, when the fluid in periphery is pushed into interface during accommodation.
- *Gravity dependent IOLs.*
- *Capsule filling lens of thermoplastic material.*

Presbyopic LASIK

It involves multifocal ablation of cornea by excimer laser system and to use central zone for distant vision and peripheral zone for near vision.

Intracorneal Inlays

The intracorneal inlays are implanted in the cornea under a microkeratome-created flap or intralase-created pocket. This small disk acts as small aperture to allow the light to pass for near vision while minimally affecting distance vision.

9

Maladies of Orbit

Symptomatic Conditions

- Proptosis
- Thyroid orbitopathy
- Ophthalmoplegia

Inflammations

- Periostitis
- Tenonitis
- Orbital cellulitis
- Orbital thrombophlebitis
- Idiopathic orbital inflammatory

Tumors and Cysts of the Orbit

- Dermoid cyst
- Capillary hemangioma
- Cavernous hemangioma
- Glioma of optic nerve
- Meningioma
- Neurofibromatosis
- Rhabdomyosarcoma
- Orbital retinoblastoma
- Metastatic neuroblastoma
- Metastatic orbital tumors
- Tumors invading orbit
- Orbital tumors of infancy and childhood
- Hydatid cyst
- Distension of paranasal sinuses
- Management of tumors and cyst of orbit

Congenital Anomalies of the Orbit

- Oxycephaly
- Hypertelorism
- Facial asymmetry

Orbital Injury

- Blow-out fracture of orbit

SYMPTOMATIC CONDITIONS

Proptosis (Fig. 9.1)

Patient presents with mild protrusion of his/her right eye. His/her friends and relatives noticed the protrusion. Patient came for cosmetic embarrassment rather than any problem in his/her eye.

Ocular examination shows mild proptosis. No other clinical finding.

Diagnosis: Mild axial proptosis

Proptosis is a passive protrusion of the eyeball. Any space occupying lesion of the orbit pushes the eyeball forward manifesting as proptosis.

Types of Proptosis

1. *Pseudoproptosis:* There is no displacement of the eyeball. The eyeball itself is larger than the normal eye, thereby gives an appearance of proptosis. It is seen in the following conditions:
   - High axial myopia
   - Buphthalmos
   - Staphyloma.
2. *Acute proptosis:* There is sudden bulging of the eyeball that is seen in cases with:
   - *Orbital emphysema* usually occurs due to rupture of the medial wall of the orbit allowing air from the sinuses to escape behind the globe which results in sudden proptosis. It is reducible by pressure.
   - *Orbital hemorrhage* during retrobulbar injection of xylocaine and trauma to orbit.

3. *Pulsating proptosis:* Patient complains of a continuous rumbling sound like that of a sound from a waterfall. On auscultation, this sound can be heard by an ophthalmologist. It is due to caroticocavernous communication between internal carotid artery and the cavernous sinus. The commonest cause for pulsating proptosis is trauma to head. Clinically, there is proptosis, vessels on the lids and conjunctiva are dilated. Proptosis is reducible. The patient complains of pain due to stretching of branches of the fifth cranial nerve.

4. *Intermittent proptosis:* Its common causes are vascular tumors and orbital varix.

5. *Unilateral proptosis:* It occurs due to orbital tumors or cysts.

   - Common tumors causing proptosis are glioma of the optic nerve, meningioma of the optic nerve sheath, hemangioma, and dermoid.
   - Common cysts of the orbit are dermoid, hydatid cyst, cysticercus and mucocele from paranasal sinuses.

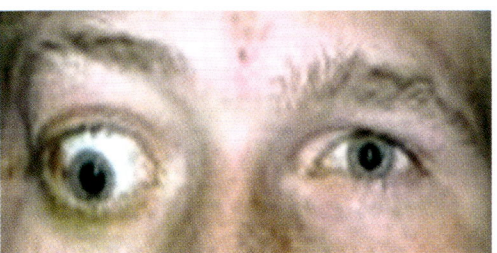

Fig. 9.1: Proptosis-down and out

6. *Bilateral proptosis:* The most common cause is thyroid orbitopathy. Other causes are leukemia, lymphosarcoma, nasopharyngeal tumors, chloroma, lymphoma and oxycephaly.

Symptoms

Usually, the only symptom is protrusion of the eyeball causing cosmetic embarrassment. If the cause is inflammatory, then there are other symptoms of pain and redness.

Signs

1. *Proptosis* may be axial or to any side depending on the site of space occupying lesion of the orbit.
2. *Limitation of ocular movement occurs* early. Usually, the limitation is towards the side of lesion.
3. *Diplopia*

Investigations

- Exophthalmometry helps in assessing the progress and prognosis.
- X-ray of the orbit
- Ultrasonography
- Carotid Doppler
- CT scan
- Magnetic resonance imaging (MRI)
- Needle aspiration
- Incisional or excisional biopsy
- Thyroid profile
- Complete blood picture
- Casoni's test for hydatid cyst
- Stool examination for ova and cyst
- Urine analysis

Management

1. Treat the cause, if amenable.
2. Surgical therapy—lateral orbitotomy

Thyroid Orbitopathy

Thyroid orbitopathy is one of the most puzzling maladies in the domain of ophthalmic cases.

Thyroid orbitopathy denotes an ocular malady that presents with lid retraction, lid lag and proptosis. This malady is usually associated with hyperthyroidism, goiter and ocular signs of lid retraction, lid lag and proptosis. It may be associated with hypothyroidism or even euthyroidism.

Etiology

It has an autoimmune basis. Thyroid orbitopathy may be a part of Graves' disease—a syndrome of hyperthyroidism, goiter and ocular signs or may be associated with hypothyroidism or even euthyroidism. There is no direct causative association between thyroid dysfunction and ocular involvement.

Pathogenesis

The pathogenesis appears to be associated with autoimmune basis. Autoimmune antibodies target extraocular muscles initiating an antigen—antibody reaction. This inflammatory reaction leads in production of mucopolysaccharides by the fibroblasts resulting in swelling followed by production of collagen that results in restriction of ocular movements. Females are more predisposed than males.

Types of Thyroid Orbitopathy

From clinical point of view, thyroid orbitopathy has been differentiated in **two types** depending on the ocular signs and symptoms.

Thyrotoxic orbitopathy *Patient in his/her forties presents with staring and frightened expression with complain of hyperanxiety and excitability. Even mobile ring makes patient suddenly alert and his/her body reacts to it.*

Patient pulse rate is high with mild tremors in hand. Thyroid profile is high or on the higher side of normal range.

Diagnosis—thyrotoxic orbitopathy.

Thyrotoxic orbitopathy is a kind of non-infiltrative ophthalmopathy.

It occurs more commonly in females with peak incidence in third to fifth decade of life while in males the peak incidence is in fourth to sixth decade of life. The onset of thyrotoxicosis may be acute or subacute and usually follows an acute illness or emotional upsurge.

It manifests with:
- General symptoms of hyperthyroidism such as loss of weight with increased appetite, sweating, intolerance to heat, tachycardia and tremors in hands.
- Patient is irritable, anxious and fatigued.
- Basal metabolic rate is high.
- Ocular signs are mild in form of lid retraction, lid lag and mild exophthalmos (Fig. 9.2).
- Most cases present with frightened and staring look due to upper lid retraction resulting in wide palpebral aperture.

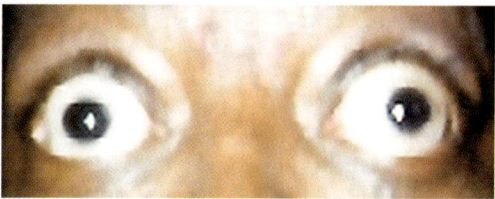

Fig. 9.2: Thyrotoxic exophthalmos

- Patient attends the clinic due to his/her staring and frightened look observed by his/her relatives.

Prognosis is very good. The malady responds well to anti-thyroid drugs orally.

Thyrotropic orbitopathy *An elderly spiritual guru presents with marked bilateral proptosis, lid retraction and congestion with ophthalmoplegia.*

His devotees narrated in praise and admiration that Guru has mastered the art of 'tratak yoga'—constant gazing without even blinking for hours since last 20 years or so. Now he cannot close his eyes, even if he desires to do so and his vision is markedly low.

In fact, guru suffered from thyrotoxicosis and devotees took his open and fixed gaze as his miracle in the art of 'tratak yoga'.

Diagnosis—thyrotropic orbitopathy/exophthalmic ophthalmoplegia.

Thyrotropic orbitopathy is a kind of infiltrative ophthalmoplegic ophthalmopathy.

It is characterized by infiltrative ocular signs and symptoms with exophthalmos and external ophthalmoplegia of varying degree. The malady affects middle-aged persons and runs a self-limiting course with remissions and relapses.

Management needs to control thyrotoxicosis, if associated and prevent ocular complications threatening the vision.

Clinical Features

1. *Exophthalmos:* Exophthalmos is an active proptosis. It is a classical sign of Graves' ophthalmopathy. As a rule, both the eyes are involved symmetrically yet it is common to find one eye showing more proptosis than the other eye or even the proptosis may remain unilateral.

2. *Retropulsion:* In early stage the exophthalmos is reducible by firm pressure and at this stage of reducibility the proptosis disappears with sleep, anesthesia and death.

3. *Lid signs:*
   - Dalrymple's sign—retraction of upper lids.
   - Normally with the eyes in primary position, the upper lid border covers the cornea for about 2 mm. When the upper lid border is resting at the level of the limbus or above the limbus, then it is true retraction of the upper lid. In a case with marked retraction, the sclera is exposed for about 5 mm. Retraction of the upper lid is usually bilateral but may affect only one eye in early stage.

     Retraction of lids gives a staring and frightened look to the patient. This look is diagnostic for *thyrotropic orbitopathy.*
   - *von Graefe's sign—lid lag:* There is failure of the upper lid to maintain its relative position with respect to the eyeball. When the patient is asked to look downwards well below the horizontal level, then the upper lid lags behind in its descent with the eyeball.
   - *Enroth's sign—puffy lids:* The lids appear full puffy and edematous due to infiltration behind the orbital septum. There is no dipping of the lid edema on pressure.
   - *Stellwag's sign—infrequent blinking reflex:* There is decreased frequency and incompleteness of the blinking reflex.

4. *Conjunctival signs:*
   - *Conjunctival hyperemia:* There is congestion of the conjunctiva especially on the temporal aspect. It is due to conjunctival venous stasis due to increased tissue pressure within the orbit.
   - *Chemosis:* The conjunctiva to begin with appears glossy, then waterlogged and finally chemosed. In a few cases of marked infiltrative ophthalmopathy, the chemosed conjunctiva may protrude between the lids usually overhanging the entire lower lid margin.

5. *Pupillary signs:* Some cases may show inequality of dilation of pupils. Some cases may show ill-sustained or jerky pupillary reaction on eliciting consensual light reflex. In late stage due to optic neuropathy the pupil reaction is sluggish or no reaction to light reflex.

6. *Ocular motility:*
   - *Moebius's sign:* There is weakness in the convergence for near work due to infiltration and fibrosis of medial rectus muscle.
   - *Ballet's sign:* There is partial or complete immobility of the eyes without internal ophthalmoplegia. To begin with, there is restriction of ocular movements which soon becomes fixed in position of depression. Usually there is limitation of elevation due to involvement of inferior rectus and inferior oblique muscles, followed by limitation of lateral movement due to involvement of medial rectus muscle, followed by fixation of the eye in position of depression due to involvement of lateral and superior rectus muscles in severe cases of thyrotropic infiltrative ophthalmopathy. The globe is fixed in position of depression mechanically as the eyes cannot be moved passively with forcep in the forced duction test. It is not unusual for ocular myasthenia to be associated with thyrotropic orbitopathy.

7. *Superior limbic keratoconjunctivitis:* Cornea is involved due to upper lid retraction, proptosis, lagophthalmos, inability to move the eye upwards, infrequent and incomplete blinking reflex.

8. *Optic neuropathy:* Optic neuropathy occurs due to direct compression of the nerve or its blood supply due to increased volume of orbital contents with increased intraorbital pressure. It is associated with slowly progressive visual loss with field defects.

Classification

Class–0 No ocular signs and symptoms.

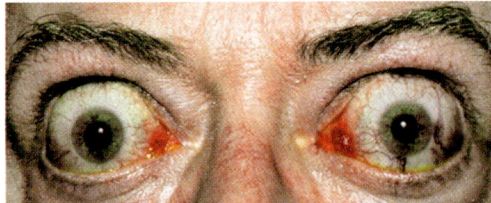

Fig. 9.3: Thyrotropic orbitopathy—class-4

Class–1 Lid signs: These are limited to upper lid retraction with or without lid lag and proptosis that may be minimal, moderate or marked.

Class–2 Soft tissue: There are signs and symptoms such as chemosis, puffy lids, extrusion of orbital fat, palpable lacrimal gland and visible extraocular muscles. These signs and symptoms may be minimal, moderate or marked.

Class–3 Proptosis: It is present in all the class from 2 to 6. Proptosis may be minimal, moderate or marked.

Class–4 Extraocular muscles: There is restriction of ocular movements that may be minimal at extreme gaze, moderate or marked with no ocular movements.

Class–5 Corneal lesion: It may be minimal in form of exposure keratitis, moderate in form of ulcer or marked in form of necrosis.

Class–6 Vision loss: It is due to involvement of optic nerve in form of optic atrophy or papilledema.

Investigations

- *Exophthalmometry:* A reading of 21 mm or more indicates proptosis. It helps to keep a watch on proptosis and prognosis.
- *Thyroid profile with antibody test and radioactive iodine uptake:* Thyroid profile is the best guide to adjust the doses to control thyrotoxicosis.
- *Ultrasonography:* It can detect even mild enlargement of extraocular muscles. And thus it is very helpful in early diagnosis.
- *CT scan:* It shows proptosis, enlargement of lateral and medial rectus muscles, thickening of the optic nerve and anterior prolapse of the orbital septum due to excess fat or swelling of muscles.
- *Magnetic resonance imaging:* It is more sensitive than CT scan. It is helpful in detecting difference between the normal and abnormal tissues.

Management

Refer the case to endocrinology or nuclear medicine to control thyrotoxicosis.

1. **Medical therapy**
   - Antithyroid drugs
   - Radioactive iodine
   - Topical artificial tear drops

   These are effective in protecting the cornea from exposure keratitis in cases of mild proptosis with retraction of the upper lid.

   - *Guanethidine 5% eye drop:* It may be effective in decreasing the retraction of the upper lid caused by over action of Müller's muscle.
   - *Systemic steroid:* It is indicated in a case with rapid progress of the exophthalmos with chemosis and optic neuropathy. Start with initial high dose of 80–100 mg of prednisolone and taper it off in about three months, if there is a favorable response.
   - *Radiotherapy:* It is indicated in cases which are unresponsive to steroids or steroids are contraindicated.

2. **Surgical therapy**
   - *Lateral tarsorrhaphy:* Tarsorrhaphy is indicated, only when there is exposure keratitis due to lid retraction. Exophthalmos and lid retraction may appear independent of each other.
   - *Extraocular muscle surgery:* It is indicated, when there is diplopia in primary position of gaze and on reading. It is done when there is no evidence of infiltrative ophthalmopathy.
   - *Blepharoplasty:* The excess of fatty tissue and redundant skin from and around the eyelids is removed.
   - *Surgery for lid retraction:* Recession of levator and Müller's muscle.
   - *Surgical orbital decompression.*

Indications

- Severe exposure keratitis due to proptosis and lid retraction.
- Optic neuropathy due to compression of the optic nerve.
- Cosmetic due to proptosis stable for long time.

Involve neurosurgeon for orbital decompression.

Two-orbital Wall Decompression (Antral-ethmoidal)

The decompression is performed by removing part of floor of the orbit and the posterior portion of the medial wall of the orbit. It achieves about 3–16 mm of retroplacement of the globe that is effective to save cornea and optic nerve. This two-wall decompression is cosmetically acceptable to the patient and the surgeon.

Note: Two-wall decompression is the best and most suitable for most cases of the proptosis. In this method, the actual space from antrum and ethmoid is provided for retroplacement of the contents of the globe. It achieves retroplacement of 3–16 mm, a wide range. It provides a better cosmetic appearance after surgery.

Ophthalmoplegia

An adult male presents with complain of mild pain in the right eye associated with diplopia, drooping of the lid and restriction of eye movements in outward direction. These symptoms manifest following a recent attack of high fever most likely due to influenza.

Ocular examination shows ptosis with involvement of sixth and third cranial nerves. Pupil reaction is normal.

Diagnosis—external ophthalmoplegia.

Ophthalmoplegia is a condition in which group of muscles are paralyzed.

Total Ophthalmoplegia

Total ophthalmoplegia is a condition in which all the extrinsic and intrinsic ocular muscles are paralyzed. It can occur as a congenital or acquired anomaly. Total congenital ophthalmoplegia is a rare condition. The acquired condition is often seen.

Internal Ophthalmoplegia

Internal ophthalmoplegia is a condition in which the intrinsic muscles are paralyzed.

External Ophthalmoplegia

External ophthalmoplegia is a condition in which the extrinsic muscles are paralyzed.

Acquired Total External Ophthalmoplegia

Total ophthalmoplegia occurs due to paralysis of third, fourth and sixth nerves.

Etiology

1. Cavernous sinus thrombophlebitis
2. Sphenoidal fissure syndrome
3. Syndrome of apex of orbit
4. Acute cranial polyneuritis
5. Diabetes
6. Acute leukemia
7. Myasthenia gravis.

Clinical Features of Total Ophthalmoplegia

1. There is complete ptosis.
2. The eyeball is slightly proptosed with slight divergence.
3. There is no ocular movement in any direction.
4. The pupil is dilated with no reaction to light, accommodation and convergence.
5. There is complete loss of accommodation.
6. The common causes for the bilateral total ophthalmoplegia are vascular or inflammatory lesion in the midbrain.
7. The common causes for unilateral ophthalmoplegia are syndrome of apex of orbit or syndrome of sphenoidal fissure.

Clinical Features of External Ophthalmoplegia

All the features of total ophthalmoplegia are present except the affection of pupillary activity and accommodation. In such a case, all the motor nuclei are affected except the

Edinger-Westphal nucleus which supplies the intrinsic muscles of the eye.

Clinical Features of Oculomotor Nerve Paralysis

- *Ptosis*—dropping of the upper lid.
- Eyeball is deviated outwards and slightly downwards due to normal action of the lateral rectus and superior oblique muscle.
- All the movements of the eyeball are limited except the outward movement.
- Pupil is dilated and not reacting to the light.
- Complete loss of accommodation.
- Intorsion of the globe on the attempted down gaze due to action of the superior oblique muscle.

Clinical Features of Trochlear Nerve Paralysis

- Limitation of the movement of the eyeball in down and in gaze.
- Eyeball is deviated upwards and inwards.
- Extorsion of the globe.
- Abnormal head posture to compensate for diplopia.

Clinical Features of Abducens Nerve Paralysis

- Limitation of the movement of the eyeball in outward direction.
- Eyeball is deviated inwards.
- Horizontal diplopia.

Investigations for Ophthalmoplegia

- History and routine examination of the eye.
- Ocular movements in all the directions of gaze.
- Visual acuity with glasses and without glasses.
- Ophthalmoscopy
- Diplopia test
- Hess screen test
- Any other investigation depending on the cause.

Treatment

Treat the cause.

INFLAMMATIONS

Periostitis

Patient presents with mild pain, tenderness and swelling at the outer aspect of right upper orbital margin. There is history of blunt trauma a few days ago.

Diagnosis—anterior superficial periostitis.

Periostitis is an inflammation of the periostium of the orbit. It is of two types: (i) Anterior superficial periostitis, and (ii) deep periostitis.

Anterior Superficial Orbital Periostitis

Anterior superficial orbital periostitis affects the orbital margin. It occurs due to injury to orbital margin, extension of inflammation from surrounding parts, tubercular and syphilitic periostitis. The usual site is outer aspect of the upper orbital margin which is most prone to trauma.

Patient complains of tenderness, pain, and swelling at the orbital margin in early stage of disease process.

On examination, there is a small area of orbital margin which is swollen with tenderness to touch and pain on deep pressure.

Tubercular anterior superficial periostitis usually manifests as osteoperiostitis with non-healing fistula.

Management

In early stage: Systemic course of broad-spectrum antibiotic gives a good response. A case with osteoperiostitis with fistula needs antitubercular treatment.

Posterior Deep Orbital Periostitis

Patient presents with deep dull orbital pain with mild proptosis and limitation of ocular movements.

Diagnosis—orbital apex syndrome.

Involvement of the apex of orbit manifests as 'orbital apex syndrome' characterized by triad of symptoms.

1. *Extraocular palsies:* One or more muscles of the eye may be involved. Usually, it is the lateral rectus which gets first involved with deviation of the eye.
2. *Trigeminal anesthesia and neuralgia:* The patient complains of severe pain in the area of the distribution of first and second divisions of the fifth nerve. There is a deep-seated pain in the eye with mild proptosis.
3. *Amaurosis:* The visual acuity is markedly reduced due to involvement of the optic nerve.

Management

Deep periostitis responds well to a course of systemic steroids covered with broad-spectrum antibiotic and supportive treatment.

Tenonitis

Patient presents with deep seated eye ache that followed an attack of mild fever and malaise. It increases on movement of the eyes and pressure touch.

Diagnosis—tenonitis.

An inflammation of Tenon's capsule is known as tenonitis.

Etiopathogenesis

Tenonitis is not a common inflammatory condition of the orbit. As a primary condition, it is usually non-suppurative in nature. It has been attributed to influenza, gout and rheumatism.

Symptoms and Signs

- Patient complains of a mild pain deep in the eyes and slight tenderness on movement of the eyeball.
- Patient presents with mild limitation and pain on the movement of the eyeball.
- Patient feels pain on pressure touch while washing his face especially closed lids.

Management

Topical and systemic steroids with cover of topical and systemic broad-spectrum antibiotics with supportive treatment give good response.

Orbital Cellulitis (Fig. 9.4)

Patient presents with marked edema of lids, congestion and chemosis of conjunctiva with restriction of ocular movements.

Diagnosis—orbital cellulitis

Orbital cellulitis is an inflammation of the cellular tissue of the orbit.

Etiology

1. *Extension of infection from surrounding structures:* The most common cause is the infection through venous stream from inflamed neighboring structures such as paranasal sinuses, boils on lids, nose or face, dental abscess or dental caries.
2. *Endogenous infection:* Metastatic infection from systemic inflammatory diseases.
3. *Exogenous infection:* Penetrating injuries especially with retained orbital foreign body.

Symptoms

- Swelling of the lids with chemosis of the conjunctiva.
- Proptosis of the eyeball with severe pain in the orbit and on movement of the eyeball.
- Fever with malaise.

Signs

- Mild proptosis in early stage. It may increase later with progress of inflammation.
- *Lids are swollen:* The upper lid may hang over the lower lid. It appears red with dilated capillaries.
- Marked conjunctival congestion with chemosis. Due to chemosis, the cornea appears like a crater surrounded by chemosed conjunctiva.
- Restriction of movement of the eyeball in all the directions. Any effort on movement gives rise to pain.
- Vision is affected if the optic nerve gets involved as optic neuritis.
- *Ophthalmoscopy:* The fundus may be normal or show features of optic neuritis.

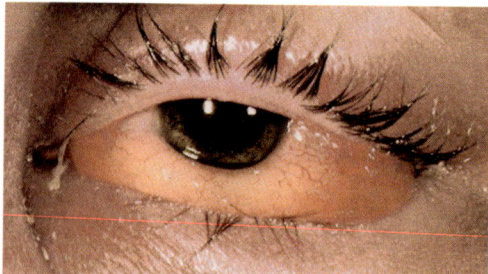

Fig. 9.4: Orbital cellulitis—edema lids and chemosis

Complications

1. *Formation of abscess:* In a delayed case, there is formation of an abscess behind the globe. The abscess usually points in the skin of lower lid near orbital margin or may empty in the lower conjunctival fornix. In a suspected case, it is better to pass a thick bore needle and aspirate it.
2. *Endophthalmitis:* Keep eye on fundus and vision.
3. *Panophthalmitis:* Rarely, it may lead to panophthalmitis.
4. *Cavernous sinus thrombosis:* Infection from orbital veins may spread to the cavernous sinus resulting in thrombosis.
5. *Optic atrophy:* Optic atrophy follows, if there had been optic neuritis.

Investigations

- Culture and sensitivity from nose and conjunctiva swabs and even blood sample.
- Geimsa and Gram's stain.
- Complete blood picture with ESR and smear.
- X-ray paranasal sinuses.
- Complete systemic check up especially ENT, dental and gynecological.
- Orbital ultrasonography
- CT scan and MRI, if needed.

Management

Intensive broad-spectrum antibiotic—topically and systemically

- Start systemic broad-spectrum antibiotic which covers large number of organisms and change according to culture and sensitivity report if necessary.

- Topical broad-spectrum antibiotic eye-drops every hourly in the day and eye ointment at night.

Supportive therapy

- Analgesic, anti-inflammatory and sedative to provide relief to the patient from pain, swelling and anxiety.
- If there is a suspicion of an abscess formation, then do not hesitate to pass a retrobulbar needle and aspirate.
- Maintain proper fluid intake
- Good nourishing diet with vitamins.
- With early, intensive and energetic treatment there are all the chances for early resolution with no complications.

Orbital Thrombophlebitis

Patient presents with marked swelling of the lids to the extent that the upper lid overhangs the lower lid margin.

Diagnosis—orbital thrombophlebitis.

Orbital thrombophlebitis denotes thrombosis of the orbital veins.

Infection may come down from cavernous sinus thrombophlebitis or infection from orbital thrombophlebitis may spread up to cavernous sinus.

Etiology

1. *Extension of infection from surrounding structures:* The infection is from venous supply from inflamed neighboring structures like paranasal sinuses, nose, face, lids, lips, dental caries or abscess, and throat. Any infection on the face or around the eye can cause orbital thrombophlebitis that may lead to cavernous sinus thrombophlebitis.
2. *Endogenous infection:* Metastasis from systemic infectious diseases, facial infection, stye, furuncles, orbital cellulitis, sinusitis, especially from mastoiditis and so on.
3. *Trauma:* Penetrating orbital injury.

Symptoms

- General symptoms *of fever and malaise.*
- *Severe pain* in the orbit and surrounding area.

- *Lid edema* to the extent that upper lid overhangs the lower lid.
- *Congestion and chemosis* of the conjunctiva.
- *Proptosis* which may increase in short time.

Signs

- Proptosis *is marked with rapid onset.*
- *Lid edema* with congestion and chemosis of conjunctiva.
- *Marked restriction of ocular movements* in all the directions. Palsy of third, fourth and sixth cranial nerves. Any attempt to move the eyes give rise to pain.
- *Optic neuritis*: Ophthalmoscopy shows optic neuritis. There is reduced vision and pupil is ill-sustained or dilated.
- *Meningitis:* Patient may show signs of meningitis, if the orbital thrombophlebitis spreads to cavernous sinus.
- *Mastoiditis*: Edema in mastoid region

Investigations

- Culture and sensitivity from nose and conjunctiva swabs and even blood sample.
- Geimsa and Gram's stain of conjunctival swab
- Complete blood picture with ESR and smear.
- X-ray paranasal sinuses especially mastoid air sinus.
- Complete systemic check up especially ENT, dental and gynecological.
- Orbital ultrasonography
- CT scan and MRI, if needed.

Management

Intensive broad-spectrum antibiotic—topically and systemically

- Start intravenous systemic broad-spectrum antibiotic which covers a large number of organisms and change according to culture and sensitivity report, if necessary.
- Topical broad-spectrum antibiotic eyedrops every hourly in the day and eye ointment at night.

Anticoagulant's role is controversial.

Supportive therapy

- Analgesic, anti-inflammatory and sedative to provide relief to the patient from pain, swelling and anxiety.
- If there is a suspicion of an abscess formation, then do not hesitate to pass a retrobulbar needle and aspirate.
- Maintain proper fluid intake and electrolytes.
- Good nourishing diet with vitamins.
- With early, intensive and energetic treatment, there are all the chances for early resolution with no complications.
- Involve neuro-physician on the slightest suspicion of cavernous sinus thrombosis or thrombophlebitis.

Idiopathic Orbital Inflammatory Disease (Ioid) (Pseudotumor)

Patient presents with severe deep seated pain, eye ache, and headache. Ocular movements are markedly restricted and painful. Imaging investigations are normal.

Diagnosis—pseudotumor.

The term 'idiopathic orbital inflammatory disease' (pseudotumor) denotes a variable and self-limiting malady that shows lymphocytic infiltration associated with polymorphonuclear cellular response and fibrovascular tissue reaction.

Etiology

- Etiology of the inflammatory process is not known.
- Inflammation may involve any or all the soft tissues of the orbit.
- Clinical picture is like that of a tumor mass.
- Usually seen in middle-aged persons, slightly more common in males.
- Usually unilateral but other eye may get involved later.
- Malady with self-limiting course with remissions and recurrences.

Signs and Symptoms

- Malady appears suddenly with an abrupt pain in the eye.

- Ocular movements are restricted and painful.
- Mild proptosis.
- Diplopia.
- Frozen orbit due to fibrosis of orbital tissues.
- Visual impairment due to involvement of optic nerve.

Complications

Optic atrophy following optic neuritis.

Management

Steroids

- *Systemic steroids:* Prednisolone 80–120 mg a day in divided doses for two weeks. Most cases show a good response. With good response, taper the steroids gradually to minimum maintenance dose for long time.
- Topical antibiotic/steroid eyedrops during day and eye ointment at night.

Supportive therapy Remember that this malady has a self-limiting course.

- Analgesic, anti-inflammatory and sedative to provide relief to the patient from pain, swelling and anxiety.
- Maintain proper fluid intake and electrolytes.
- Good nourishing diet with vitamins.
  With early, intensive and energetic treatment, there are all the chances for early resolution with no complications.
- Refer to neurophysician and neurosurgeon.

TUMORS AND CYSTS OF THE ORBIT

Dermoid Cyst

- Dermoid cyst is congenital in origin.
- Because of its small size, it remains undetected during early years of life. Gradually, it enlarges in a smooth painless swelling in the upper temporal or nasal quadrant of the orbit (Fig. 9.5).
- Cyst is usually free. It may be attached to orbital bones. Sometimes it is connected to the intracranial dura through a stalk-like extension of the cyst passing through an opening between the orbital bones.

- Cyst is lined with keratinizing epithelium and contains dermal adenexal structures such as hair follicles and sebaceous glands.
- Surgical removal is rewarding with good results.

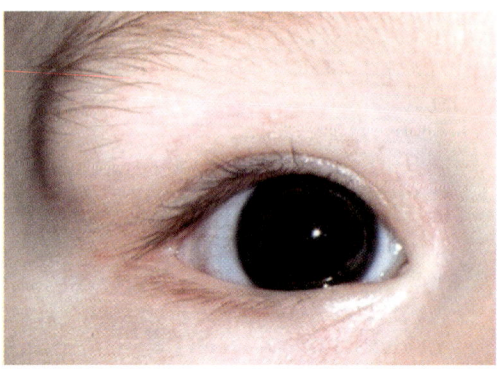

Fig. 9.5: Dermoid at outer upper angle of orbit

Capillary Hemangioma

- Capillary hemangioma is the most common tumor of the orbit in infancy and childhood.
- Manifests as an ill-defined bluish mass usually in the upper nasal quadrant of the orbit. It becomes more prominent, when the infant cries.
- Compressible and has a tendency for a spontaneous regression.
- Irradiation and steroids have been used to induce early regression.

Cavernous Hemangioma

- Cavernous hemangioma is a common orbital tumor in muscle cone.
- Well encapsulated malady of reddish or bluish in color without large feeding vessels.
- Common cause of unilateral proptosis that is slowly progressive and axial in character.
- Surgical removal with good results without hemorrhagic complications.

Glioma of Optic Nerve

- Glioma is the primary ectodermal tumor of the optic nerve.
- Non-neoplastic and self-limiting tumor with good prognosis for life.

- Common in children and usually manifests in first decade of life.
- Surgical removal is safe in early stage.

Meningioma

- Meningioma is a primary mesodermal tumor of the meninges.
- Arises around the optic nerve in the orbit or from intracranial meninges and invades the orbit.
- *Most commonly the tumor arises from the lateral portion of the sphenoid ridge which causes unilateral proptosis and visual loss.*

Neurofibromatosis (Plexiform Neuroma)

- Neurofibromatosis affects both the lids and orbit.
- Neurofibromatous proliferations extend anteriorly causing deformation of lids. In a typical case, the temporal region is also affected.
- Swollen lid and temporal region form a characteristic clinical picture.
- Neurofibroma is due to proliferation of all the various components of the peripheral nerves.
- *On palpation, hypertrophied nerves can be felt as hard cords or knobs, a feeling which is pathognomonic for neurofibroma.*

Rhabdomyosarcoma

- Rhabdomyosarcomas are extremely malignant tumors and occur in the first decade of life.
- Arise from voluntary muscles, grow rapidly, extend in all directions and produce rapidly increasing proptosis.
- Treated by a combination of chemotherapy and radiotherapy.

Orbital Retinoblastoma

- Orbital retinoblastoma occurs due to extension of the retinoblastoma in the orbit through the choroidal emissary or optic nerve.
- Incidence of orbital retinoblastoma has decreased due to early detection and treatment of retinoblastoma.

Metastatic Neuroblastoma

- Neuroblastoma is one of the common malignant tumor of the infancy and the childhood.
- Neuroblastoma is a tumor of embryonic neuroblastic tissue and usually arises in the adrenal medulla.
- Commonly metastasizes to both the orbits.
- *Presence of a bilateral hemorrhagic proptosis with facial masses in an infant or a child is pathognomonic for metastatic neuroblastoma.*
- Radiography shows osseous lesions.
- Increased catecholamines in the urine.

Metastatic Orbital Tumors

Common metastatic orbital tumors are:
- Metastatic neuroblastoma from the adrenal medulla.
- Metastatic orbital retinoblastoma
- Metastatic carcinoma from the breast of females
- Metastatic carcinoma from the lungs of males.

Tumors Invading Orbit

Common tumors invading orbit are:
- Carcinoma from the sinuses
- Nasopharyngeal carcinoma
- Intracranial meningioma
- Retinoblastoma from the eyeball.

Tumors of Infancy and Childhood

Common tumors of infancy and childhood are:
- Capillary hemangioma
- Metastatic neuroblastoma
- Neurofibromatosis
- Rhabdomyosarcoma
- Glioma of the optic nerve.

Hydatid Cyst

- Hydatid cyst is due to parasitic infestation 'Taenia echinococcus'.
- Natural host for this tapeworm is the intestines of the dog.
- Hydatid cyst occurs due to ingestion of poorly cooked meat containing the encysted form of the larvae.

- Causes unilateral proptosis that is rapidly progressing.
- Treatment is the total removal of cyst by lateral orbitotomy.

Distention of Paranasal Sinuses

- Orbit is surrounded by paranasal sinuses— *the frontal, ethmoid, maxillary and sphenoid.* These drain in the nose through their orifices. Orifices are likely to be blocked by catarrh, polypi or growth, therefore, may result in distention of the paranasal sinuses which shall affect the orbit.
- *Distention of the frontal sinus* causes bulging at the upper and inner part of the orbit displacing the eyeball downwards and outwards.
- *Distention of the ethmoid* also causes proptosis and displacement of the eyeball. Other features may be diplopia, venous congestion and ptosis.
- *Distention of the maxillary sinus* results in upward displacement of the eyeball with diplopia and proptosis.
- *Distention of the sphenoid sinus* may be responsible for optic neuritis.

Management of Tumors and Cysts of Orbit

Lateral orbitotomy (Kronlein's operation):
- Surgical removal of the lateral half of the supraorbital margin with the quadrilateral piece of bone from the lateral orbital wall to expose the orbital contents for dissecting off the retrobulbar mass causing proptosis.
- Lateral orbitotomy provides adequate exposure of the tumor behind the globe.
- Excision of tumor is easy with minimum of manipulation.
- Lateral approach provides better dissection of tumor in the anteroposterior plane with reduced risk of damage to orbital vessels and nerves.

CONGENITAL ANOMALIES OF ORBIT

Oxycephaly

- Skull is short with high vault, therefore, also known as 'Tower skull'.

- Oxycephaly is due to premature synostosis of the bones at the base of skull and also of transverse sutures.
- Orbits are shallow and placed laterally.
- Gives an appearance of an exophthalmos and divergent squint.
- Some cases may show optic atrophy due to papilledema which is due to raised intracranial pressure.
- X-ray shows a "silver beaten" appearance of the vault of the skull due to raised intracranial pressure.

Hypertelorism

- Forehead is prominent with broad bridge of nose and widely separated orbits.
- Associated ocular features may be divergent squint and optic atrophy.

Facial Asymmetry

- Minor degree of facial asymmetry is common and is due to effects of molding of the head during birth.
- Usually not associated with any ocular complications.
- Marked facial asymmetry shows squint and relative proptosis.

Management

Treat the cause with supportive therapy.

ORBITAL INJURY

Blow-out Fracture of Orbit

The term "blow-out fracture of the orbit" covers a specific condition, wherein there is a fracture of the floor of the orbit without a fracture of the orbital rim, usually caused by a blow from front of the eye.

Etiology

A blow-out fracture occurs following an injury to the orbit by a blunt object that is bigger in size than the diameter of the orbital margin. An injury by a smaller object shall produce a severe contusion or concussion causing even rupture of the globe. The most common mode is a blow from a fist, a tennis ball or rounded blunt object. It mainly involves orbital floor and medial wall.

Pathogenesis

Hydraulic theory: Smith and Began in their 'Hydraulic theory' postulated that when a blunt object strikes the orbit, the eyeball along with its soft tissues are pushed posteriorly, thereby suddenly increasing the intraorbital pressure. This increased intraorbital pressure is relieved by fracture of the posterior orbital floor. The posterior orbital floor is very thin (0.5 to 1.0 mm), has a slight convexity and is inclined superiorly and is further weakened by infraorbital groove and canal. All these factors contribute to its fracture.

Buckling force: A blow to the inferior orbital margin produces a 'buckling force' on the floor of the orbit. The force is transmitted directly to the thin orbital floor, buckling it and fracturing it downwards into the maxillary antrum.

Clinical Features

- *Proptosis* follows immediately after the injury due to marked orbital hemorrhage or emphysema. The real picture manifests after the subsidence of emphysema and absorption of hemorrhage.
- *Emphysema of the eyelids*: Emphysema can be diagnosed easily by putting mild pressure on the swollen lids. On pressure, there is a feeling of air in the lids being displaced.
- *Enophthalmos* is due to fracture of the floor of the orbit and damage to supporting ligaments of the globe. The herniation of the soft tissues of the orbit in the maxillary sinus further contributes to an appearance of enophthalmos. If the enophthalmos is marked, then there is a noticeable superior sulcus deformity.
- *Globe-ptosis* occurs in a large fracture of the floor of the orbit. The ptosis of the globe can be assessed by placing a scale across the medial canthi and compare the position of the two eyes.
- *Diplopia* is the most common presenting symptom in all the cases. Any patient who complains of diplopia in any field two weeks after injury must be explored for orbital floor fracture.
- *Paresthesia:* There is an infraorbital paresthesia due to the involvement of the infraorbital nerve which supplies the skin over the region and oral mucosa.

Investigation

- Plain X-rays
- CT scan and MRI

Management

Surgical repair depends on the degree of enophthalmos, globe-ptosis, diplopia and tissue incarceration.

10

Maladies of Lacrimal Apparatus

Symptomatic Disorders

- Lacrimation
- Epiphora

Maladies of Lacrimal Gland

- Dry eye syndrome
- Sjögren's syndrome
- Mikulicz's syndrome
- Dacryoadenitis
- Mixed tumor of lacrimal gland

Maladies of Lacrimal Apparatus

- Eversion of the lower punctum
- Occlusion of the punctum
- Occlusion of the canaliculus
- Congenital dacryocystitis (dacryocystitis neonatorum)
- Acute dacryocystitis
- Chronic dacryocystitis

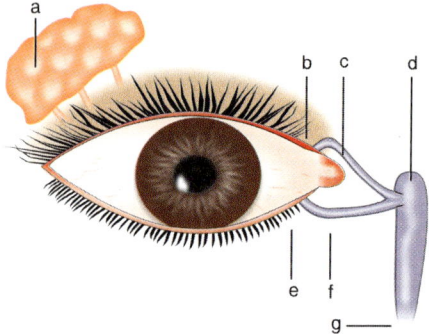

Fig. 10.1: Lacrimal apparatus (a: lacrimal gland; b, e: Punctum; c, f: canaliculi; d: sac; g: naso-lacrimal duct)

Lacrimal apparatus (Fig. 10.1) consists of two parts:

1. The lacrimal gland and the accessory glands which secrete the tear fluid.
2. The lacrimal drainage system that comprises the punctum, the canaliculi, the lacrimal sac and the nasolacrimal duct. This system drains the tear fluid from the conjunctival sac to the nose.

SYMPTOMATIC DISORDERS

Lacrimation

Lacrimation is an active process of excessive secretion of tear fluid. Though the lacrimal drainage system is functioning normally yet it is not *able to drain the excessive secretion of the tear fluid, therefore, there is overflow of tears resulting in an annoying symptom of epiphora—the watering of the eye.*

Lacrimation can occur in the following conditions:

- Irritation of cornea due to foreign body or distorted lashes.
- Inflammation or ulceration of cornea.
- Irritation of conjunctiva
- Inflammation of conjunctiva
- Uveitis
- Reflex irritation due to diseases of nose and sinuses
- Emotional factors.

Treat the cause.

Epiphora

Epiphora is a passive process in which though the secretion of tear fluid is normal yet the lacrimal drainage system is not able to drain the tear fluid due to obstruction in the drainage system resulting in overflow of tear fluid causing an annoying symptom of epiphora—the watering of the eye.

Etiological Factors

- Eversion of lower punctum
- Occlusion of lower punctum
- Occlusion of canaliculi
- Congenital dacryocystitis
- Acute dacryocystitis
- Chronic dacryocystitis
- Functional insufficiency of lacrimal drainage system.

Any obstruction in the lacrimal drainage system can be diagnosed by regurgitation test or syringing of the lacrimal sac.

Treatment of epiphora is to treat the cause to achieve clear passage of lacrimal drainage system.

MALADIES OF LACRIMAL GLAND

Dry Eye Syndrome (Keratoconjunctivitis Sicca: KCS)

Patient presents with complaints of mild itching, photophobia, burning and sandy feeling in the eyes with annoying mucoid filamentary discharge especially on near work and outdoors.

Slit-lamp shows lusterless cornea with mild haze and absence of lower lid marginal tear film. Tear film break up time is reduced.

Diagnosis—dry eye syndrome.

Dry eye syndrome is a symptom complex that occurs as sequelae to deficiency in any component of precorneal tear film.

Deficiency in any of the components of the precorneal tear film results in dryness of the eye due to the appearance of dry spots on the corneal and conjunctival epithelium.

Dry eye syndrome is a disease of the ocular surface exposed to different disturbances of the natural function and protective mechanism of the external ocular surface leading to an unstable tear film during open eye.

It is important to realize that the external ocular surface has to maintain the integrity during force of blinking, air currents, humidity, minute foreign bodies and microorganisms.

Etiology

- *Aqueous deficiency dry eye:* It occurs in Sjögren's syndrome, sarcoidosis, lymphoma, leukemia and amyloidosis. Aqueous deficiency can occur in idiopathic hyposceretion and affection of the lacrimal glands.
- *Mucin deficiency dry eye:* It occurs, when goblet cells are damaged as in xerophthalmia and conjunctival scarring which may be due to trachoma, Stevens-Johnson syndrome, ocular pemphigoid, chemical burns, chronic bacterial or viral conjunctivitis and irradiation.
- *Lipid deficiency dry eye:* Lipid deficiency is rare. Lipid abnormality is seen in patient with chronic blepharitis and meibomitis.

Miscellaneous Factors

- Effect of drugs like atropine and diuretics
- Mumps
- Deficient blinking
- Lid surgery not allowing proper polishing.
- Impaired eyelid function as in cases of Bell's palsy, symblepharon, pterygium, lagophthalmos and ectropion.
- Exposure keratitis

Symptoms

- Foreign body sensation—scratchy or a sandy feeling in the eye
- Excessive secretion of mucus
- Burning sensation especially under the fan, air-conditioning, watching television, study and on exposure to heat
- Difficulty in opening the eyelids as if they are stuck up
- Itching
- Photophobia
- Mild pain
- Mild redness
- Less secretion of tears even when exposed to irritant odors, fumes and emotional turmoil.

Signs

- Lusterless ocular surface
- Conjunctival xerosis
- Mild redness of the conjunctiva with mucus in fornix
- Mild blepharitis
- Punctate epithelial erosions on the lower part of cornea taking fluorescein stain
- Filaments on the cornea moving with each blink and takes rose bengal stain
- Deficient or absent lower lid marginal tear strip.

Test

- Tear film break-up time reduced or even less than 10 seconds.
- Rose bengal staining shows devitalized epithelium of conjunctiva in the inter-palpebral area and mucus plaques on the cornea.
- Schirmer's test-I is positive.
- Giemsa staining of the conjunctival scraping may show increased number of goblet cells as in a case of Sjögren's syndrome.

Management

- Artificial tear eyedrops—the mainstay in the management of dry eye syndrome
- Topical cyclosporine 0.05 to 0.1% eyedrops
- Acetylcysteine 5% eyedrops as mucolyte
- Topical retinoids
- Cool and humid environment
- Protective goggles
- Punctum occlusion.

Sjögren's Syndrome

Sjögren's syndrome is characterized with **triad** *of:*

i. Keratoconjunctivitis sicca.
ii. Xerostomia (dry mouth) with or without enlargement of salivary glands.
iii. Rheumatoid arthritis.

Keratoconjunctivitis sicca appears in the fourth to sixth decade of life.

Treatment is to provide relief to ocular symptoms of dryness. Systemic steroids are helpful in cases with rheumatoid arthritis.

Mikulicz's Syndrome

Mikulicz's syndrome is characterized by a symmetrical enlargement of the lacrimal and salivary glands.

- Etiology is not clear.
- Swelling of glands is of lymphomatous nature.
- Enlargement of parotid and lacrimal glands in uveoparotid inflammation known as "uveoparotitis or Heerfordt's disease".

Dacryoadenitis (Fig. 10.2)

Patient presents with painful swelling involving outer third of the upper lid.

- Dacryoadenitis occurs occasionally in general infectious diseases like mumps, influenza and infectious mononucleosis.
- Painful swelling at the outer third of the upper lid. It may be associated with follicular conjunctivitis, periorbital edema, uveitis or optic neuritis.
- Rarely it may suppurate and the abscess so formed may burst on the surface forming a fistula.
- In early case, a course of broad-spectrum antibiotic systemically along with analgesics and hot compresses takes care. If an abscess has formed, then it is better to drain it.

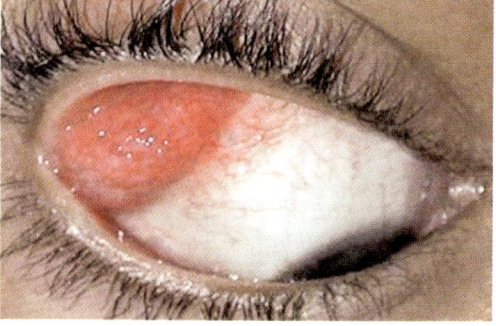

Fig. 10.2: Acute dacryoadenitis

Mixed Tumor of Lacrimal Gland

The most common tumor of the lacrimal gland is the "Mixed tumor", a pleomorphic adenocarcinoma.

Benign Mixed Tumor of the Lacrimal Gland

Patient presents with slowly progressive painless swelling in the upper lid with watering and diplopia.

- Occurs in the middle span of life.
- Pushes the eye downwards and medially.
- *Treatment:* Surgical removal with good results.

Malignant Mixed Tumor of the Lacrimal Gland

Patient presents with fast growing painful and tender swelling in the upper lid with watering and diplopia.

- Pushes the eye downwards and medially.
- Extends to the lower temporal quadrant of the orbit.
- *Treatment:* Radical surgery with poor prognosis.

MALADIES OF LACRIMAL APPARATUS

Eversion of the Lower Punctum

Patient presents with eversion of the lower punctum that causes epiphora as the tear fluid cannot be drained though the lacrimal passage is normal.

Etiopathogenesis

- Laxity of the lids in old age
- Chronic conjunctivitis
- Blepharitis
- Ectropion.

On examination, normally the lower punctum is not visible without slight retraction of the lower lid.

If the lower punctum is visible without retraction of the lid then it is said to be a case of eversion of the lower punctum.

With eversion, the punctum does not dip in the lacrimal lake, therefore, there is improper or no drainage of tear fluid resulting in epiphora—watering of the eyes.

Management

- Three snip surgery is the ideal choice for all the cases of eversion of lower punctum.
- In an early case and in aged, the eversion may be corrected by cautery punctures

along the whole length of the lower tarsus at its lower border. In a few weeks with cicatrization, the lid punctum should be pulled back to its normal position.

Eversion of the lower punctum due to ectropion of the lower lid needs correction of ectropion by surgery.

Occlusion of the Punctum

Patient presents with epiphora—the annoying symptom with social and cosmetic embarrassment.

Congenital occlusion of the punctum is rare.

Cicatricial occlusion of the punctum causes epiphora.

On examination, if there is an occlusion of the lower punctum, then it is essential to verify the patency of the lacrimal drainage system by syringing through the upper punctum.

If the lacrimal drainage system is patent on syringing, then open the stenosed punctum by a point of canaliculus knife under operating microscope.

Occlusion of Canaliculus

Patient presents with epiphora—the annoying symptom with social and cosmetic embarrassment.

- Occlusion of the canaliculus can occur due to a scar, foreign body or due to fungal infection with *Actinomyces*.
- Eyelash is a rare foreign body that can be removed easily. Fallen eye lash in the lower fornix can be sucked in the canaliculi, the end is projecting giving rise to feeling of foreign body with each blink. Slit-lamp examination shows the projecting end.
- Concretions or *Actinomyces* can be removed by dilating the canaliculus, slitting and curetting it.
- Occlusion due to the cicatrization needs a plastic repair.

Congenital Dacryocystitis

Young mother with her two months old baby presents with watering in both the eyes of her infant since a month or so.

Ocular examination shows epiphora in both the eyes.

Regurgitation test is negative. Syringing shows regurgitation of clear fluid in both the eyes from upper punctum.

Diagnosis—congenital dacryocystitis

Etiopathogenesis

- Dacryocystitis in infants may be unilateral or bilateral and occur due to non-canalization of the nasolacrimal duct.
- Lumen of the duct is filled by epithelial debris.
- There is either non-canalization or delay in canalization of the nasolacrimal duct which persists for a few months after birth.

Symptoms

- Infant is brought to the eye clinic with a complaint of watering since birth in one or both the eyes.
- Some cases report conjunctival discharge with a history of sticking of the lids.

Signs

- Watering from the eye or eyes with mild mucus or mucopurulent discharge.
- Regurgitation test may be positive or negative.
- Syringing shows regurgitation of fluid from the upper punctum.

Management

Topical and systemic therapy

- If there is no regurgitation of either mucus or mucopurulent discharge on regurgitation test and regurgitation of clear fluid on syringing, then advise parents to keep the eyes clean and use topical broad-spectrum antibiotic eyedrops to prevent infection.
  This treatment can be continued until the age of about 4 months. There are all the chances that the normal and natural canalization shall be complete. If epiphora persists, then it is rewarding to perform probing of nasolacrimal duct without any further delay.

- If there is an infection of the lacrimal sac with regurgitation test positive with regurgitation of mucopurulent discharge, then syringe daily for 3–5 days with topical broad-spectrum antibiotic eyedrops along with topical instillation of eyedrops and ointment four to six times daily.
  Systemic broad-spectrum antibiotic for short duration shall be rewarding in controlling the infection.
  Once the infection is well under control, then it is better to perform probing of nasolacrimal duct without delay.

- Probing of the nasolacrimal duct is rewarding, if performed before the age of 4 months.

Surgical therapy *Probing of the nasolacrimal duct:* It is an operation in which a lacrimal probe is passed down the nasolacrimal duct to canalize it.

- It is advisable to perform probing early so that the obstruction of the duct may not become fibrotic due to chronic infection or unnecessary delay.
- Results of probing are 100% provided the probing has been performed early say within the age of 4 months. With delay, the result also gets delayed.

Acute Dacryocystitis (Fig. 10.3)

Patient presents with intense pain with cyst like swelling near the inner canthus since yesterday.

Ocular examination shows red, hot, firm, vertically oval globular swelling with radiating pain and tender to touch in the lacrimal sac region.

Diagnosis—acute dacryocystitis.

Acute dacryocystitis is an acute suppurative inflammation of the lacrimal sac or its pericystic tissue.

Etiology

- Causative organisms are *Staphylococcus, Streptococcus* and *Pneumococcus*.
- Acute exacerbation of the chronic dacryocystitis.
- Acute pericystitis due to acute suppurative inflammation of pericystic tissue usually due to endogenous or systemic source of infection.

Symptoms

- Severe pain with radiation over frontal region.
- Epiphora with conjunctival congestion and discharge.
- Swelling at the lacrimal sac area which may extend downwards and laterally towards the lower lid.
- Swelling is red, hot, firm and tender to touch.
- Some cases may show a pus point on the summit of the swelling.

Signs

- Marked conjunctival congestion and muco-purulent discharge.
- Swelling in the region of lacrimal sac which may extend towards the lower lid.
- Diffuse or nodular red, hot, firm and tender swelling with severe pain and tenderness.
- Abscess formation with pus point.
- Discharging external or internal fistula.

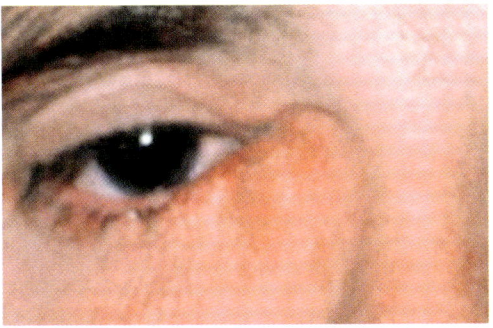

Fig. 10.3: Acute dacryocystitis

Complications

- General malaise with fever
- Orbital cellulitis
- Hypopyon corneal ulcer
- Cavernous sinus thrombophlebitis
- Osteomyelitis of the lacrimal bone
- External or internal fistula.

Management

Systemic and topical antibiotics In early stage before formation of a lacrimal abscess, systemic and topical broad-spectrum anti-biotics instillation of eyedrops and ointment may be effective to cause resolution.

Malady usually ends up as chronic dacryocystitis.

Supportive therapy

- Analgesics and anti-inflammatory to provide relief from pain.
- Hot compresses are helpful.
- If there is either a formation of an abscess or there is a pus point, then it is better to incise and drain the abscess for early resolution.

Surgical therapy Dacryocystorhinostomy should be performed after complete resolution to eradicate the source of chronic infection and the annoying symptom of epiphora.

Chronic Dacryocystitis (Fig. 10.4)

An adult female patient presents with constant watering since four years in her left eye. No relief by topical eyedrops.

Ocular examination shows a small globular swelling at the lacrimal sac region. The lacrimal lake is full of tears. Regurgitation test is positive.

Diagnosis—chronic dacryocystitis.

Chronic dacryocystitis is a primary chronic inflammation of the lacrimal sac and not secondary to acute dacryocystitis.

Etiopathogenesis

- Most common organisms responsible for chronic dacryocystitis are *Pneumococcus, Streptococcus* and *Staphylococcus.*
- Affects people of middle age and seen predominantly in females.
- Incidence is higher in persons with low socioeconomic status and poor environmental hygienic conditions.
- Incidence is higher in persons in whom there is recurrent inflammation of the nose, sinuses and the conjunctiva.
- Stasis of the lacrimal fluid in the lacrimal sac due to some kind of obstruction in the nasolacrimal duct.

Nasolacrimal duct is surrounded by a rich capillary plexus with character of an erectile tissue, therefore, it can cause obstruction of the duct even with slight engorgement of vessels due to even mild inflammation of the nose or sinuses.

Nasal polypi, hypertrophied inferior turbinate and deviated nasal septum result in mild obstruction to drainage.

With slight stasis due to obstruction of the nasolacrimal duct, there is epiphora and if stasis is not relieved, then stasis provides a ground for bacteria to grow and multiply to manifest as chronic suppurative inflammation of the sac.

Epiphora, swelling and unilateral conjunctivitis are pathognomonic and diagnostic for chronic dacryocystitis.

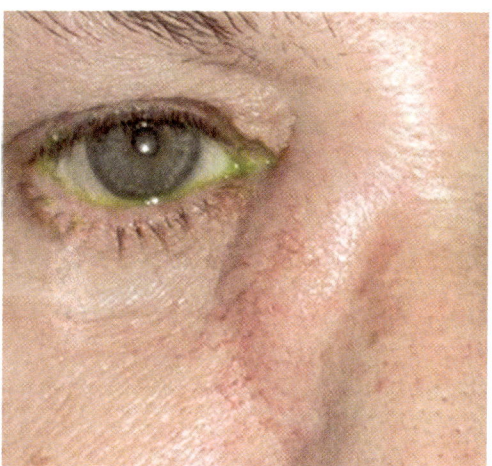

Fig. 10.4: Chronic dacryocystitis

Clinical Features

- Swelling in the lacrimal sac region below the level of inner canthus.
- Tenderness is absent and no complaint of pain.
- Swelling is not freely mobile.
- Skin over the swelling is free and normal.
- Regurgitation test is positive.
- Syringing shows regurgitation of clear fluid or mucopus from the upper punctum.
- Dacryocystgraphy shows a dilated sac with smooth outline.
- It is most suitable for dacryocystorhinostomy operation.

Clinical Types and Features

1. *Chronic dacryocystitis with encysted lacrimal sac* In a few cases of chronic dacryocystitis, both exit; the canaliculi and the nasolacrimal duct get blocked, thereby forming a cyst of the lacrimal sac with mucus.
   - Swelling at the lacrimal sac region below the level of inner canthus.
   - No pain or tenderness.
   - Swelling is not freely mobile.
   - Skin over the swelling is free and mobile.
   - Regurgitation test is negative.
   - Syringing test shows regurgitation of fluid back through the same punctum indicating block at the sac—canaliculus junction.

   It is most suitable case for dacryocystorhinostomy.

2. *Chronic dacryocystitis with fibrotic lacrimal sac:*
   - Patient complains of watering.
   - No swelling at the lacrimal sac region on inspection.
   - No swelling felt even on palpation.
   - Regurgitation test is negative.
   - No history of recurrent unilateral conjunctivitis.
   - Syringing test shows regurgitation of clear fluid from the upper punctum.
   - Dacryocystogram shows only the canaliculi and small sac.

   Dacryocystorhinostomy can be performed as fibrotic sac gives thick sac flaps for suturing.

3. *Chronic dacryocystitis with functional block:*
   - Swelling in the lacrimal sac region below the level of inner canthus.
   - Tenderness is absent and no complaint of pain.
   - Swelling is not freely mobile.
   - Skin over the swelling is free and normal.
   - Regurgitation test: The lacrimal sac empties partly in the nose and partly in the conjunctival sac. Usually, the patient is able to demonstrate this phenomenon that has been learned by experience. He/she has learned to empty the sac contents to get relief from epiphora for a few hours until the sac refills.

- Syringing shows partial patency.
- Dacryocystogram shows dilated sac with dye in the duct and nose.

Pathogenesis of the functional block lies in the flbroelastic nature of the lacrimal sac and rich venous capillary plexus around the naso-lacrimal duct. Engorgement of the venous plexus of the duct results in partial block causing retention of fluid in the sac which dilates to accommodate it. In course of time with repeated attacks of partial block, the lacrimal sac becomes dilated and atonic. Though the duct is partially open yet the sac is unable to discharge its contents in the nose due to failure of its normal tone. But with pressure by the patient thumb, the sac gets empty in the nose.

It is a case of functional block of the sac.

It is most suitable for dacryocystorhinostomy.

Complications of Chronic Dacryocystitis

- It is a common cause for chronic conjunctivitis.
- It may exacerbate in acute dacryocystitis.
- It is a common cause for hypopyon ulcer.
- It is a source of infection for any intraocular surgery.

Diagnosis

- A case of unilateral epiphora with unilateral conjunctivitis is enough to diagnose chronic dacryocystitis.
- In all the cases of unilateral conjunctivitis and epiphora, syringing is a must before excluding chronic dacryocystitis as the regurgitation test may be negative.

Management—Surgical Therapy

Dacryocystectomy is an operation in which the entire sac is excised.

Dacryocystorhinostomy is an operation in which an anastomosis is made between the lacrimal sac and the mucous membrane of the middle meatus of the nose to relieve the patient of his source of repeated infection, annoying symptom of epiphora and social embarrassment.

- Topical broad-spectrum antibiotic eye-drops to treat associated conjunctivitis.
- Dacryocystorhinostomy is the first choice unless there is an absolute contraindication for it.
- Plan for dacryocystorhinostomy in every case and terminate in dacryocystectomy, if there is surgical problem.

11

Maladies of Lid

Congenital Anomalies

- Epicanthus
- Distichiasis
- Microblepharon
- Coloboma of lid
- Cryptophthalmos

Symptomatic Conditions of Lid

- Ptosis (Blepharaoptosis)
  - Congenital simple ptosis
  - Myasthenic ptosis
  - Other types of ptosis
- Bell's palsy
- Ecchymosis of lids
- Xanthelasma

Inflammation of Lid

- Blepharitis
- Molluscum contagiosum
- External Hordeolum
- Hordeolum internum
- Chalazion

Maladies of Lashes and Lids

- Trichiasis
- Entropion
- Ectropion
- Symblepharon
- Lagophthalmos
- Retraction of lid
- Blepharochalasis
- Blepharophimosis
- Ankyloblepharon

Benign Tumors of Lid

- Nevus or mole
- Capillary hemangioma

- Neurofibromatosis
- Dermoid cyst

Malignant Tumors of Lid

- Squamous cell carcinoma (epithelioma)
- Basal cell carcinoma (rodent ulcer)
- Sebaceous gland carcinoma

Lid Injury

- Contusion
- Wounds
- Burns

CONGENITAL ANOMALIES

Epicanthus

Young mother with her 1-year-old baby presents with complain of mild inward deviation of both the eyes since birth. It is more apparent now.

Epicanthus gives an impression of apparent convergent squint.

Hirschberg's test is normal. Pull up the skin at root of nose by thumb and index finger in a fold and deviation disappears.

Assure the mother that it shall be normal within a few months with the growth of the bridge of nose.

Diagnosis: Epicanthus.

- Epicanthus is a bilateral anomaly and characteristic of mongolian race.
- Epicanthus appears as a semilunar fold of skin extending from the root of nose to the inner end of the lower eyelid.
- Concavity of the fold is towards the eye and it tends to conceal the inner canthus and caruncle.

- Clinically, the child gives an appearance of pseudoconvergent squint that alarms the parents.
- Epicanthus may exist in infantile life usually up to the age of 6 months.
- Epicanthus disappears with the development of the bridge of nose.

Management

If epicanthus persists, then it can be treated surgically by removal of an elliptical fold of skin from root of nose and suture the skin with subcutaneous suture.

Distichiasis

Congenital distichiasis is a rare anomaly in which there is an extra row of eyelashes occupying the position of meibomian glands which open into cilia follicles as ordinary sebaceous glands. These may be misdirected and rub against the cornea.

Management

Electroepilation or cryoepilation.

Microblepharon

Microblepharon is a condition in which the lids are abnormally small. It is rare and is usually associated with microphthalmos or congenitally small eye, or anophthalmos.

Coloboma of Lid

- Coloboma of lid is a condition in which there is a full thickness triangular notch at the edge of the lid.
- Notch is usually situated at the inner side of the midline of the lid generally affecting the upper lid.
- Two or more notches in the same lid.
- May be associated with dermoid or other defects of the eye.

Management

Plastic surgery for cosmetic embarrassment.

Cryptophthalmos

Cryptophthalmos is a condition in which the skin is continuous from eyebrow to cheek passing over the eye. It is usually associated with other defects of the eye.

SYMPTOMATIC CONDITIONS OF LID

Ptosis

Ptosis is a term given to a condition of drooping of the upper lid, when the eye is open.

Congenital Simple Ptosis (Fig. 11.1)

Young lady with child in her lap presents with complaint of drooping of left lid in her child since birth.

Ocular examination shows drooping, smooth, unwrinkled left lid with no tarsal fold and covering the pupil.

Diagnosis—congenital unilateral simple ptosis.

Congenital unilateral or bilateral simple ptosis is the most common type of ptosis covering about 77% cases of ptosis.

- Congenital simple ptosis may manifest as uncomplicated ptosis or with paresis of the ipsilateral superior rectus muscle.
- Strong hereditary tendency.
- Ptosis remains stationary for the whole life.
- Drooping of the lid since birth.
- Lid is smooth, unwrinkled, and thin, without tarsal fold and may cover the pupil.
- If the pupil is partially covered then the patient adopts a characteristic posture in which chin is raised, head is tilted backwards, and the forehead on the affected side shows horizontal furrows with raised eyebrow. This posture is adopted in attempt to have vision in the affected eye.
- It is most amenable to resection of the levator muscle surgery.

Etiopathogenesis

- *Congenital simple ptosis is due to failure in the differentiation of the muscles.*
- Levator palpebrae superioris and the superior rectus muscles are closely associated, therefore, the congenital anomaly frequently involves both the muscles.
- Hereditary with autosomal dominance with a relatively high penetrance.

- Affects both the sex and transmits the condition equally.

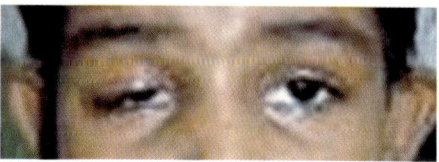

Fig. 11.1: Congenital simple ptosis

Symptoms

1. *Drooping of lid:* It is the parents who bring the patient usually a child with a complaint that the child is unable to lift the lid of one eye. In most cases, it is since birth. It is a cosmetic embarrassment for the child and parents, both.
2. *Diplopia:* Patient with partial ptosis usually complains of diplopia.
3. *Characteristic posture:* Patients adopt a characteristic posture, if the ptosis covers the pupil partially interfering with vision.

Signs

1. *Drooping of upper lid:* There is a drooping of the upper lid. The lid is smooth, unwrinkled, and inert with no tarsal fold.
2. *Characteristic posture:* A characteristic head posture shows a raised chin, head tilted backwards, eyes being rotated downward, eyebrow is raised with horizontal furrows on the forehead. The raised eyebrow and horizontal furrows on the forehead are due to forced contraction of the frontalis muscle in an attempt to raise the lid to uncover the pupil. This posture is adopted only when the pupil is partially covered causing diplopia.
3. *Amblyopia exanopsia:* It may occur if the ptosis covers the pupil completely.

Tests for Planning Ptosis Surgery

1. *Measurement of amount of ptosis:*
   - The central palpebral width in the primary position of gaze gives the amount of ptosis.
   - *In a case of unilateral ptosis,* the amount of ptosis is the difference between the palpebral fissure widths on each side with fixation of the frontalis muscle.
   - *In a case of bilateral ptosis,* the amount of ptosis is difference between the normal average palpebral fissure width of 10 mm and the width actually measured. To measure the amount of ptosis, it is essential to lift the lid of one eye so that the patient is able to fix his/her gaze in the primary position, and measurement is taken of the opposite eye. Repeat the process for the other eye.

2. *Measurement of levator muscle function:* With Burke's method, the patient is asked to look to extreme down gaze. The zero mark of the millimeter ruler is placed adjacent to the central upper eyelid margin. The frontalis muscle is fixed with direct pressure on the eyebrow by the surgeon. Keeping the frontalis muscle fixed, the patient is asked to look in extreme up gaze. Measure directly on the ruler the excursion (movement) of the lid from down gaze to up gaze position. The normal levator movement ranges from 15 to 18 mm.

Grading of levator function:
- Normal—15 mm
- Good—8 mm or more
- Fair—5 mm or more
- Poor—4 mm or less

In all cases of primary congenital simple ptosis, the levator resection operation is indicated, if the levator muscle shows movement of 4 mm or more.

3. *Measurement of the eyelid crease:* To give a better cosmetic result, it is essential to measure the 'margin crease distance' (MCD) preoperatively. The margin crease distance is the distance from the center of the upper eyelid margin to the center of the upper eyelid crease, when the eye is in down gaze position. If the eyelid crease is not visible, then the skin of the upper lid may be slightly elevated to expose the lid crease. At the time of surgery, the site of the crease is chosen that corresponds to the measurement.

4. *Photographic record:* In the present era of mobile photography, it is advisable to

maintain a photographic record of the ptosis in its primary position as well as in up and down gazes to have a better assessment and plan surgery accordingly.

Management

Surgical therapy is the only choice.

1. *Resection of levator muscle:*
   - Conjunctival approach (Blaskowic's operation)
   - Skin approach (Everbusch's operation) is preferred for the following reasons:
     - Exposure of the levator is easy.
     - Extensive exposure can be achieved for large resection of the muscle.
     - It is easy to identify all the attachments of the levator muscle.
     - It is easy to attach the resected muscle at the site of insertion, the anterior surface of the tarsal plate.
     - Levator can be resected to about 28 to 35 mm, in cases with poor action of the levator muscle.

2. *Frontalis sling operation:* It is indicated in congenital ptosis with less than 4 mm of levator function, ptosis with external ophthalmoplegia and ptosis due to third nerve paralysis. *An autogenous facia lata* is better tolerated and is the choice for frontalis sling procedure in cases of congenital ptosis. Some surgeons use supramid for sling surgery.

Myasthenic Ptosis (Fig. 11.2)

Patient presents with complain of drooping of both the lids by evening and recovers by next morning since last two years or so. Now the lids droop even after a few hours of near work.

Patient shows an expressionless face with mild drooping of both the lids.

Diagnosis—ocular myasthenia gravis.

Myasthenia gravis is a disease characterized by generalized muscular weakness and rapid onset of fatigue. It is an autoimmune disease caused by an abnormality at the neuromuscular junction, some dysfunction or blockage at the neuromuscular endplate.

Early symptoms are difficulty in reading and writing for long hours, diplopia and bilateral ptosis. These symptoms are more pronounced by evening, when the patient is tired from the full day work. The patient shows a bilateral ptosis with expressionless face. Even on effort, the frontalis muscle fails to show any action that is the forehead remains smooth and unwrinkled.

Patient responds well to medical therapy.

Prostigmine test for myasthenia gravis: In a case of a bilateral ptosis due to myasthenia gravis, the patient shows a marked improvement in ptosis, ocular movements and the facial expressions. Inject intramuscular prostigmine methyl sulfate combined with atropine and watch for the response. The ptosis due to organic lesion remains unaffected but the ptosis due to myasthenia gravis shows improvement after a few minutes. Remarkable temporary improvement in the action of muscles is obtained by injection of prostigmine intramuscularly. Within half an hour, the ptosis disappears with return of facial expressions and ocular movements.

The positive response is diagnostic for myasthenia gravis.

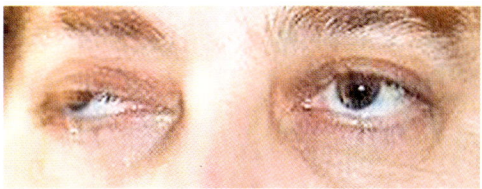

Fig. 11.2: Ocular myasthenic ptosis

Other Types of Ptosis

1. **Pseudoptosis:** An apparent or a pseudoptosis is due to lack of support to the upper lid seen in the following conditions: Phthisis bulbi, enophthalmos, small prosthesis and facial hemiatrophy. It is also seen in old age due to loss of orbital fat. It is also seen after prolonged bandaging due to loss of tone of muscles.

2. **Traumatic ptosis:** Any trauma to the levator muscle or to the tendon of the muscle or

to the nerve supplying the muscle results in ptosis.

3. *Mechanical ptosis:* It is due to increased weight of the lid usually seen in the cases of trachoma and tarsitis. In trachoma, the ptosis is due to fibrosis and involvement of the levator and Müller's muscle.

4. *Ptosis with congenital sympathetic lesion:* Sympathetic lesion central or in its course results in ptosis with other signs of sympathetic paresis like narrow palpebral aperture, relative miosis and enophthalmos. All these features are of Horner's syndrome.

5. *Neurogenic ptosis:* Any lesion in the pathway of the nerve supplying the levator muscle at any level can cause ptosis. Ptosis can occur as a part of symptom complex involving the oculomotor nerve. An isolated ptosis due to involvement of the levator muscle only can occur from the lesion of supranuclear pathways as the levator is the only extraocular muscle having a separate representation in the cortex.

6. *Synkinetic ptosis (jaw winking or marcus gunn phenomenon):* It is congenital and unilateral. On asking the patient to move the jaw laterally right and left or open and shut the mouth, the affected drooping lid shoots upwards with the movement of the jaw.

It is due to abnormal nervous connection in the central nervous system between the nerve supply to the levator muscle and associated muscles.

A case of ptosis with jaw winking phenomenon can be treated by excision of levator muscle on both the sides and giving a frontalis sling. Results are gratifying.

Bell's Palsy (Fig. 11.3)

A young adult male presents with complain of water escaping from right angle of his mouth and cannot close the right upper lid properly since this morning, when he came after early morning walk in cold and windy weather.

Ocular examination shows lagophthalmos of left lid.

Diagnosis—Bell's palsy neurogenic lagophthalmos.

Etiology

The term Bell's palsy is used for cases of isolated facial palsy of unknown origin manifesting as lagophthalmos.

- Bell's palsy occurs due to edema, ischemia and compression of the facial nerve in its canal usually following an exposure to cold weather, wind or mild fever.
- A viral infection has been suggested as an etiological factor since minor epidemics of Bell's palsy occurs occasionally.
- The compression of the facial nerve results in paralysis of the function of the nerve which if not relieved early may sometimes leads to Wallerian degeneration of the nerve.
- There may be an associated history of mild trauma to mandible close to exit of the stylomastoid foramen and tympanitis.

It affects young and elderly people of both the sexes.

Clinical Features

- Unable to close the eye on the affected side.
- While drinking the fluid escapes from the angle of mouth on the affected side.
- Numbness on the affected side.
- The facial expression is lost on the side affected.
- Patient is unable to wrinkle the brow and forehead.
- Patient is unable to retract the angle of mouth.
- Patient is unable to whistle.
- There is paralysis of the upper and lower parts of the affected side of face.

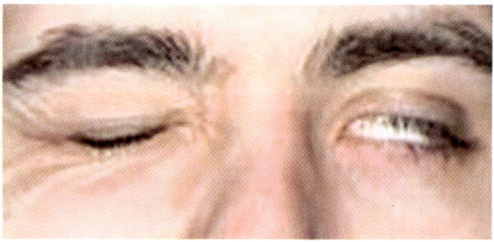

Fig. 11.3: Bell's palsy

Management

The main role of the ophthalmologist is to treat the Bell's palsy and manage ocular complications caused by lagophthalmos as a result of facial palsy.

- About 75 to 90% of the patients recover spontaneously and completely. The prognosis is good, if the patient is young and the palsy is incomplete. The signs of recovery are seen within the first 2 to 3 weeks and full recovery occurs within few months. About 10 to 25% patients do not show full recovery.
- Systemic steroids and supportive treatment are rewarding.
- Lubricants such as artificial tears to be used frequently.
- A thin strip of tape can be used to close the palpebral aperture especially during sleep.
- Goggles or spectacles with temporal shields shall help protect the cornea from wind and dust.
- Tarsorrhaphy is the treatment of choice in the cases with anticipated delayed recovery or cases with no recovery.

Ecchymosis of Lids (Fig. 11.4)

A male patient presents with right eye covered by hanky and palm of his right hand. He got injury to his right eye by fist only two hours ago.

Inspection shows swollen black lid of right eye.

Slit-lamp shows marked conjunctival ecchymosis.

Diagnosis—ecchymosis of lid.

The most common cause for lid ecchymosis is concussion or contusion injury usually by a fist or any blunt object.

In ecchymosis of the lids, the blood tends to diffuse through the loose connective tissue of the lids. The blood is checked from further spread to the forehead by the firm adhesion of the fascia at the eyebrows and cheek by the firm adhesions at the nasojugal and malar folds. The lid becomes swollen and the eye is closed. The upper lid may overhang the lower lid.

On the second day, the patient and his relatives get worried by observing the black swelling of the right lid spreading to the opposite lid also.

The blood has an easy way to cross-over the nasal bridge and spread into the tissue of the opposite eyelid. The skin over the bridge of the nose is thick, therefore, the skin over the bridge of nose appears normal. This is nature's natural phenomenon to diffuse the blood and reduce the swelling in the affected lid.

Clinical Features

- Lid is swollen and tense.
- Upper lid overhangs the lower lid.
- Use lid retractor to examine the eye.
- Bulbar conjunctiva may show minor or large ecchymosis.
- Cornea is normal.
- Pupillary reaction is normal.
- Ocular movements may show restriction due to ecchymosis.
- Fundus is normal.

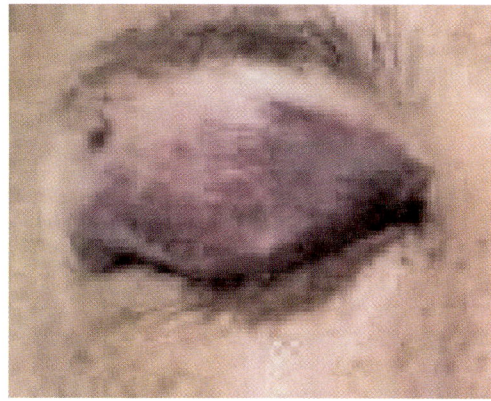

Fig. 11.4: Ecchymosis of lids

Management

- Assure the patient.
- Assure the patient and his relative that the edema and blood of the injured eye may spread to the opposite eye. It is normal phenomenon to diffuse the edema and blood.
- Topical broad-spectrum antibiotic as eye drops during day and ointment at bedtime.

- Ice-packs, if large ecchymosis.
  Systemic broad-spectrum antibiotic as prophylaxis against infection of hematoma in the lid.
- It will take minimum 3 weeks to resolve.

Xanthelasma (Fig. 11.5)

An elderly female patient presents with yellow flat symmetrical plaques near inner canthus of both the lids.

Diagnosis—xanthelasma.

Xanthelasma manifests as slightly raised creamy yellow plaque-like lesions near inner canthus often symmetrical in both the lids and both the sides.

Etiopathogenesis

These are common in elderly females. These can manifest as an isolated phenomenon in the skin of lids with or without hypercholesterolemia. These may be associated with diabetes, hypertension and occlusive vascular disease.

Clinical Features

1. Characteristically, it manifests as round or oval yellowish flat plaque with smooth surface or slightly raised surface near inner canthus.
2. Usually, it starts at the inner canthus of upper lids, followed by the involvement of lower lids symmetrically.
3. Investigate the case for systemic disease and lipid profile.
4. There are no other signs or symptoms except cosmetic embarrassment.

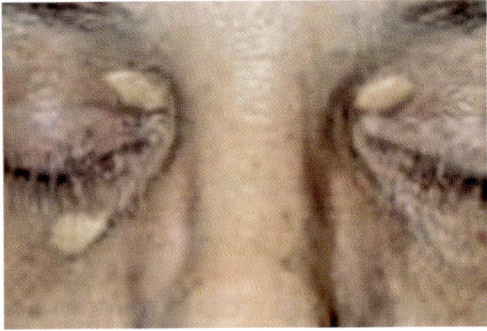

Fig. 11.5: Xanthelasma

Management—Surgical Therapy

- Surgical removal of the patch of skin.
- It has tendency to recur.
- It is better to perform surgery in early stage with small plaques with gratifying results.

INFLAMMATION OF LID

Blepharitis

A male patient presents with scanty eyelash, itching and collection of whitish crust at lid margin. Itching is intense and patient is forced to scratch it with nail of his little finger.

Slit-lamp shows edema, redness with crusts and ulcers at lid margin.

Diagnosis—blepharitis squamous and ulcerative.
    Blepharitis is a chronic inflammation of the lid margins.

Clinical Type with Etiopathogenesis

1. *Squamous blepharitis:* It is due to constitutional or metabolic factor or of the nature of seborrhea usually associated with dandruff of the scalp.
2. *Ulcerative blepharitis* (Fig. 11.6) usually follows untreated and unattended squamous blepharitis for long time.
3. *Parasitic blepharitis* is caused by the following parasites: *Demodex folliculorum* and *Phthiriasis palpebrum* (crab louse and rarely head louse).

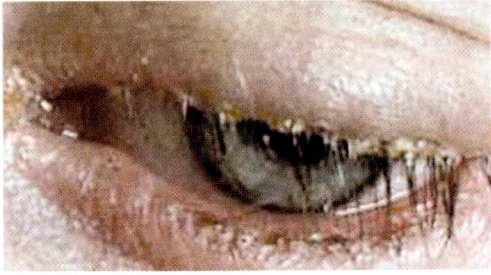

Fig. 11.6: Parasitic blepharitis

A young lady from high socioeconomic status presents her child with anxiety and points towards the eye lashes which are laden with peculiar knots. My child is constantly rubbing the eyes.

Slit-lamp shows crab louse nits on the lashes.

Diagnosis—parasitic blepharitis crab louse infestation.

Crab louse is normally an infestation of pubic hairs—hairs around the genitals. Crab louse infestation can occur even in children from high socioeconomic status due to transmission of infestation from maid handling the kids in high society or for working moms. The patient could not believe about crab louse infestation.

Ocular examination shows a large number of crab louse gripping onto the roots of eyelashes or eyebrows with their claws. The ovas are deposited on eyelashes. These ovas appear as nits of dark color almost involving all the lashes. Patient feels itching and tends to scratches the lid margin with finger nails.

Head louse can infest the lashes along with the infestation of the scalp. The head louse bites to suck the blood from the lid margin. This results in itching and scratching leading to secondary infection of the lid margin.

Symptoms

- Mild itching at the lid margin. Patient is forced to scratch the lid margin with the nail of his little finger to get temporary relief.
- Crusts formation of whitish material at the lid margin.
- Swollen and hyperemic lid margins.
- Scanty eyelashes.
- Mild and photophobia and lacrimation.
- Nits on lashes.

Signs

- Lid margins appear hyperemic and swollen. The posterior lid margin which is normally sharp now looks rounded due to swelling, therefore, there is epiphora— scanty eyelashes.
- *Squamous blepharitis:* There is an accumulation of white scales among the lashes which are matted. On removal of the scales, the underlying lid margin is hyperemic but no ulcers or bleeding spots.
- *Ulcerative blepharitis*: There is a formation of thick crust on the lid margin. The eyelashes are glued together with mucus

discharge. On removal of crusts, the underlying lid margin shows small ulcers with bleeding spots.

- *Parasitic blepharitis:* There are typical nits and parasites can be seen by slit-lamp biomicroscopy. There is always a history of infestation with crab louse or head louse in the patient or any member of the family.

Sequelae of Ulcerative Blepharitis

1. *Chronic conjunctivitis:* It may be the cause for blepharitis or the blepharitis may lead to chronic conjunctivitis. It is extremely chronic and requires treatment for a long period with regular follow-up.
2. *Madarosis:* It is a condition in which there are only a few small, scattered and distorted cilia visible on the lid margin. It is due to infection of the lid margin destroying the hair follicles so that the lashes fall out. These may not grow, if follicles are completely destroyed or only a few small lashes grow from follicles which have been spared.
3. *Poliosis:* Grey eyelashes.
4. *Trichiasis:* The ulcers on the lid margin heal with cicatrization giving rise to a condition of trichiasis.
5. *Tylosis:* Due to cicatrization, the lid becomes hypertrophied and shows drooping due to its weight resulting in a condition of tylosis.
6. *Epiphora:* The posterior margin of the lid is sharp and is in close contact with the globe which helps in drainage of tear fluid. In blepharitis, the posterior lid margin losses its sharpness and close contact with the globe due to edema and cicatrization. Because of this, there is improper drainage of tear fluid resulting in epiphora.
7. *Ectropion:* Due to constant epiphora, the patient is constantly wiping the tear fluid from the eyes. It causes ectropion of lower lid. Thus epiphora leads to ectropion and that leads to further epiphora thus vicious circle is set up.

Management

Blepharitis needs early, energetic and long treatment for complete cure and prevention of the sequelae of ulcerative blepharitis.

- Examine the case thoroughly after cleaning the lid margin of its scales and crusts under slit-lamp biomicroscopy specially to exclude any infestation with parasites.
- Remove the scales and crusts by a pledget of wet cotton wool rubbing slowly over the lid margin.
- Epilate the loose, diseased and distorted eyelashes.
- Remove nits and parasites with forceps slowly and carefully. It is rather difficult, painful and a tiring job.
- *Trim eyelashes*: It is advisable to trim the lashes for proper cleaning the lid margin of its scales, crusts and parasites. It is easy to remove the entire nits in one shot and clean the margin easily. Eyelashes grow fast within 2 to 3 weeks.

Topical therapy

- Broad-spectrum antibiotic eyedrops four times daily and eye ointment at bedtime.
- Broad-spectrum antibiotic and steroid eye ointment three times daily in squamous blepharitis.
- Advise patient to massage the ointment on the lid margin to achieve better results.

Supportive therapy

- Vitamins and good diet shall help.
- Look for a septic focus in the system and treat it accordingly.
- Correct refractive error, if any.
- Treat the dandruff of the scalp.
- Take care to delouse the source the maid handling the child.
- Explain the hygiene of the eyes and body to the patient and parent.

Molluscum Contagiosum (Fig. 11.7)

A young girl presents with mild discomfort, itching, photophobia and watering in both the eyes since 2 months or so.
Slit-lamp shows few tiny pale waxy globular mass with umbilicated top and tiny dark spot in the center on both the lids and surrounding area.
Diagnosis—molluscum contagiosum.

Molluscum contagiosum is a contagious viral infection of the skin characterized by appearance of small globular umbilicated epithelial tumors.

Etiology

It is caused by a filterable virus which mostly affects children and young adults. Infection spreads by direct contact or fomites with incubation period of about 35 days.

Symptoms

- Small discrete nodules on lids and surrounding area.
- Mild discomfort, itching, watering and photophobia.

Signs

Slit lamp shows small, multiple, elevated, nodular, pale white waxy globular mass with umbilicate top and a tiny dark spot in the center on both the lids and surrounding area.

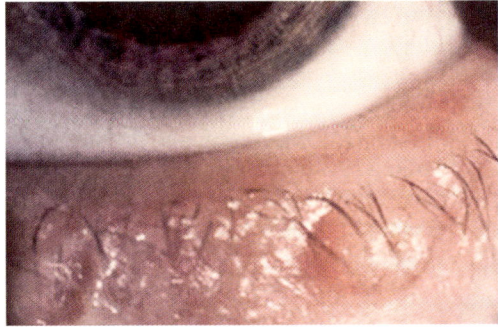

Fig. 11.7: Molluscum contagiosum

This characteristic appearance is pathognomonic and diagnostic.

Course

To begin with, the nodules are firm and solid. Later these become soft and on squeezing there is exudation of waxy looking material. Sometimes these may disappear spontaneously also. These may persists for months without any symptom except cosmetic embarrassment. Sometime these may break down, suppurate but heal without scar.

Complications

A small nodule near the lid margin may not be visible. The chronic shedding of cells laden with virus particles may induce chronic follicular conjunctivitis and superficial keratitis. It may not respond to any therapy.

Management

- Incise or puncture each nodule with sharp pointed knife and evacuate the contents by squeeze out the sebum-like material from it. Follow with cauterization of inside of nodule with tincture of iodine.
- Does not recur, if all the tumors have been adequately dealt with.
- With disappearance of these tumors, the intractable follicular conjunctivitis and superficial keratitis also resolves soon.
- Results are gratifying.

External Hordeolum (Stye)

Patient presents with localized tenderness with slight edema at specific point along the lid margin.

Slit-lamp shows a localized hard, red, tiny non-suppurative point at the lid margin.

Diagnosis—external hordeolum or stye (Fig. 11.8).

External hordeolum or stye is an acute localized suppurative inflammation at the lid margin involving the ciliary follicle and associated gland of Zeis.

Etiology

The common causative organism is *Staphylococcus aureus*.

Predisposing Factors

- Eye strain due to muscle imbalance or refractive error.
- If stye occurs in crops that is one after the other then investigate the case for diabetes.
- It can occur in crops in chronic debility, metabolic factors, habitual rubbing of eyes or fingering of nose.

Symptoms

In early stage, the patient complains of an *acute pain and tenderness* at a particular point on the lid margin. Soon there is edema of the lid followed by a suppurative point.

Signs

- Localized hard, red, tender point at the lid margin with mild edema.
- Soon an abscess forms pointing near the base of the cilia on the lid margin.
- Swelling and abscess may increase, if the abscess does not discharge or pus is not evacuated. Pain subsides soon on evacuation of pus.

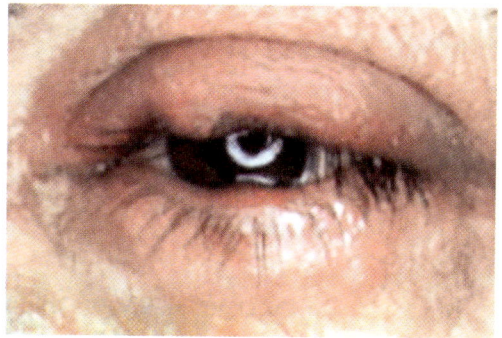

Fig. 11.8: Stye

Management

Systemic and topical broad-spectrum antibiotic

- Systemic broad-spectrum antibiotic to control the acute infection.
- Topical broad-spectrum antibiotic eye-drops and eye ointment to prevent conjunctivitis and spread of infection.

Supportive therapy

- Hot compresses are helpful.
- Analgesic to provide relief to the patient from acute pain.
- Epilate the affected eyelash for drainage of pus from gland of Zeis.
- If an abscess has formed, then evaluate it by surgical incision.
- Improve general resistance with good nourishing diet with vitamins.
- Exclude diabetes, if it occurs in crop.
- Exclude a septic focus in the system.
- Explain hygiene of the eyes to the patient.

Hordeolum Internum (Acute Meibomitis)

Patient presents with localized, hard and tender nodule in the lid away from lid margin.

Inspection and palpation reveals localized, hard and tender to touch nodule in the substance of the lid away from the lid margin.

Diagnosis—hordeolum internum.

Hordeolum internum is an acute suppurative infection of the meibomian gland associated with blockage of the gland duct.

Etiology

- It is less common as primary infection and occurs usually due to the secondary infection of the chalazion.
- The causative organism is *Staphylococcus aureus*.

Predisposing Factors

- Eye strain due to muscle imbalance or refractive error.
- If it occurs in crops that is one after the other, then investigate the case for diabetes.
- It can occur in crops in chronic debility, metabolic factors, habitual rubbing of eyes or fingering of nose.

Clinical Features

- The symptoms and signs of inflammation are much more than in a stye as the meibomian gland involved is larger and embedded in a thick layer of fibrous tissue the tarsal plate.
- Localized hard, tender nodule in the lid away from lid margin with edema of lid.
- On examination, there is a large and hard tender nodule in the lid.
- The pus point appears as a yellow spot shining through the conjunctiva. The abscess usually bursts through the conjunctiva.

Management

Systemic and topical broad-spectrum antibiotic

- Systemic broad-spectrum antibiotics
- Topical broad-spectrum antibiotic in form of eyedrops during the day and eye ointment during night.

Supportive therapy Analgesics and anti-inflammatory to provide relief from pain.

Surgical therapy If there is no resolution and an abscess has formed, then only treatment is the evacuation of pus by surgical incision through the conjunctival side.

Chalazion (Meibomian Cyst)

Patient presents with a small hard and painless nodule in the upper lid.

Nodule is visible on inspection. Palpation demonstrates a small hard nodule in the lid. It is neither tender on touch nor painful on pressure.

Diagnosis—chalazion.

Chalazion (Fig. 11.9) is a chronic non-infective granulomatous inflammatory manifestation of the meibomian gland.

Etiopathogenesis

Chalazion may occur as a solitary nodule or multiple nodules or nodules in crops. It is common in adults. The glandular tissue is replaced by granulations containing giant cells probably due to chronic irritation by an organism of low virulence.

Predisposing Factors

- Eye strain due to muscle imbalance or refractive error.
- If it occurs in crops that is one after the other, then investigate the case for diabetes.
- It can occur in crops in chronic debility, metabolic factors, habitual rubbing of eyes or fingering of nose.

Symptoms

The patient complains of a small nodular or multiple nodules in the lid. There are no signs of any inflammation. The patient reports for cosmetic disfigurement of the lids.

Signs

- A small nodule may not be visible. In such a case, it is the patient who points the site of nodule. It is advisable that the lid should be palpated by passing the finger over the skin of both the lids. By this method, even a small nodule can be appreciated.

- A large nodule is easily felt as a hard painless nodule by palpating finger.
- On eversion of the lid, the conjunctiva over the nodule is red, purple, grey or even yellow. Grey color of the conjunctiva indicates that the granular mass has been converted into a jelly-like mass.
- A yellow point indicates that it has been infected and now it is hordeolum internum.
- Some cases may show a granular mass sprouting through the opening in the conjunctiva through which the contents of the chalazion have been discharged spontaneously.
- A large nodule in the upper lid may give rise to drooping of the lid—mechanical ptosis because of its weight.

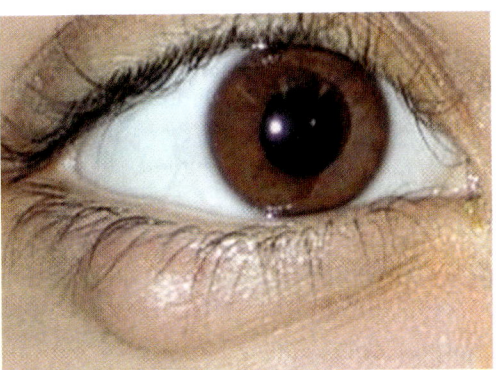

Fig. 11.9: Chalazion

Management

- *Intralesional injection* of long-acting steroid—*triamcinolone* can cause resolution in about 50% cases especially in small and soft nodules.
- *Incision and scrapping* of the chalazion is the treatment of choice. Thorough scrapping is required to prevent sprouting of granulation tissue later through the incision. The inside of the nodule should be touched with carbolic acid.
- *Histopathology* is needed in a case of recurrent chalazion in an elderly patient.

MALADIES OF LASHES AND LIDS

Trichiasis

Trichiasis is a condition of inward misdirected cilia rubbing against the cornea with normal position of the lid margin. The inward turning of lashes along with lid margin as seen in entropion is called *pseudotrichiasis.*

Etiology

- Any condition causing entropion causes trichiasis. The most common cause for entropion is trachoma and spastic entropion. In both the conditions, the whole margin of the lid is involved.
- It is seen in congenital distichiasis.
- Other conditions in which a few cilia are distorted backwards and rub against the cornea are blepharitis, stye, hordeolum internum, burns, operations and injuries. In all of these conditions, the primary factor is cicatrization which results in inward distortion of the cilia.

Symptoms

- Foreign body sensation due to continuously rubbing of inward directed cilia against the sensitive cornea and lower bulbar conjunctiva.
- Irritation, redness of the eye, lacrimation and reflex blepharospasm.

Signs

- There may be entropion, therefore, the whole lid margin is turned inwards and so all the lashes are rubbing against the cornea.
- Presence of ciliary congestion with photophobia and reflex blepharospasm indicates involvement of the cornea with superficial keratitis.
- Slit-lamp shows superficial corneal opacities and vascularization. Fluorescein staining is helpful.

Complications

Trichiasis can cause superficial corneal erosions, opacities and vascularization.

Management

- Electrolysis for few isolated cilia. It causes destruction of the hair follicle. A current of 3–5 mA for 10 seconds is enough.
- Entropion operation is the choice where the whole lid margin is involved.
- Epilation of cilia by the patient himself should be discouraged.

Entropion

Entropion is a condition of rolling inwards of the lid margin.

Types and Etiopathogenesis

Spastic or senile entropion It is invariably restricted to the lower lid. It is commonly seen in old and debilitated persons in whom there is lack of orbital fat and skin of the lids is redundant. It is also seen following a tight bandaging after ocular surgery.

Spastic entropion occurs due to spasm of the orbicularis muscle associated with degeneration of the palpebral connective tissue. Degeneration of Müller's muscle which is a lower lid retractor also plays a part. Degeneration of the inferior lid aponeurosis also plays a part in occurrence of lower lid entropion. All these factors cause entropion of the lower lid particularly when there is insufficient support to the eyeball in cases with phthisis bulbi or the eyeball is deeply set due to lack of the orbital fat.

Cicatricial entropion It is caused by cicatricial contraction of the palpebral conjunctiva. It is seen typically in the fourth stage of trachoma mostly affecting the upper lid. In fourth stage of trachoma, the tarsal plate is distorted by atrophic or hyperplastic changes. Rolling of the lids inwards may be extreme to result in trichiasis.

Cicatricial entropion can also occur following injury and burns.

Symptoms and Signs

Spastic or senile entropion

- Rolling inwards of the whole lid margin of the lower lid. The lashes are rubbing against the cornea and conjunctiva.

- Irritation and conjunctival congestion of the lower bulbar conjunctiva is due to foreign body sensation caused by lashes.
- Epiphora is due to improper drainage of the tear fluid due to inturning of the lid margin.
- Superficial erosions or opacities on the lower margin of cornea.

Cicatricial entropion

- Trachomatous cicatrization; thickening of the lid margin, Arlt's line and scarring of the palpebral conjunctiva results in entropion and trichiasis.
- Irritation, congestion, mild discharge, vascularization, and watering of the eye.

Management

Spastic or senile entropion If there is an obvious cause like tight bandaging, then remove the bandage. If the spastic entropion of the lower lid is due to age, then it needs a surgical correction.

Cicatricial It is due to trachoma needs surgical correction. There are various types of operations for this. The basic principle is to alter the shape of the tarsal plate so that lid margin is brought to its normal position there by eyelashes should be placed normally. The common operations performed for entropion are Burrow's and Jaesche-Arlt's operation or some modification of these operations.

Ectropion

Ectropion is a condition of rolling outward of the lid margin.

Types and Etiology

Senile ectropion It is common in elderly persons and it affects only lower lid. It is due to loss of tone of the orbicularis muscle. In early stage, there is sagging of the lid in its inner (nasal) aspect causing eversion of the lower punctum. Gradually, the whole lid sag causing epiphora and exposure of the conjunctiva. Epiphora is due to eversion of the lower punctum.

Spastic ectropion It is seen in prominent eyes in which the lids are well supported. A spasm of orbicularis muscle can lead to ectropion of lower lid in a prominent eye with good support to the lids.

Paralytic ectropion It affects lower lid in cases of facial nerve paralysis.

Cicatricial ectropion It occurs due to lacerating injury, thermal or chemical burns or scarring of the lids by any factor.

Symptoms and Signs

- *Epiphora* is due to eversion of the lower punctum and sagging of the lower lid, thereby there is loss of capillary action produced by sharp posterior border of the lid, when in close contact with the globe.
- *Exposure of the conjunctiva* due to sagging of the lower lid. The lower palpebral conjunctiva, lower fornix and lower bulbar conjunctiva are exposed.
- *Keratinization and xerosis of conjunctiva* due to constant exposure of the conjunctiva induces changes leading to keratinization and xerosis of the exposed conjunctiva.
- *Exposure keratitis* of the lower part of the cornea may occur.

Management

1. *Early senile ectropion* of the inner part of the lid may be treated by a few diathermy applications to the palpebral conjunctiva behind the punctum and fornix. Cicatrization pulls the lid back to its normal position.
2. *Spastic or senile ectropion* involving the whole lid margin needs surgical correction by horizontal lid shortening by full thickness pentagonal excision.
3. *Paralytic ectropion* causing exposure keratitis needs tarsorrhaphy.
4. *Cicatricial ectropion* needs plastic surgery.

Symblepharon

It is a condition wherein lid gets adherent with the eyeball as a result of adhesions between the palpebral and bulbar conjunctiva.

Types

- *Anterior symblepharon:* Lid margin gets adherent to the bulbar conjunctiva.
- *Posterior symblepharon:* Adhesions in the fornix.
- *Total symblepharon:* Adhesions of palpebral conjunctiva to the bulbar conjunctiva.

Symblepharon is not only restricted to these types. There is a large variation depending upon the types and extent of the part of the conjunctiva lining the globe and lids get adherent and the causative factors; thermal, chemical, injury or inflammation.

Etiology

Formation of raw areas on opposite surfaces is essential. Raw areas on the opposite conjunctival surfaces; palpebral and bulbar can occur in the following conditions:

- Thermal or chemical burn
- Ulceration in membranous conjunctivitis
- Raw surfaces on the conjunctiva due to injury or operation and inflammation.
- Ocular pemphigus
- Stevens-Johnson syndrome.

Symptoms

- *Diplopia:* Patient complains of seeing a double image of an object on restricted movement of the eyes.
- *Lagophthalmos:* Patient is unable to close the lids properly as the movement of the lid is absent or restricted due to adhesion.
- *Cosmetic:* Cosmetic embarrassment to the patient due to restricted movement of the lid and eye with alteration in the shape and size of the palpebral aperture.

Signs

- Adhesion of the palpebral conjunctiva to the bulbar conjunctiva.
- Bands of fibrous tissue can be seen stretching between the lid and the globe.
- Restriction of movement of the eyes.

Treatment

Surgical therapy

- Excision of fibrous bands with mucous membrane graft.

- Prevention by use of contact lens or application of eye ointment.

Lagophthalmos (Fig. 11.10)

Young mother with her daughter of about 8 years presents with complain that her daughter's eyes remain slightly open during sleep. Other kids have normal closure of lids in sleep.

On asking the baby girl to close the eyes forcefully, she could not close the eyes even by squeezing the eyes.

On asking to close the eyes softly, there was improper closure of the eyes. The cornea was not visible. Only small portion of bulbar conjunctiva was visible.

Diagnosis—physiological lagophthalmos.

Lagophthalmos is a condition of incomplete closure of the palpebral aperture during sleep and even when an attempt is made to close the eyes forcefully by squeezing the lids.

Etiology

Lagophthalmos is seen in the following conditions.

Physiological lagophthalmos: It is a condition wherein people sleep with eyes slightly open. It is compensated by Bell's phenomenon which protects the cornea from exposure. The nature's natural phenomenon 'Bell's phenomenon' provides protection to the entire humanity by virtue of upturning the eyeball during sleep or on closing the lids. It saves the lower part of cornea from exposure and desiccation even in cases with mild lagophthalmos. Only lower bulbar conjunctiva below the cornea is exposed. Conjunctiva can withstand the exposure for a long period without being affected by xerosis.

- Paralytic lagophthalmos—seen in Bell's facial palsy.
- Mechanical lagophthalmos—seen in proptosis and exophthalmos.
- Functional lagophthalmos—seen in extremely ill and unconscious patients due to absence of reflex blinking.
- Congenital deformity of the lid.

- Cicatricial contracture of lids due to injury or burn.
- Ectropion of lower lid.

Symptoms and Signs

- Incomplete closure of the eye.
- Conjunctival congestion in the lower palpebral conjunctiva.
- Lower part of cornea shows erosions or opacities.
- Keratinization and xerosis of lower bulbar conjunctiva.
- Constant epiphora.

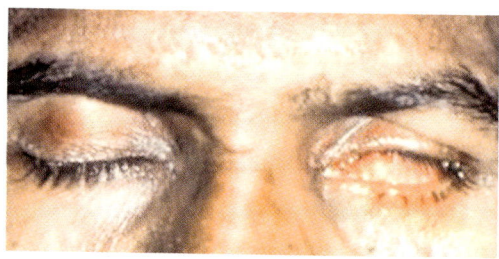

Fig. 11.10: Lagophthalmos

Complications

- Exposure keratitis
- Keratinization and xerosis of the exposed conjunctiva
- Ectropion of the lower lid.

Management

- Treat the cause.
- Tarsorrhaphy is the operation of choice, if needed.

Retraction of Lid

Retraction of lid is a condition in which the upper lid is retracted to expose the sclera above the upper margin of the cornea.

Etiology

- Congenital in a normal eye.
- Thyroid orbitopathy—staring or frighten look.
- Cicatricial scars of lids due to injury or operation.
- When staring or in anger.

Management

- Treat thyrotoxicosis.
- Cicatrization needs plastic surgery.

Blepharochalasis

Blepharochalasis is a condition of redundancy of the skin of the upper eyelid forming a fold of skin to hang over the upper lid margin.

It is seen in elderly and usually obese people. It does not interfere with vision.

Management

Excision of the excess skin of the lid.

Blepharophimosis

Blepharophimosis is a condition wherein the palpebral aperture appears to be contracted at the outer canthus.

Etiology

- Adhesion of the lid margin at the outer canthi following ulcerative conditions of skin, lid margin or conjunctiva.
- Congenital and may be associated with epicanthus. In such cases, the total outline of palpebral fissure is narrow than normal.

Management

- No treatment for congenital condition.
- Plastic surgery for acquired blepharophimosis.

Ankyloblepharon

Ankyloblepharon is a condition in which there is an adhesion of the margins of the two lids.

Ankyloblepharon may be congenital or acquired, partial or complete.

- In congenital cases, one or more tags of skin may be there extending from one lid margin to the other.
- In acquired ankyloblepharon, the adhesion may be at places or along the whole lid margin.
- Most common cause is chemical burns with acid. Other causes may be symblepharon and ulcerations of lid margin.

Management

Plastic repair with mucous membrane graft.

BENIGN TUMORS OF LID

Nevus or Mole (Fig. 11.11)

Young professional lady presents and points towards black blue nodule on the lower lid since her childhood. She has come due to cosmetic embarrassment.

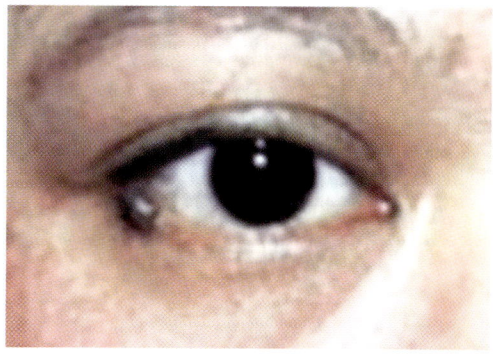

Fig. 11.11: Nevus—mole lower lid

Slit-lamp shows a nevus/mole
Diagnosis—nevus/mole.

- Nevus or a mole occurs on the lid margin involving both the skin and the conjunctiva.
- Two moles may be symmetrically situated on the lids of the same eye indicating their origin at a time, when the lids were still united.
- Tendency for growth at puberty.
- Rare to change in malignancy.
- Best is to leave these alone and undisturbed.

Management

If you treat, then treat by complete and extensive excision including normal tissue.

Capillary Hemangioma

A young lady presents with her newborn baby of about 1 year and points towards the peculiar and conspicuous dark red areas covering the lid and face.

Palpation shows that the areas are not compressible.

Diagnosis—capillary hemangioma.

Capillary hemangioma typically presents at birth or soon after as a periocular swelling in the anterior part of the orbit. It may show increase in size during crying and straining. There is no pulsation or a bruit.

- Capillary hemangioma appears as dark red slightly elevated areas covering variable part of the lid and face.
- Involves the area covered by distribution of one or more branches of fifth cranial nerve.
- May affect only a small area of one lid or may cover large area of lid and face covering even the entire area supplied by fifth nerve.
- May also appear as one or more bright red, soft and globulated masses known as 'strawberry' marks.
- Tumor grows in the first year of life then stabilises and eventually shows regression and disappearance by the age of 5 years.
- *Pathologically*: It is made up of superficial dilated capillaries with little connective tissue-stroma.
- No symptoms of any kind except cosmetic embarrassment.

Neurofibromatosis (von Recklinghausen's disease, Plexiform neurofibroma)

Patient presents with thick, flabby, pendulous, drooping left upper lid covering the eyeball and overhanging over the lower lid. Patient is unable to lift the lid.

Palpation of the lid gives a feeling of a bundle of hard cords in the lid.

Diagnosis—neurofibromatosis (Fig. 11.12)

The neurofibromata represent a developmental defect of the neuroectodermal tissue. It is dominantly inherited.

- *Palpebral form* involving the upper lid is the most characteristic manifestation of the neurofibroma.
- It involves lid, temporal region and orbit.
- Lesion is present at birth and grows slowly and increases rapidly with onset of puberty.

- Most common site is within the distribution of the trigeminal and cervical nerves.
- Supraorbital branch of the fifth nerve is the most commonly involved nerve.
- Neurofibroma represents a proliferation of all the various components of the peripheral nerve, i.e. the axon, its sheath and its supporting connective tissue cells.

When the tumor is well evolved then:

- Involved upper lid appears drooping, thick, flabby, pendulous, covering the eyeball and overhanging the lower lid.
- Patient is unable to lift the involved lid.
- Palpation does not demonstrate any tenderness.
- Tendency to penetrate in the orbit causing proptosis.
- Overlying skin is normal and moves freely over the growth.
- Some cases may show thick, hyperelastic and coarse skin.
- Mass of the lid is soft to feel and deeply fixed.
- Swollen lid and temporal region form a characteristic picture.
- Hypertrophied nerves can be felt through the skin like hard cords.
- On palpation, the cord-like masses in the lid feels like a 'bag of worms', a feeling once felt cannot be mistaken.

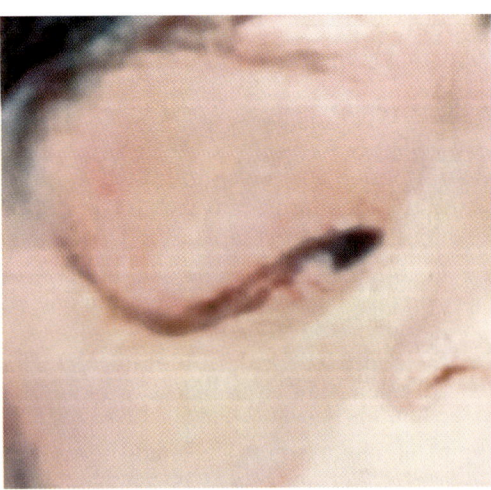

Fig. 11.12: Neurofibromatosis—right lid

Management

Operative measures are not satisfactory. If the surgical removal of the mass is not complete then it can recur. Problematic, if there is deep penetration in the orbit.

Dermoid Cyst

- Dermoid cysts are congenital in origin believed to result from an embryonic displacement of epidermis to a sub-cutaneous location.
- Remains unnoticed during the early years of life because of its small size.
- Later it enlarges to form a smooth, painless swelling located in the upper nasal or upper temporal quadrant of the orbit or supraorbital margin involving lid.
- Overlying skin is free.
- Cyst may be attached to the underlying bones giving support to the theory that dermoid cysts represent the sequestration of surface ectoderm owing to closure of suture lines of the bony orbit.
- Sometimes there may be a stalk connecting the cyst to intracranial dura through the opening in the bone.
- Deep seated dermoid cyst must be evaluated with X-ray and CT scan.

Management

Surgical removal of the cyst without any rupture as the cheesy material in the cyst is irritating to the orbital tissue.

MALIGNANT TUMORS OF THE LID

Squamous Cell Carcinoma

- Squamous cell carcinoma is derived from the epithelial cells of the skin.
- Clinically, it appears as a small nodule at the lid margin where the character of the epithelium changes.
- Nodule soon ulcerates and grows as a fungating mass.
- Low grade of malignancy and metastasis is rare.
- *Histology:* It is characterized by the presence of *'cell nests'* which show a small

mass of keratin in the center surrounded by immature epithelial cells.

Management

- Surgical removal of the tumor mass.
- It is radiosensitive so radiotherapy may be used where surgery is not possible and also following surgery.

Basal Cell Carcinoma (Rodent Ulcer)

An elderly patient presents with an ulcerated nodule in the lower lid near inner canthus.

Slit-lamp shows that the ulcer has indurated base, raised margins and satellites.

Diagnosis—basal cell carcinoma (Fig. 11.13).

Basal cell carcinoma arises from the basal cells of the epidermis.

- It shows predilection for the lower lid near inner canthus.
- It commences as a small shiny translucent nodule or cyst which ulcerates.
- On removing the scab, the ulcer shows raised margins with indurated base.
- The ulcer extends slowly by formation of small pearly satellite nodules.
- The epithelial growth extends under the skin in all the direction like fingers and also deeply destroying the lid, orbit and bone.
- It is a locally malignant tumor with no metastasis.
- Lymphatic nodes are not involved.

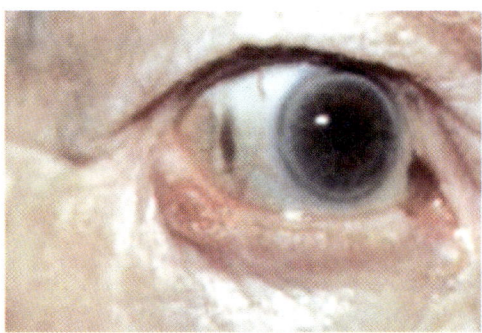

Fig. 11.13: Basal cell carcinoma

Management

- Excision biopsy with frozen section or Moh's micrographic surgery.
- It should be removed, when it is a small nodule or ulcer.
- Later it is difficult to eradicate it completely and require extensive surgery with radiation.

Sebaceous Gland Carcinoma

- It arises as isolated or multicentric from the meibomian glands.
- Appears as a discrete, yellow, firm nodule on the lid.
- Associated with chronic blepharitis.
- Likely to be mistaken for chalazion.
- Nodule in elderly must be seen with suspicion and if there is recurrence then histopathology is a must.
- Treat by local excision.

LID INJURY

Contusion

- Most common injury to lid is the *contusion injury* which occurs due to a blow by hand or injury due to stone or with any hard object.
- Immediate manifestation is ecchymosis of lids and conjunctiva. Lids are swollen with hemorrhage in the conjunctiva with chemosis. Soon the lids appear black due to the presence of hemorrhage in the subcutaneous tissue of lids. Black eye is alarming to the patient.
- Cold compresses give relief. It takes about 3 weeks for the hemorrhage to absorb.

Wounds

A wound in the direction of the fibers of orbicularis muscle shows a little gap and heals without obvious scarring.

That is why surgical incisions in the lids are made in the direction of fibers of the orbicularis muscle.

Burns

- *First degree burns* of lids require only cleaning and application of penicillin gauge.
- *Second degree burns* require cleaning and opening of any vesicles, removal of dead epithelium, and dressing with penicillin gauge.
- *Third degree burns* require cleaning with skin graft.

Management

Later some cases may need temporary tarsorrhaphy to prevent exposure keratitis due to cicatricial ectropion.

12

Maladies of Conjunctiva

Infective Types of Conjunctivitis

- Acute mucopurulent conjunctivitis
- Acute purulent conjunctivitis
- Ophthalmia neonatorum
- Acute membranous conjunctivitis (diphtheritic conjunctivitis)
- Chronic conjunctivitis
- Angular conjunctivitis

Chlamydial Follicular Conjunctivitis

- Trachoma
- Inclusion conjunctivitis

Viral Conjunctivitis

- Epidemic keratoconjunctivitis
- Pharyngoconjunctival fever
- Acute herpetic conjunctivitis

Allergic Conjunctivitis

- Acute allergic conjunctivitis
- Phlyctenular conjunctivitis
- Vernal conjunctivitis (spring catarrh)

Degenerative Conditions

- Concretions
- Pinguecula
- Pterygium

Symptomatic Conditions of Conjunctiva

- Subconjunctival ecchymosis
- Epithelial xerosis

Cysts

- Retention cyst
- Epithelial implantation cyst

Tumors

- Epibulbar dermoid
- Dermolipoma
- Papilloma
- Simple granuloma
- Epithelioma (squamous cell carcinoma)
- Nevi or mole

INFECTIVE TYPES OF CONJUNCTIVITIS

Patient presents with red eye, i.e. intense conjunctival congestion, mucopurulent discharge, matting of eyelashes, swelling of lids, chemosis, petechial ecchymosis, true or pseudomembrane formation.

Ocular examination shows intense conjunctival congestion of bulbar and tarsal conjunctiva, mucopurulent discharge flowing from angles, red and swollen lids, chemosis of conjunctiva, petechial hemorrhages and a few cases may show membrane formation.

Patient needs intensive broad-spectrum antibiotics; systemic and topical along with energetic supportive therapy and to keep the discharge flowing and preventing the matting of lashes.

Incidence of infective types of conjunctivitis has markedly reduced due to awareness, antibiotics, improved social status, clean environmental living conditions and good protein-energy intake.

Diagnosis—infective conjunctivitis.

Acute Mucopurulent Conjunctivitis
(Fig. 12.1)

It often occurs in epidemic form and is called pink eye or red eye by the patients. It is contagious and spreads directly by the conjunctival secretion and indirectly by flies, fingers and common towels. The disease reaches its height in 3–4 days and if not properly treated, it passes into a chronic condition. There is a tendency for spontaneous recovery.

Etiology

The common causative organisms are: *Staphylococcus aureus*, Koch-Weeks bacillus or *Haemophilus aegyptius*, *Pneumococcus and Streptococcus*. Mucopurulent conjunctivitis generally accompanies exanthemata such as measles, chickenpox, flu, etc.

Predisposing Factors

- Contact with infected individual.
- Oculogenital spread with sexual abuse.
- Concomitant bacterial otitis media, sinusitis, pharyngitis, nasopharyngeal bacterial colonization, foreign body.

Symptoms

- *Red eye with discharge:* Conjunctiva is fiery red as all the conjunctival vessels are congested. Conjunctival discharge may be watery, mucus, mucopurulent or purulent and that is seen in the fornix or at the margins of the lids.
- *Feeling of grittiness:* Feeling of foreign body sensation as if lot of sand is present in the eyelids. This sensation is due to marked hyperemia of the conjunctiva.
- *Photophobia:* Patient is unable to keep the eyes open in bright light due to hyperemia of the conjunctiva.
- *Matting of eyelashes:* Due to thick mucoid or mucopurulent discharge, there is sticking of the lid together and there is matting of eyelashes with dirty yellow crusts. The mother has to clean the eyelashes in the morning so that the child can open his/her eyes.

- *Lid edema:* There is marked lid swelling of the upper lid.

Signs

- *Intense conjunctival congestion:* Conjunctival congestion involving the whole conjunctiva from limbus to fornix.
- *Conjunctival discharge:* Discharge may be watery, mucus, mucopurulent or purulent depending on the virulence of the causative organisms.
- *Lid edema, chemosis and ecchymosis:* In a pneumococcal conjunctivitis, there is marked swelling of the lids, chemosis, petechial ecchymosis and sometimes pseudomembrane formation.

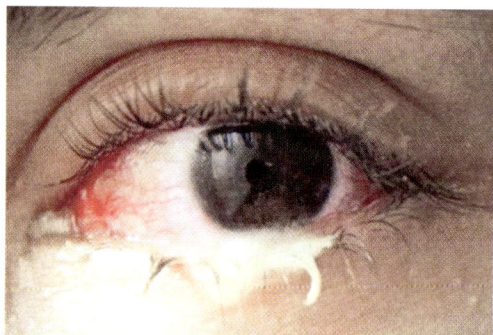

Fig. 12.1: Acute mucopurulent conjunctivitis

Complications

- Superficial punctate keratitis
- Marginal corneal ulcers

Management

Culture and sensitivity test of conjunctival discharge.

Antibiotics

- Topical broad-spectrum antibiotic eyedrops every half an hour for first few hours and thereafter every hourly until there is reduction in the formation of conjunctival discharge followed by 4–6 times a day.
- Topical broad-spectrum antibiotic eye ointment three times a day to prevent sticking of lids together in children is necessary. Application at bedtime is a

must to avoid early morning stickiness of the lids.

- Systemic broad-spectrum antibiotics, if the conjunctivitis is severe with no or poor response to topical therapy.

Supportive therapy

- *Saline lavage of conjunctival sac:* Irrigate the eyes with sterile lukewarm twice a day or more to washout the conjunctival discharge.
- *Wipe off* the discharge frequently by sterile swab to keep the eye clean.
- *Dark goggles*
- *Examine for any septic focus and treat.*

Acute Purulent Conjunctivitis

Incidence of gonococcal conjunctivitis has been markedly decreased rather eradicated due to awakening, antibiotics and overall improved socio-economic status.

In adults, it occurs due to direct infection from genitals usually affecting males affecting right eye first in a right-handed individual.

Etiology

Most cases are caused by the *Gonococcus*. The other organisms involved giving rise to clinically the same picture are staphylococci, streptococci or mixed infection. There is an incubation period of a few hours to three days.

Predisposing Factors

- Contact with infected individual.
- Oculogenital spread with sexual abuse.
- Concomitant bacterial otitis media, sinusitis, pharyngitis, nasopharyngeal bacterial colonization, foreign body.

Symptoms

- *Lid edema*: Lids are markedly swollen and tense.
- *Intense conjunctival congestion:* Fiery red from limbus to fornix.
- *Purulent discharge:* Copious purulent discharge.

Signs

- *Lid edema:* The lids are swollen, tense, showing blood vessels over them, warm

and tender to touch to such an extent that the examination of the eyeball is not possible. Use lid retractor to examine the cornea and conjunctiva. The upper lid usually overhangs the lower lid with pus discharge at the lid border. On separation of lids by fingers or lid retractor, one can see purulent discharge flowing out from the conjunctival sac.

- *Intense conjunctival congestion with chemosis:* On separation of lids by a lid retractor, the conjunctiva appears intensely congested. There is marked chemosis to the extent that the cornea may appear as a crater, i.e. deep seated surrounded by raised chemosed conjunctiva.
- *Pseudomembrane:* Some cases may show pseudomembrane over the palpebral conjunctiva. It peels off readily without leaving any bleeding points.
- *Preauricular lymphadenopathy:* Preauricular lymph nodes are enlarged and tender to touch.
- *Malaise and fever:* Patient may have mild temperature and body ache.

Complications

- *Corneal ulcer:* Occurrence of a corneal ulcer is a rule and constitutes a common cause for blindness due to conjunctivitis. There may be a diffuse haziness of the whole cornea with grey or yellow spots in the central part due to direct invasion of the organisms causing necrosis of corneal epithelium. There may be marginal ulcers extending completely round the cornea due to retention of pus and organisms in the angle (gutter) formed at the periphery of the cornea by the chemosed conjunctiva. Once the ulcer has formed, then it progresses rapidly going deep and usually perforates with all the complications of perforation of a corneal ulcer. Keeping the above complication in view it is essential to handle the case very gently with energetic treatment.
- *Anterior uveitis:* It may be independent of corneal ulcer. The *Gonococcus* and its toxins can penetrate the intact corneal

epithelium to enter the anterior chamber and induce *uveitis*.

- *Gonorrheal arthritis:* Occurrence of gonorrheal arthritis is not uncommon.
- *Endocarditis and septicemia:* With affection of genitourinary tract, there may be endocarditis or septicemia as systemic complications.

Management

Broad-spectrum antibiotics

- Topical antibiotic eyedrops every 15 minutes for first few hours and thereafter every hourly until there is reduction in the formation of conjunctival discharge followed by 4–8 times a day.
- Topical antibiotic eye ointment three times a day to prevent sticking of lids together in children is necessary. Application at bedtime is a must to avoid early morning stickiness of the lids.
- Systemic antibiotics in full dose for a few days.

Supportive therapy

- *Saline lavage:* Irrigate the eyes with sterile lukewarm saline twice a day or more to washout the conjunctival discharge. Wipe off the discharge frequently by sterile swab to keep the eye clean.
- *Atropine eyedrops* 1% once a day to keep the pupil dilated as a prophylaxis for prevention of complications of *anterior uveitis*.
- *Culture and sensitivity test*: Change the antibiotic depending on the report.
- *Refer to urologist* for treating genitourinary tract infection.
- *Analgesic* and antipyretic, if needed.
- *Dark goggles.*

Ophthalmia Neonatorum

Incidence of ophthalmia neonatorum is rare due to awakening with effective pre- and postnatal care, antibiotics and improved socioeconomic status.

Ophthalmia neonatorum is a preventable conjunctivitis. It occurs in newborn infant due to maternal infection of genital organs.

Etiology

- Ophthalmia neonatorum due to gonococci. Its incidence has markedly declined due to effective methods of prevention and treatment.
- Ophthalmia neonatorum due to serotypes D to K of *Chlamydia trachomatis* and due to *Streptococcus* and other organisms.
- Ophthalmia neonatorum caused by herpes simplex-II virus in 80% cases occurs due to direct transmission via infected birth canal.

Predisposing Factors

- Vaginal delivery by infected mother.
- Inadequate prenatal, perinatal and postnatal care.

It occurs due to direct infection during delivery from the genital infection. It is essential that mother is examined before and treated early to prevent the occurrence of ophthalmia neonatorum. Any discharge from the infant's eye during first week should arouse suspicion as tears are not secreted in the first week of life.

Symptoms

1. Intense conjunctival congestion.
2. Watery discharge to begin with which may later turn in a purulent discharge.
3. Watering of the eyes in the first week of life.

Signs

1. *Lid edema:* Lids are swollen and tender to touch.
2. *Conjunctival congestion and chemosis.*
3. *Conjunctival discharge* may be mucus or purulent.
4. *Cornea involvement* in form of superficial punctate keratitis especially in herpes simplex ophthalmia neonatorum.
5. *Vesicular skin eruptions.*

Complications

Every case of ophthalmia neonatorum is prone to develop a corneal ulcer. Even slightest haziness of the cornea should be viewed with suspicion.

Management

Antibiotics
- Treat bacterial ophthalmia with broad-spectrum antibiotics and herpes simplex viral ophthalmia with antiviral topical eye ointment.
- Topical instillation of broad-spectrum antibiotic eyedrops and ointment 3 to 4 times a day to prevent matting of eyelashes and provide proper antibiotic concentration in the conjunctival sac.
- Systemic broad-spectrum antibiotic.

Supportive therapy
- *Culture and sensitivity test.*
- *Preventive care:* Adequate care and prophylactic treatment at antenatal, prenatal, perinatal and postnatal periods is better than curative treatment.
- *Frequent lavage* of the conjunctival sac with normal saline.

Acute Membranous Conjunctivitis
(Diphtheritic Conjunctivitis)

The incidence is rare due to awakening with effective immunization against diphtheria and improved nutritional and living environment.

It is characterized by formation of a membrane usually in the palpebral conjunctiva.

Etiology
- Causative organisms, which can form a fibrinous membrane over the conjunctiva are *Corynebacterium diphtheriae, Pneumococcus and Streptococcus.*
- Mild cases may be diphtheritic and severe cases may be non-diphtheritic hence every case should be labeled as diphtheritic membranous until a bacteriological examination has been done.
- It is more common in children who have not been immunized and are weak, malnourished and have suffered from some ailment specially measles.

Pathogenesis

Corynebacterium diphtheriae causes violent inflammation of the conjunctiva with fibrinous exudates on the surface and within the conjunctiva resulting in formation of a membrane. Healing occurs by granulation tissue.

Symptoms and Signs
- *Swelling of lids:* Lids are swollen, red and tender to touch.
- *Conjunctival congestion with discharge:* Marked congestion of the conjunctiva with watery or mucus discharge.
- *Membrane formation:* On eversion of upper lid, there may be a membrane formation. If the membrane peels off easily without any bleeding points, then it is a *pseudomembrane*. If the membrane is sticking firmly and on peeling it off, the underlying conjunctiva shows bleeding points, then it is a membrane due to diphtheria bacillus. The membrane may be patchy or continuous.
- *Pre-auricular glands* are enlarged and tender.
- *Associated infection of throat.*
- *Fever and malaise.*

Complications
- *Corneal ulcer:* Corneal ulcer can occur in the first 6 to 10 days due to secondary infection.
- *Anterior uveitis:* The toxins can penetrate through the intact corneal epithelium and cause uveitis.
- *Symblepharon:* After the separation of membrane or slough, there is a danger of adhesions forming between the palpebral and the bulbar conjunctiva.
- *Xerosis:* Due to destruction of the conjunctiva, there may be occurrence of xerosis.

Management
Antibiotics
- *Culture and sensitivity:* Every case of membranous conjunctivitis should be treated as a case of diphtheritic conjunctivitis unless proved otherwise by bacteriological examination with culture and sensitivity test.

- *Intensive topical and systemic* administration of penicillin together with antidiphtheritic serum in consultation with physician or pediatrician.
- In membranous conjunctivitis due to other organisms, the topical and systemic treatment should be given depending on the sensitivity report.
- Topical penicillin eye ointment twice a day and especially at bedtime.

Supportive therapy
- IV fluids and vitamins.
- Manage fever and malaise.
- Isolate the patient from other members of the family especially infants and children.
- If unilateral, then protect the other by early prophylactic local treatment and by use of a protective eye shield.
- Repeat the culture and bacteriological examination every third day to assess the progress and prognosis of the infection.

Chronic Conjunctivitis

Patient presents with mild itching, grittiness, burning, congestion, watering, and mucus discharge with tiredness even after study for a few hours.

Slit-lamp shows mild congestion in fornix, papillae, redness and swelling of the lid margin with a little mucus discharge at canthus.

Diagnosis—chronic conjunctivitis.

Etiology

Acute conjunctivitis ends up into chronic conjunctivitis due to improper treatment or sometimes even with intensive treatment.
- Continuous exposure to smoke, dust, heat, wind, foul air, chemical irritants and sandy atmosphere.
- Irritation due to concretions, misdirected eyelash, chronic dacryocystitis and chronic rhinitis.
- Hypersensitivity to an allergen is common cause.
- Among systemic factors, the dandruff and chronic sinusitis are important.
- Uncorrected refractive error especially astigmatism is an important factor.

Symptoms
- *Burning of the eyes* by evening or after a few hours of near work. Patient complains in his/her own words that the eyes are burning like a hot coal (*angare ki tarah jal rahi hai*).
- *Feeling of grittiness*: Foreign body sensation in the eyes on blinking.
- *Edges of the lids feel hot.*
- *Mild mucus discharge* due to increased secretion from the meibomian glands.
- *Feeling of sleepiness* and tiredness by the evening and usually after near work.

Signs
- Congestion of the fornix and the palpebral conjunctiva.
- Papillae in the palpebral conjunctiva giving it a velvety and rough appearance.
- Lid margin appear red and slightly swollen.
- Slight mucus discharge at the canthus usually seen in the early hours or late evening.

Management

Antibiotic and astringents
- *Topical and systemic antibiotics.*
- Anticongestion and astringents to provide symptomatic relief.

Supportive therapy
- Eliminate and treat the causative factor.
- Protective glasses to avoid exposure to irritants.
- Look for a foreign body, misdirected eyelash, concretions and treat accordingly.
- Eliminate the allergen.
- Correct any refractive error.
- In a case with abnormal secretion from meibomian glands, treat by repeated massage of the lids to squeeze out the glands.
- General improvement of health by physical exercise, good diet and vitamins.

Angular Conjunctivitis

A young adult presents with complain of mild itching, discomfort while working and embarrassing collection of frothy discharge at both the outer canthus angles.

depressions in the connective tissue of the limbocorneal junction. These are filled with epithelium and look like small lucid circles or semicircles in a semi-opaque limbus.

- *Minute corneal erosions:* These are usually present at the advancing edge of the progressive pannus. These can be diagnosed by slit-lamp examination with fluorescein stain.

The World Health Organization (WHO) classification (FISTO)

- *Trachomatous follicles (F):* There are five or more follicles of at least 0.5 mm diameter on the upper tarsal plate with visible palpebral conjunctival blood vessels. A few papillae may be visible. Treatment at this stage leaves no scarring or minimal scarring.
- *Trachomatous inflammation intense (I):* More than 50% of the palpebral conjunctival blood vessels are not visible due to numerous follicles and papillae. This stage indicates high risk of serious complications.
- *Trachomatous scarring (S):* There is scarring of the tarsal conjunctiva with white fibrous bands.
- *Trachomatous trichiasis (T):* It shows presence of at least one trichiatic eyelash.
- *Trachomatous corneal opacities (O):* Presence of corneal opacity covering part of pupillary region resulting in blurred vision.

Complications and Sequelae

- *Pannus:* There is vascularization of the cornea from periphery usually affecting the upper part of the cornea, but later it may involve the whole corneal periphery.
- *Corneal erosions:* These are seen at the advancing edge of the progressive pannus.
- *Herbert's pits:* These are seen at the superior limbus, as small lucid circles or semicircles in a semiopaque cornea.
- *Trachomatous ptosis:* Due to thickening of the tarsal plate and infiltration of the conjunctiva and tarsal plate, the lids become thick and heavy. These thick and heavy lids give an appearance of ptosis.

- *Entropion and trichiasis:* Due to cicatrization of the tarsal plate, the lid margin rolls inwards leading to a condition of entropion. If the rolling in of the lid margin is more, then the eyelashes rub the cornea and the conjunctiva, the condition is known as trichiasis.
- *Trachomatous xerosis:* Due to cicatrization, the bulbar conjunctiva appears dry and lusterless.

Diagnosis

Clinical diagnosis The presence of any two sets of signs out of the following four signs is diagnostic for trachoma.

1. Follicles and papillae in the fornix and tarsal conjunctiva.
2. Superficial epithelial erosions on the cornea usually at the advancing edge of the progressive pannus.
3. Pannus in any stage whether progressive, regressive or under resolution.
4. Minute star-shaped scars in the tarsal conjunctiva.

Pathological diagnosis

- *Conjunctival cytology:* Giemsa stained conjunctival smear shows predominantly polymorphonuclear reaction with presence of plasma and leber cells.
- **Detection of inclusion bodies** in conjunctival smear.
- **Microimmunofluorescence (micro-IF)** method to detect the specific antibodies by serotyping of TRIC agents.
- **Direct monoclonal fluorescent antibody microscopy** of conjunctival smear.

Management

Systemic and topical antibiotic therapy

- *Topical antibiotic therapy:* Tetracycline or erythromycin 1% eye ointment four times a day for 6 weeks or sulfacetamide 20% eyedrops three times a day with tetracycline 1% eye ointment at bedtime for 6 weeks.
- *Intermittent regime:* This continuous topical treatment should be followed by intermittent regime in endemic areas by

applying 1% tetracycline eye ointment twice a day for 7 days in a month for at least 6 months.

- *Systemic therapy:* Tetracycline or erythromycin 250 mg four times a day for 3–4 weeks or doxycycline 100 mg twice a day for 3–4 weeks.
- *Combined therapy:* Trachomatous intense follicular inflammation needs combined topical and systemic therapies with intermittent regime.

Supportive therapy

- Improve environment.
- Improve diet. Add vitamins and protein.
- Use separate towels or hanky.
- Insist for follow-up to watch for reinfection and for abandon of the treatment.
- Explain the visual hygiene to children themselves. They are very receptive and understanding to their own problems.
- Explain to elders as well about the visual hygiene and how the spread of trachoma can be prevented.
- Take help of village elders, Sarpanch, Govt officers, etc. to undertake and follow the treatment regularly.

Inclusion Conjunctivitis (Fig. 12.3)

Its incidence has been almost eradicated due to awakening, antibiotics and improved socioeconomic and educational status.

It is a type of acute follicular conjunctivitis. It affects young adults during their sexually active period.

Etiology

It is caused by the serotype D, E, F, G, H, J and K of 'Chlamydia trachomatis'.

The conjunctivitis manifests after a week of sexual exposure and may be associated with non-specific urethritis in males and cervicitis in females. The infection may be transferred from the genitals by the fingers. Another common mode of infection is through the water of the swimming pools, which may cause local epidemics known as **'swimming bath conjunctivitis'.**

Clinical Features

- It is an acute bilateral mucopurulent conjunctivitis.
- Follicles are seen in the lower fornix. Later these appear on upper fornix and upper tarsal plate.
- Preauricular lymph node is enlarged and tender.
- Epithelial keratitis is seen in the upper part of cornea.
- Micro-pannus may be there.
- It runs a benign course and often evolves in chronic follicular conjunctivitis.

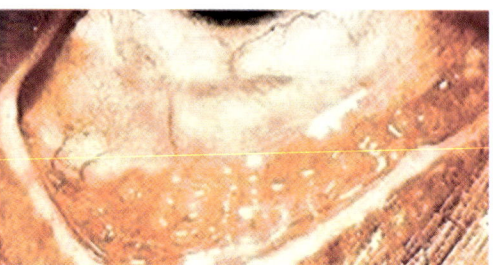

Fig. 12.3: Inclusion conjunctivitis

Special Investigation

- *Giemsa staining* of conjunctival scrapings.
- *FTA-ABS test* (fluorescent treponemal antibody absorption): This is a specific test to detect antitreponemal antibodies. Once positive, the test remains positive for the rest of life. This test should be done seeing the venereal nature of the disease.
- *VDRL* (venereal disease research laboratory): This is non-specific test useful for screening.
- *Gram staining:* Gram staining of the smear of the pus discharge from urethra will show the organism.
- *Urine examination with culture and sensitivity:* It is required to diagnose or exclude gonorrhea.

Differential Diagnosis

Adult inclusion conjunctivitis is to be differentiated from viral follicular conjunctivitis (Fig. 12.1).

Table 12.1: Differences between inclusion conjunctivitis and viral conjunctivitis

	Inclusion	*Viral*
Incubation	2–3 weeks	3–7 days
Age	Young adult	Any age
Systemic disease	Genitourinary	Upper respiratory
Discharge	Mucopurulent	Watery
Preauricular lymphadenopathy	Present	Present
Follicles	Fornices	Fornices
Keratitis	Present	Present
Cytology	Inclusion bodies	No inclusion bodies
Polymorphs	Mononuclear cells	
Response to tetracycline	Good	No response

Management

Systemic and topical antibiotic

- *Topical therapy:* Application of tetracycline 1% eye ointment in the eyes four times a day for 6 weeks.
- *Systemic therapy:* Any broad-spectrum antibiotics such as:
  - Tetracycline 250 mg four times a day for 3–4 weeks.
  - Doxycycline 100 mg twice a day for 1–2 weeks.
  - Erythromycin 250 mg four times a day for 3–4 weeks only in pregnant and lactating females.
  - Ofloxacin 200 mg twice a day for 7 days.

Supportive therapy

- Counseling
- Improve environment.
- Improve diet. Add vitamins and protein.
- Use separate towels or hanky.
- Insist for follow-up to watch for reinfection and for abandon of the treatment.

VIRAL CONJUNCTIVITIS

Patient presents with mild discomfort, photophobia, and watering of the eyes especially while engaged in near work and/or outdoors in bright light.

Slit-lamp shows follicles in the tarsal conjunctiva, mild congestion and a few spots of superficial punctuate keratitis.

Diagnosis—viral conjunctivitis (Fig. 12.4).

Epidemic Keratoconjunctivitis (EKC)

Etiology

It is a type of follicular conjunctivitis. It has been associated with several types (3, 7, 8 and 19) of the adenoviruses. An immune-fluorescent test detects the adenoviral group antigen in conjunctival secretions. It is highly contagious and occurs in epidemics.

Symptoms and Signs

- Patient presents with pain, lacrimation, redness and photophobia and lid edema.
- Ocular examination shows conjunctival congestion, follicles more in the lower lid, lid edema and watery or mucus discharge.
- Sometimes there may be a pseudomembrane formation.
- Preauricular lymphadenopathy.

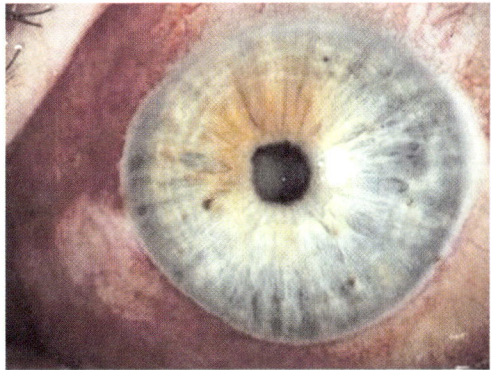

Fig. 12.4: Viral conjunctivitis

- Superficial punctate keratitis is a common complication.
- Subepithelial opacities associated with photophobia persists for months or years though the conjunctival follicles diminish and later disappear.
- Systemic features like fever, headache, myalgia, pharyngitis.

Management

- Topical antibiotic and steroid eyedrops and ointment. Taper with response.
- Artificial tear eyedrops
- Supportive therapy

Prevent transmission as it is highly contagious. Good diet with vitamins.

Pharyngoconjunctival Fever

It is an adenoviral infection associated with subtypes 3 and 7. It usually affects children in epidemic form.

Symptoms and Signs

It is characterized by the following symptoms and signs.

- Acute follicular conjunctivitis
- Pharyngitis
- Fever
- Preauricular lymphadenopathy
- Superficial punctuate keratitis in some cases.

Management

It is transient in nature. It needs only supportive treatment for conjunctivitis, pharyngitis and fever.

Acute Herpetic Conjunctivitis

It occurs as a primary manifestation of herpes. It usually affects children who are infected by carriers of the virus. It occurs in two clinical forms—in a typical form with vesicular lesions of face and lids and in atypical form without any vesicular lesions.

It is commonly caused by herpes simplex virus type1.

Symptoms and Signs

It is characterized by the following symptoms and signs.

- Large follicles in the conjunctiva.
- Presence of preauricular lymphadenopathy.
- Reduced corneal sensation.
- Corneal involvement in the form of dendritic figure is common.

Management

Topical application of acyclovir eye ointment 3% five times a day for 7 to 12 days.

ALLERGIC CONJUNCTIVITIS

Acute Allergic Conjunctivitis

Patient presents with complain of mild itching, watering and photophobia especially during outdoor engagements.

Slit-lamp shows mild conjunctival congestion with follicles on tarsus.

Diagnosis—allergic conjunctivitis (Fig. 12.5).

Etiology

It is an acute or subacute allergic or hypersensitive reaction of the conjunctiva to an allergen.

- Allergen is a bacterial protein of endogenous nature, the most common being the *Staphylococcus* in the upper respiratory tract and nasal cavity.
- Allergens are exogenous protein such as animal dandruff, house dust mites, pollens, flowers and grass.
- Commonly associated with hay fever-allergic rhinitis. There is elevation of IgE levels in plasma and tears.
- Use of some cosmetics, chemicals and dyes.
- Instillation of eyedrops such as atropine and its preservatives.

Symptoms

- Fiery red eye in no time due to acute hyperemia of the conjunctiva.
- Chemosis may be mild or severe.
- Copious watery discharge.
- Intense itching of the eyelids.

Signs

- *Congestion:* Intense conjunctival congestion involving the whole conjunctiva or the conjunctiva of the lower fornix depending on the allergen. Some cases may show marked chemosis.

- *Watering of the eyes:* Copious flow of tears from the eyes.
- *Allergic dermatitis of skin of lids:* Allergic dermatitis of the skin of the lids and surrounding area.

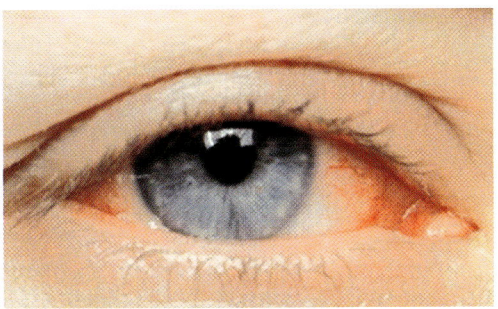

Fig. 12.5: Allergic conjunctivitis

Management

1. *Elimination of causative factor:*
   - Avoid exposure to an allergen
   - Avoid contact with animals, pollen, flower, dyes, chemicals, cosmetics, drugs
   - Use protective glasses.
2. *Local instillation of eyedrops*
   - Disodium chromoglycate—a weak mast cell inhibitor; 2% eyedrops four times a day for 2–4 weeks or until symptoms subside and clears off.
   - Steroid eyedrops and ointment should be instilled and applied, if poor or no response.
3. *Systemic:*
   - Steroids may be given orally or intramuscularly for a short period to provide quick relief to the patient from the symptoms in an acute case.
   - Antihistaminic drugs as required.

Phlyctenular Conjunctivitis (Fig. 12.6)

Mother presents with her female child with complain of two nodules near the black diamond of left eye since a week or so.

Slit-lamp shows two nodules at the limbus with localized congestion, mild watering of the eyes, flowing of the nose and rhagades at the outer canthus of left eye.

Diagnosis—phlyctenular conjunctivitis.

Etiology

- Allergic condition caused by endogenous bacterial protein the most common being the tubercular.
- Next common bacterial protein is from *Staphylococcus* or *Streptococcus*. The site of infection is the tonsils or adenoids.

Predisposing Factors

- Children below 12 years of age.
- Children who are ill-nourished.
- Children who have tonsils and adenoids of long standing.
- An attack of measles, influenza, fever, and diarrhea, i.e. any disease which lowers the vitality or immunity of the child.

Symptoms

- *Nodule in the eye:* Congestion is limited around the nodule.
- *Discharge from the eyes:* Usually, watery-serous.
- *Photophobia:* Marked, if the cornea is involved.
- *Pain:* Only when the cornea gets involved.
- *Eczema around the eye, on the lids and near the nose:* With a general look one can see a few patches of eczema around the eye and near the nostril with flowing nose, tear flow and mild photophobia.

Signs

- *Nodule in the eye:* One or more nodules in the eye located slightly away from the limbus with congestion around it. In some cases, the nodules may be close to the limbus or even astride the limbus, i.e. riding on the cornea.
- *Congestion:* Limited around the nodule. In a case with associated conjunctivitis, the congestion may be marked involving the whole conjunctiva.

- *Eczema:* Eczema around the lids, face, lips and near the nostrils.
- *Rhinitis:* Usually free flowing nasal discharge.
- *Watering:* Watering of the eyes.
- *Pre-auricular gland*: Enlarged

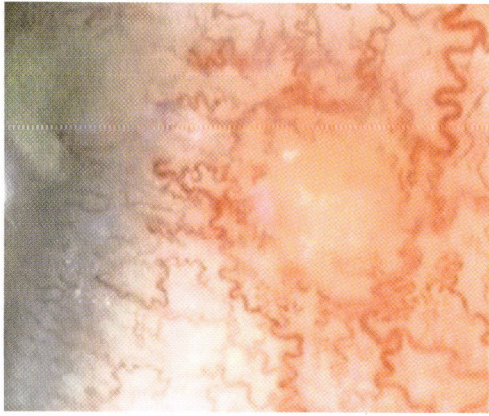

Fig. 12.6: Phlyctenular conjunctivitis

Course

It responds very well to topical steroids used as drops and ointment. Recurrence is common until the resistance of the child is improved with good diet.

Pathology

A phlycten is an infiltration of mononuclear lymphocytes. Phlycten resembles a bleb so there is a true vesicular stage. In later stage, the epithelium over the surface of a phlycten becomes necrotic forming small ulcers of conjunctiva which heals quickly without any scar. These minute ulcers on the conjunctiva have no significance, but the same minute ulcer of the phlycten on the corneal margin manifests by increase of symptoms of pain, photophobia, and watering of the eyes. In an untreated case, this minute ulcer progresses towards the center of cornea followed by a leash of blood vessels known as *fascicular ulcer*. The phlycten on the conjunctiva does not leave a scar on healing. The ulcerated phlycten on the corneal limbus *heals with a triangular scar the base being at the limbus*.

Complications

- *Phlyctenular keratoconjunctivitis:* A simple phlycten astride the limbus does not give rise to many symptoms. Once the epithelium over the nodule is necrosed, then this ulcerated phlycten gives rise to marked symptoms of pain, photophobia, and watering of the eyes.
- *Scar at the limbus*: A corneal phlycten heals with formation of a triangular scar, the base towards the limbus and apex towards the center of the cornea. It may show degenerative changes later in life.
  A triangular scar with base towards the limbus is diagnostic for phlyctenular keratitis.
- *Conjunctivitis:* Phlycten may follow conjunctivitis or it may be complicated by occurrence of conjunctivitis due to secondary infection. The symptoms are more pronounced, when associated with conjunctivitis.

Management

Topical steroids and antibiotic

- Steroid in the form of eyedrops and eye ointment gives dramatic response. The patient is normal in a few days.
- Antibiotic eyedrops and eye ointment if there is associated conjunctivitis.

Supportive therapy

- Treat tonsils and adenoids by systemic administration of antibiotics.
- Investigate for any tubercular focus in the system and treat accordingly.
- Improve general health by good diet rich in proteins, vitamins, iron and calcium.

Vernal Conjunctivitis (Spring Catarrh)

Young mother enters the clinic holding the hand of her male child about ten years in age. The child is vigorously rubbing his eyes with one hand. The mother complains that there is a reddish-white-grey membrane around the black diamond of both the eyes of her son. There is great itching in the eyes with sticky (chip-chipaa) discharge.

Slit-lamp shows jelly-like semitranslucent raised pinkish-white-grey mass of hypertrophic conjunctiva over riding the limbus. There is intense conjunctival congestion especially in the palpebral area on both the sides of cornea. There is thread-like sticky discharge that moves up and down with the movement of lid.

Diagnosis—vernal conjunctivitis (Fig. 12.7) bulbar type.

Etiology

- Vernal conjunctivitis is a recurrent bilateral allergic conjunctivitis occurring with onset of Summer and subsides with onset of Winter.
- Vernal conjunctivitis is a hypersensitive reaction to exogenous allergens and is mediated by IgE as indicated by the accompanying eosinophilia and increased serum IgE levels.
- Affects young people usually boys from all classes and is sporadic and non-contagious.
- Strong sunlight plays a part as exciting factor.

Types of Vernal Conjunctivitis

Palpebral vernal conjunctivitis

- *Cobble stone appearance:* Palpebral conjunctiva is hypertrophied and mapped out like cobble-stones as raised polygonal area. The flat raised nodules are hard and the epithelium covering them is thick giving it a milky hue. These nodules are hypertrophied papillae and not follicles.
- *Upper bulbar congestion* of conjunctiva.

Bulbar vernal conjunctivitis

- *Limbal nodules:* Limbal nodules appear as whitish-yellow jelly-like elevated lumps. There may be just one limbal nodule or crop of nodules. One nodule or one crop of nodules may recede and other nodule or other crop of nodules may appear at different sector of limbus.
- *Gelatinous ring around the limbus:* Typical raised ring of jelly-like semitranslucent hypertrophic conjunctiva about 1 to 3 mm broad all around the limbus or in the sector of limbus.
- *Bulbar congestion of conjunctiva:* With the appearance of limbal nodules, there is simultaneous congestion of the conjunctiva

in the same sector. With the development of confluent gelatinous ring around the limbus, there is intense conjunctival congestion in the palpebral area on both sides of cornea.

Mixed type of vernal conjunctivitis
Raised flat nodules in the palpebral conjunctiva with nodules or gelatinous hypertrophic conjunctiva affecting a sector or entire limbus.

Symptoms

- Itching, redness, burning, lacrimation, photophobia and ropy-sticky discharge.
- *Characteristic symptoms*: **'No itching, no vernal conjunctivitis'.**
- *Ropy discharge:* Patient complains that the discharge which collects at the canthi is sticky. On wiping the discharge, it stretches like a thread. Quite often the mucoid discharge is drawn like a thread in the conjunctival sac due to movement of lids. This thread-like discharge moves up and down across the cornea like a thread.

Signs

1. Raised, flat, polygonal nodules in the upper palpebral conjunctiva.
2. There is a gelatinous thickening of the conjunctiva around the limbus astriding the corneal periphery.
3. *'The presence of ropy discharge is diagnostic'.*

Course

It may persist for years recurring at the onset of Summer and subsiding in Winter but ultimately the prognosis is good. The child is

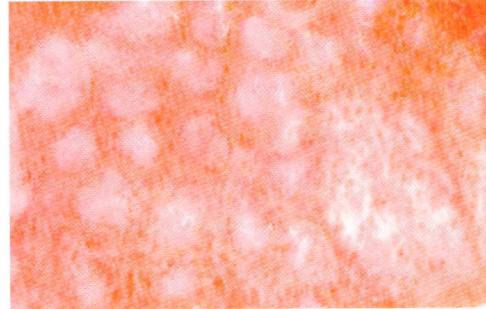

Fig. 12.7: Vernal papillary conjunctivitis

unable to read and write due to constant itching, watering and feeling of grittiness. He lags behind in his studies. Therfore, continuous treatment in consultation with eye clinician is essential.

Complications

Vernal conjunctivitis is often accompanied by occurrence of superficial punctate keratitis, thereby increasing the intensity of symptoms of burning, itching watering and photophobia and blepharospasm. It causes much discomfort to the patient.

Management

Topical steroids and mast cell stabilizer

- *Topical steroids:* Topical instillation of steroids in the form of eyedrops four to six times a day and eye ointment at bedtime, until the symptoms are controlled usually in a week's time. Thereafter reduce the instillation gradually to keep the patient free of his annoying symptoms.

  A prolonged use of steroids should be avoided since it is often followed by herpes simplex keratitis, cataract, glaucoma, fungal and other opportunistic corneal ulcers. That is why either reduce the frequency of instillation or dilute the drops to reduce its concentration for long time use.

- *Olopatidine 1% twice daily:* It has dual action. It acts by stabilizing the mast cells and prevents release of histamine as well as binding with the H1 receptors preventing the effect of histamine already released.

- *Epinastine:* It is also a dual action drug with better antihistaminic than a mast cell stabilizer.

- *Mast cell stabilizer—sodium cromoglycate 2% eyedrops:* Topical use as an adjuvant to steroids four times a day. Its only action is to prevent release of the vasoactive amines. It must be used for several days before it shows a positive response in providing relief to the patient of his embarrassing and annoying symptoms.

- *Acetyl cysteine 2% eyedrops:* It is useful in controlling excess mucus formation, thereby providing relief to patient from

ropy discharge and annoyance of wiping the discharge repeatedly.

- *Topical cyclosporine 1% eyedrops:* Effective in some unresponsive cases.

Supportive therapy

- *Cryotherapy:* It is helpful in a case with large raised nodules and hypertrophic conjunctiva around the limbus.

- Vasoconstrictor, antihistamine, cold compresses, ice-packs and cool environment are helpful in providing relief from the annoying symptoms.

- Desensitization has been rewarding in some cases.

DEGENERATIVE CONDITIONS

Concretions

An elderly couple enters the clinic with a sweet broad smile. The elderly grand-mama complains of grittiness off and on for the last one year or so in spite of using various eyedrops prescribed.

No other symptom of any kind.

Slit-lamp shows yellow spots in large number on the everted upper tarsus. A few of these are projecting through the conjunctiva.

Diagnosis—conjunctival concretions.

Any elderly patient who complains of grittiness or foreign body sensation in the eyes should be examined for concretions usually in the upper palpebral conjunctiva.

Conjunctival concretions are visible even in a diffuse light as minute hard yellow spots usually in the upper palpebral conjunctiva in elderly people.

Pathogenesis

Concretions are formed due to the accumulation of inspissated mucus and debris of dead epithelial cells into the conjunctival depressions called *Henle's loops*. Concretions are formed slowly by accretion and eventually project out of the Henle's loops and thereby give rise to feeling of grittiness or foreign body sensation to the patient with each act of blinking. Quite often, the depressions of Henle's loops get closed by mass of cells, therefore, such concretions lie dormant in the conjunctiva and do not give rise to grittiness or foreign body sensation in the eyes.

Clinical Features

- *Diffuse light*: Concretions are visible in rows or scattered all over the conjunctival surface.
- *Slit-lamp* shows that most of these concretions are covered by epithelium. A few of these are projecting through the conjunctiva. These projecting concretions give rise to feeling of grittiness or foreign body sensation to the patient with each act of blinking.
- *Fluorescein stain* may demonstrate fine epithelial erosions on the cornea.

Management

Projecting concretions can be easily shelled out with a sharp needle after local anesthesia providing a complete relief to the patient from his/her annoying symptom of grittiness or foreign body sensations in the eyes with each blink.

The concretions under the cover of epithelium need no treatment.

Formation of concretions is a continuous process. Advise the patient to report whenever there is grittiness in the eyes.

Pinguecula

A young smart professional enters the clinic with anxiety on her face. She immediately points towards a small round yellowish raised spot on the nasal side of the cornea in her left eye. She noticed it in the mirror yesterday while.......!

Slit-lamp shows a small yellow raised nodule nasal to limbus in the palpebral aperture.

Diagnosis—pinguecula.

Pinguecula appears as a raised yellowish triangular patch in the bulbar conjunctiva on either side of the cornea in the palpebral aperture. There are no symptoms of any kind. Patient consults primary for cosmetic purpose.

Clinical Features

- Affects young people
- Appears first on the nasal side and thereafter on the temporal side.

- Appears on either side of the limbus in a triangular form with the base towards the limbus.
- Moderate size and stationary.
- Yellowish in color and there are many yellowish spots as satalites.
- Occasionally, it gets inflamed due to inflammation of the overlying epithelium.

According to Wilson (1949), both the pinguecula and pterygium fluorescein ultraviolet light. This phenomenon is used to differentiate these from malignant epithelioma.

Pathogenesis

It is of a degenerative nature. There is an elastotic degeneration of collagen fibers of the substantia propria of conjunctiva coupled with deposition of amorphous hyaline material in the substance of conjunctiva.

Treatment

It does not require any treatment.

It can be excised or destroyed by cautery for cosmetic purpose.

Pterygium (Fig. 12.8)

An adult farmer enters the clinic pointing towards the peculiar growth-like a wing of a small butterfly in his left eye since last six months or so noticed by his family members and friends.

No other symptom except cosmetic embarrassment.

Slit-lamp shows thin, pale, atrophic triangular encroachment of the bulbar conjunctiva over the periphery of the cornea on the nasal side of his left eye.

Diagnosis—non-progressive inactive pterygium —left eye.

Pterygium is a triangular or wing-shaped fold of bulbar conjunctiva encroaching on the cornea from either side within the interpalpebral fissure.

Etiological Factors

- Environmental factors like exposure to sun rays, dust and wind.
- Hot and sandy climate favors its growth.
- Chemical irritants like fumes, gases and smoke, etc.
- Decrease of lacrimal secretion.

- Exposure to ultraviolet rays in solar radiation.

All the factors do not explain its occurrence on the nasal side of the eye and no progress beyond the middle of cornea.

All the factors do not explain its bilaterality and its occurrence on both sides of cornea. It occurs first on the nasal side and later on the temporal side.

Clinical Features

- Early change is the *appearance of grey opacities* in the cornea near the limbus with shrinkage of the conjunctiva. Some cases may show a *pigmented line* just ahead of the superficial opacity.
- As it grows, there is a triangular apex which is blunt. In front of the apex, there are small irregular opacities at the level of Bowman's membrane as seen by the slit-lamp.
- The rest of pterygium appears as a triangular fold of the conjunctiva with overhanging upper and lower borders and the base merging into the bulbar conjunctiva.
- There are no specific symptoms except cosmetic embarrassment.
- Can cause astigmatism.
- Dim vision, when it reaches the pupil.
- Diplopia due to limitation of abduction.

Progressive Active Pterygium

- Fleshy, thick and vascular with presence of white subepithelial fibrotic lesions at the head of pterygium called *Foch's spots*.
- Usually, on the nasal side of cornea.

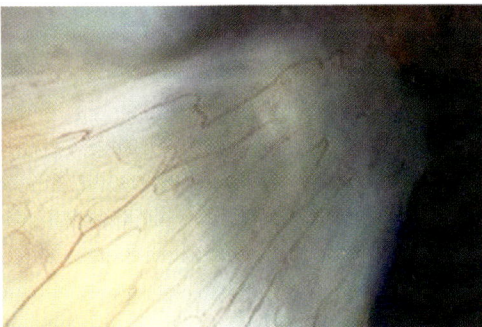

Fig. 12.8: Pterygium—non-progressive

Non-progressive Inactive Pterygium

Appears thin, pale and atrophic with little vascularity and often shows a pigment line at the head of pterygium called—*Stocker'line*.

Natural Pterygium and its Pathogenesis
(Fig. 12.8)

It is firmly fixed with the corneal tissue throughout its extent. It occurs only on the nasal or temporal side of the cornea and only in the palpebral aperture. It has overhanging upper and lower borders and base merging into the underneath bulbar conjunctiva.

It is a degenerative and hyperplastic condition of conjunctiva. The subconjunctival tissue undergoes elastotic degeneration and proliferates as vascularized granulation tissue under the epithelium. It encroaches on to and into cornea, thereby destroys corneal epithelium, Bowman's layer and superficial stroma of the cornea.

Pseudopterygium and its Pathogenesis

It is firmly fixed to the cornea only at the apex forming a bridge over the limbus under which a probe can be passed. It can occur anywhere around the cornea.

It follows an occurrence of corneal ulcer. In a case of an acute mucopurulent conjunctivitis, there is marked chemosis. Due to chemosis, there are chances for development of a marginal corneal ulcer in the gutter formed by chemosed conjunctiva around the cornea. The chemosed conjunctiva gets adherent to the marginal ulcer. The ulcer is progressive towards the center of cornea, therefore the adherent conjunctiva is dragged across the cornea to some extent before it heals. Thus it leaves a gap at the limbus through which a probe can be passed.

Management

- *Non-progressive pterygium* needs no treatment except assurance to the patient that it shall neither grow nor cause any dim vision.
- Avoid direct exposure to sunlight by using good quality of sun glasses to avoid exposure to ultraviolet rays.

- *Progressive pterygium* needs surgical removal for marked symptoms and cosmetic purpose.

A recurrent pterygium tends to grow more aggressively and faster than the primary lesion. Therefore, treat the patient with vasoconstrictors and steroids for a few weeks to reduce its vascularity so as to make it appear thin, pale and atrophic and to halt its growth before surgical procedure. Patients usually respond well.

Pterygium needs removal for the purpose of cosmetic and for providing a smooth surface over which lid movement can give proper polished cornea.

SYMPTOMATIC CONDITIONS

Subconjunctival Ecchymosis (Fig. 12.9)

Senior citizen couple enters the clinic with great anxiety and the lady points towards the big red patch in the right eye of her oldy boy friend, noticed today morning soon after he came out of toilet and sat for morning cup of tea.

Ocular examination shows a big patch of subconjunctival hemorrhage on the outer bulbar conjunctiva close to limbus.

Diagnosis—subconjunctival ecchymosis.

Ecchymosis or subconjunctival hemorrhage is common and varies in extent from a minute petechial to extensive hemorrhage spread under whole of the bulbar conjunctiva.

Etiology

- Local minor trauma is the commonest cause for subconjunctival ecchymosis. Sometimes even rubbing the eyes for itching is enough to produce ecchymosis.
- Petechial hemorrhage in pneumococcal conjunctivitis.
- Acute febrile systemic infections such as influenza, measles, typhoid, malaria can produce petechial hemorrhages.
- Cases have been seen without any apparent cause.
- Systemic vascular diseases like arteriosclerosis, hypertension, nephritis and diabetes mellitus can present with ecchymosis especially after straining during toilet or violent cough, sneeze or vomit.
- Blood dyscrasia as purpura, thrombocytopenia and leukemia.
- Sudden and severe venous congestion of head and thorax in the people who are engaged in the profession wherein they have to force the thorax to blow out, e.g. workers in glass factory and people blowing the trumpet.
- *Children with whooping cough:* Child with whooping cough is usually brought for the first time to the eye clinic for subconjunctival ecchymosis. It is the eye clinician who directs the patient to child specialist to treat whooping cough. Parents fail to understand and digest the idea of associating eye hemorrhage with cough. The ecchymosis in these cases is usually bilateral and profuse even to the extent to force out the lower fornix.

Incidence of whooping cough is almost eradicated with awakening and early treatment for cough.

- Fits and forceful compression of thorax in a stampede.
- Severe injury to the orbital structures:
  - In fracture of the roof of orbit, the blood tracks along the levator muscle to upper fornix and lids.
  - In fracture of the floor of orbit, the blood tracks along in lower fornix and lids.
  - In fracture of the apex of orbit, the blood tracks along the lateral rectus muscle.
  - In fracture of the orbital plate of sphenoid, the blood tracks along the temporal aspect of the globe.
  - In fracture of the base of skull, the blood tracks along the floor of the orbit then to fornix and finally to conjunctiva. Usually it takes 12 to 24 hours for the blood to reach the conjunctiva.

Clinical Features

- Ecchymosis as such is symptomless except cosmetic and social embarrassment.
- A patch of ecchymosis looks flat, bright red in color and well-defined margins.

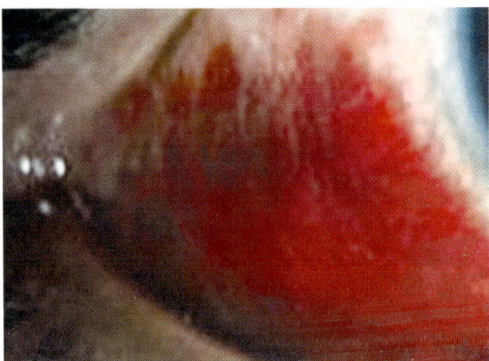

Fig. 12.9: Conjunctival ecchymosis

- There is change in the color during absorption from red to orange to yellow. It is a good sign.
- It takes one to three weeks for absorption even of a tiny spot of ecchymosis.

Investigation

Angiography, platelet count, total blood profile, blood sugar-fasting and postprandial and complete cardiovascular system check-up and as required.

Management

Supportive therapy
- Counseling and assurance that nothing is going to happen to the vision and inform that even a small patch of ecchymosis takes about one to three weeks to absorb.
- Supportive eyedrops such as mild astringents or artificial tear eyedrops.
- Cold packs applied to the eye with closed lids, if large hemorrhage.
- Large patch of ecchymosis may take longer time about 4–6 weeks to absorb.
- Report soon, if there is any increase in ecchymosis.
- Complete eye examination with ophthalmoscopy is mandatory, especially if the patient is elderly with no history of trauma of any kind.
- Any patient presenting even with a tiny spot of ecchymosis should be subjected to a thorough check-up of cardiovascular system and for the blood dyscrasia.

Epithelial Xerosis

A young girl enters the clinic with complain of white patches on outer side of cornea in her both the eyes since her early childhood. She is keen to get rid of these for cosmetic embarrassment.

Slit-lamp shows white foamy patches on temporal side of both the cornea close to limbus.

Diagnosis—epithelial xerosis—Bitot's spot.

Epithelial xerosis is a dry lustreless condition of the conjunctiva. It occurs in two groups of cases:

Parenchymatous xerosis—as a sequelae of a local ocular affection:
- Following trachoma, pemphigus, and diphtheritic conjunctivitis and burns—thermal, chemical or radiational.
- Following exposure of the conjunctiva in ectropion, severe proptosis, facial palsy and lagophthalmos.

It is due to cicatricial degeneration of the conjunctiva. The main changes occur in the epithelium which becomes epidermoid like that of skin with granular and horny layers and ceases to secrete mucus.

Epithelial xerosis—due to hypovitaminosis-A: The epithelial xerosis due to vitamin A deficiency is characterized by three cardinal signs:

Lack of conjunctival luster
- Wrinkling of conjunctiva near limbus
- *Bitot's spots:* Bitot's spots appear as small triangular white patches with base towards the limbus on either side of the cornea, more commonly on temporal side and frequently symmetrical. These are covered by a material resembling dried foam and not wetted by tear fluid. Bitot's spot may not disappear even after administration of vitamin A. Bitot's spots are associated with general nutritional deficiency rather than deficiency of vitamin A only in early childhood.

Malnourished child may present with epithelial xerosis associated with *night blindness.*

Infants who are malnourished and had an attack of severe diarrhea usually present with necrosis of the cornea known as *keratomalacia*. *Keratomalacia*—cornea appears dull, hazy or cloudy but there are no signs of inflammation, i.e. there is absence of congestion, lacrimation and pain.

It should be kept in mind that a failure of lacrimal secretion does not produce xerosis but the xerosis develops, if the secretory activity of the conjunctiva itself is hampered even with normal lacrimal secretion.

Management

- Treat the parenchymatous xerosis due to local cause in the conjunctiva, if possible by surgical method. If not possible, then only treatment available is artificial tears and protective goggles.
- Treat the epithelial xerosis due to deficiency of vitamin A by systemic injection of vitamin A (aqueous form) three lac units followed by oral vitamin A for a month in a dose of 5000 units daily. Supplement the therapy with good diet rich in protein, fruits, green vegetables. Replace fluids, if lost in diarrhea.
- Topical instillation of tear substitutes 2–4 times daily.
- Bitot's spot can be removed surgically to provide cosmetic improvement.
- Keratomalacia shows a marked improvement with vitamin A given intramuscularly. If there is no improvement in the appearance of the cornea in 3 days, revise the opinion and treatment.
- Night blindness due to vitamin A deficiency disappears with first injection of vitamin A—three lac units. The patient must receive vitamin A, regularly thereafter orally with protein rich diet.

CYSTS

Epithelial Implantation Cyst

- Implantation cyst occurs due to implantation of a few cells from epithelium in the subconjunctival tissue usually following a trauma or surgery.
- These cysts are lined with stratified squamous epithelium and contain clear fluid.

- Cysts appear as a small round swelling painless but causing discomfort to the patient.
- Cyst can be removed surgically.

Retention Cyst (Fig. 12.10)

- Retention cyst results due to obstruction of the duct of an accessory lacrimal gland or of a mucous gland.
- These are lined with the same kind of epithelium which lines the affected gland.
- Cysts contain clear fluid, and appear like a small swelling painless but give rise to discomfort.
- Cyst can be removed surgically.

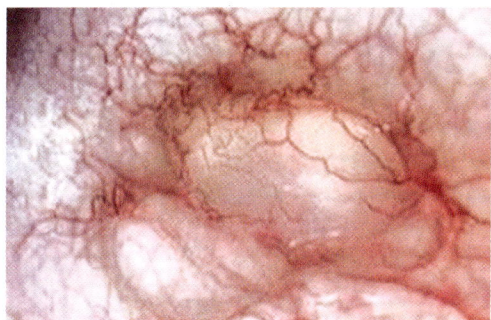

Fig. 12.10: Retention conjunctival cyst

TUMORS

Epibulbar Dermoid

- Epibulbar dermoids consist of collagenous connective tissue, sebaceous glands and hairs lined by epidermoid epithelium.
- Epibulbar dermoid tumor is a small non-progressive tumor usually at the limbus (Fig. 12.11) astriding the corneal margin mostly on the outer side.
- Only treatment is surgical removal.

Dermolipoma (Fig. 12.12)

- Dermolipomas consist of fibrous tissue and fat with dermoid tissue on the surface and are not encapsulated.
- Fat is continuous with the orbital fat.
- Dermolipomas are congenital tumors usually situated at the limbus or outer canthus.

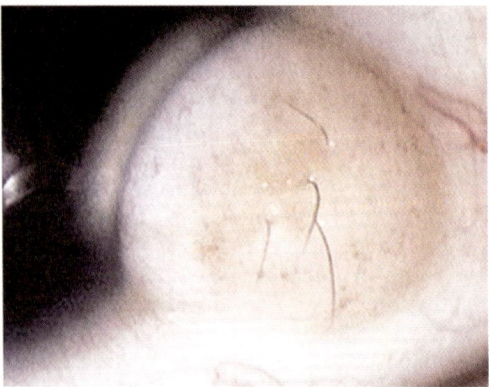

Fig. 12.11: Dermoid at limbus

- Dermolipomas appear as soft, yellowish white movable mass under the conjunctiva.
- Treat by surgical removal of the main mass.

Papilloma

Papillomas occur commonly at the inner canthus, fornices and at the limbus. As there is a tendency to become malignant, therefore, the surgical removal is the best treatment.

Simple Granuloma

- Simple granuloma consists of excessive growth of granulation tissue and is usually polypoid—cauliflower in form.
- Commonly seen following the incision and scrapping of the chalazion and at the site of wound and foreign body.
- Remove surgically and cauterize the stump.

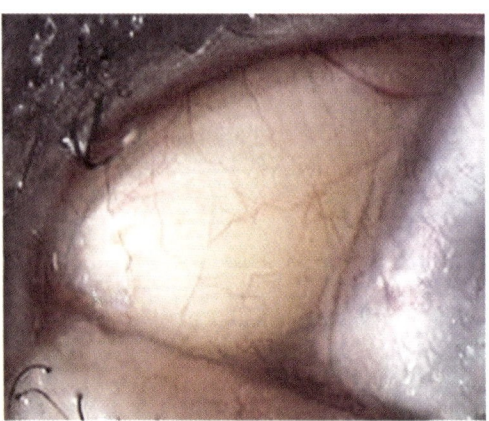

Fig. 12.12: Dermolipoma

Epithelioma (Squamous Cell Carcinoma)

- Common site for its occurrence is a transitional zone where one kind of epithelium passes into another, therefore, the limbus and the lid margin are the favorable sites.
- Usually associated with old age and UV-B exposure.
- Epithelioma presents as raised, pearly grey or pink well demarcated mass with feeder vessels.
- Spreads over the surface and in the fornices but does not penetrate globe.

Slit-lamp shows:

- Fine keratin nodules
- Intrinsic tumor vessels
- Feeder vessels to neoplasm
- Rose bengal or lissamine green staining helps to delineate the extent of tumor mass.

Management

- Surgical excision with wide margins.
- Remove the tumor freely and cauterize the edge with cryotherapy.
- Mitomycin C drops are used in cases with corneal involvement.

Nevi or Mole

Nevus or mole is seen as pigmented patch or nodule near the limbus (Fig. 12.13) or near the plica semilunaris.

Congenital and have tendency to grow at puberty.

These can be left as such unless it shows a growth.

Once decide to excise then excise completely including a healthy area.

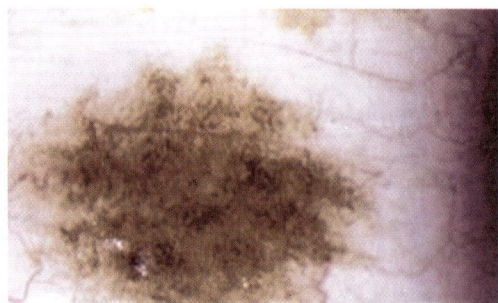

Fig. 12.13: Nevus at limbus

13

Maladies of Cornea

Corneal Ulcer (Infective Keratitis)

- Bacterial corneal ulcer
- Hypopyon corneal ulcer
- Mycotic corneal ulcer
- Marginal catarrhal corneal ulcer
- Herpes simplex keratitis
- Herpes zoster ophthalmicus
- Mooren's corneal ulcer (ulcer serpens, rodent ulcer, idiopathic ulcer)

Superficial Keratitis

- Exposure keratitis
- Neuroparalytic keratitis
- Superficial punctate keratitis (recurrent corneal erosion)
- Phlyctenular keratitis

Deep Keratitis

- Interstitial keratitis
- Disciform keratitis

Degenerative and Dystrophic Conditions

- Arcus senilis
- Arcus juvenilis
- Band shape keratopathy
- Salzmann's nodular degeneration
- Reis-Buckler's corneal dystrophy
- Fuch's endothelial dystrophy

Ectatic Conditions

- Keratoconus
- Keratoglobus

Corneal Pigmentation

- Blood staining of cornea
- Krukenberg's spindle
- Wilson's disease

Symptomatic Conditions

- Corneal opacity
- Xerophthalmia
- Photophthalmia
- Corneal vascularization
- Corneal staphyloma
- Cystoid cicatrix and fistula

CORNEAL ULCER (Infective Keratitis)

Corneal ulcer denotes discontinuation in normal corneal epithelial surface associated with edema, cellular infiltration and necrosis of corneal tissue. Cornea is constantly exposed to all kinds of environmental changes in the surrounding atmosphere, hence prone to infection easily. At the same time, cornea is protected moment to moment from minor infection and minute abrasions by its natural defense mechanism of blinking and tear fluid due to effective washing and polishing with presence of lysozyme, betalysin and other protective proteins.

Corneal ulcer usually develops, when the defense mechanism becomes ineffective with low immunity and exposure to virulent organisms of any kind.

Bacterial Corneal Ulcer

Patient presents with red eye, pain, lacrimation, photophobia and blepharospasm.

Slit-lamp shows corneal ulcer with edema, infiltration and necrosis with intense circumciliary congestion and mild vascularization.

Diagnosis—bacterial corneal ulcer.

Etiology

Organisms

It is always due to exogenous infection from pyogenic organisms, namely *Gonococcus, Corynebacterium diphtheriae, Pneumococcus, Staphylococcus aureus, Streptococcus, Moraxella Pseudomonas pyocyanea, E. coli,* etc.

Incidental factors

- The common sources of these organisms gaining entry in the conjunctival sac may be a foreign body, infection of the conjunctiva, chronic dacryocystitis, etc.
- The gonococcus and diphtheriae can penetrate the intact normal corneal epithelium.
- The virulent organisms are not always present in the conjunctival sac, therefore, ulceration is not so common.
- An abrasion of the cornea is of a common occurrence but the normal corneal tissue offers a good resistance and the virulent organisms are not always present to produce an ulcer.
- A diminished resistance of the corneal epithelium and presence of virulent organisms in the conjunctival sac favors the growth of these organisms and occurrence of corneal ulcer. The most important cause for low resistance of the corneal epithelium is the corneal edema due to any factor such as debility, chronic illness, general malnutrition and old age.

Keeping the above factors in view, a corneal ulcer occurs due to:

- Low resistance of corneal epithelium.
- Presence or entry of virulent organisms in the conjunctival sac.
- Favored by minute abrasions which occurs commonly.

Pathogenesis

Progressive stage To begin with, there is a localized necrosis in the most superficial layers of the cornea involving the epithelium and Bowman's membrane. The necrosed tissue, the *sequestrum,* is partly disintegrated and cast off into the conjunctival sac. Some part of necrosed tissue sticks to the base of the ulcer. After casting off the sequestrum, the ulcer appears larger as epithelium is cast off from a larger area than the area of the ulcer. The ulcer appears as *saucer-shaped* with the edge of the ulcer projecting above the normal surface of cornea due to edema of corneal lamellae. There is a grey zone of infiltration with leukocytes surrounding the saucer-shaped ulcer.

Regressive stage The second zone of infiltration is formed by the polymorphs while the lymphocytes are carrying out their digestive function of macerating and dissolving the necrotic tissue in the base of the ulcer. After the necrotic, tissue has been cast-off, the ulcer looks larger in size but the floor and the edges of the ulcer are smooth and transparent.

Cicatrization The minute superficial vessels grow in from the part of the limbus which is close to the ulcer. These vessels supply the pabulum to restore the loss of substance and antibodies to help in fighting the bacterial invasion. Sometimes the growth of these superficial vessels exceed far more than requirement and one can see a leash of vessels reaching the ulcer which is now labeled as *fascicular ulcer.* The healing occurs by formation of fibrous tissue which results in an opaque scar on the cornea.

Symptoms

- *Pain, blepharospasm, photophobia and lacrimation* are due to exposed nerve endings of the ophthalmic division of the fifth nerve.
- *Circumciliary congestion* around the cornea is due to dilation of the anterior ciliary vessels.
- *Dim vision* if the ulcer is centrally placed involving the pupillary area.

Signs

- *Blepharospasm with edema of lid* is due to reflex irritation of exposed nerve endings of ophthalmic division of fifth nerve
- *Circumciliary congestion*
- *Saucer-shaped ulcer*
- *Vascularization of corneal ulcer*

- *Toxic anterior uveitis with secondary glaucoma* is due to absorption of toxins secreted by bacteria through the cornea.

Complications

Corneal facet

In a corneal ulcer, the superficial epithelium is destroyed and cast-off in the conjunctival sac. On healing the ulcer may not heal up to the surface level of the cornea leaving a depressed but transparent area of the size of the ulcer. This depressed and transparent area on the cornea in place of an ulcer is known as *facet*. The facet in the pupillary area results in a marked loss of vision. It can be diagnosed by a slit-lamp and keratoscope. On slit-lamp examination, the beam of the light gets depressed, when passing over the facet. On examination, with keratoscope, the circles appear irregular at the site of facet.

Corneal opacity
A corneal scar in the center of cornea covering the pupillary area causes marked loss of vision.

A thin diffuse nebular opacity of the cornea covering the pupillary area interferes more with the vision due to irregular refraction of the light rays than a localized macular opacity which stops all the light rays.

A dense macular or leukomatous scar on the cornea is cosmetic embarrassment for the patient. It causes marked loss of vision.

In due course of time, there is a tendency for the corneal opacity to get thinner especially in young patients.

Descemetocele
The herniation of the Descemet's membrane through the base of the corneal ulcer is known as *descemetocele.* It is seen in the cases wherein the whole thickness of the substantia propria has been destroyed and cast-off, thereby the Descemet's membrane forms the base of the ulcer. The Descemet's membrane is unable to withstand the normal intraocular pressure and, therefore, it bulges forward through the base of the ulcer herniating and appearing as a transparent vesicle *descemetocele.*

Ulcer threatening to perforate
At this stage, the ulcer seems to be threatening the patient and the surgeon that 'if you both do not take care and treat me with respect then I am going to perforate', therefore, at the stage of a descemetocele or keratocele, the ulcer is known as "ulcer threatening to perforate".

It should be treated on following lines:

- Ask patient not to strain suddenly as any strain such as cough, sneeze, straining during toilet, etc. increases the blood pressure and this is reflected in the eye as sudden rise of intraocular pressure. Any sudden rise of the intraocular pressure can be a cause of perforation of the ulcer.
- Complete bed rest.
- Maintain low intraocular pressure by systemic use of diamox tablets.

Perforation of Ulcer

With the perforation of the corneal ulcer, there is a sudden escape of aqueous humor, thereby lowering the intraocular pressure and the iris and the lens move forward and come in contact with the ulcerated area. It disturbs the normal physiology, the optics and the metabolism of the eye. The perforation is attended with many complications. The complications vary depending on the site, size and the force with which the ulcer perforates. Obviously, a small perforation in the periphery with slow or a little escape of the aqueous humor causes fewer disturbances in the eyeball than in comparison to a large central perforation with sudden and forceful escape of aqueous humor.

Beneficial Effect of Perforation

- Better nutrition of cornea
- Early healing of the ulcer
- Immediate relief from the unbearable pain.

All these beneficial effects are due to lowering of the intraocular pressure. The low intraocular pressure provides immediate relief from pain and better diffusion of tissue fluid through the corneal lamellae, thereby enhances the healing process. This beneficial effect on relief of pain and early healing of the corneal ulcer has been utilized to benefit the patient by a surgical method of the *paracentesis.* In paracentesis, the aqueous is allowed to flow out guarded with a paracentesis needle providing relief to the patient from the pain and early healing.

Complications of Perforation of Corneal Ulcer

a. *Anterior synechia:* The adhesion of the iris to the posterior surface of the cornea is known as anterior synechia.

In a small perforation in the periphery of cornea, the iris comes in contact with the posterior corneal surface at the site of the ulcer. It gets attached to it resulting in anterior synechia. Later synechiotomy can be performed to free the iris. The synechiotomy operation is required, if there is a raised intraocular pressure or the case needs keratoplasty for vision or cosmetic purpose.

b. *Prolapse of iris:* It is a condition wherein iris protrudes through the perforated ulcer.

If the perforation is in the periphery, then the prolapse of the iris appears hemispherical in shape. If the perforation is in the central part of the cornea, then the iris lies free over the cornea. In either case, it is advisable to let the ulcer heal with iris incarcerated in it. Later on synechiotomy may be done, if needed.

c. *Adherent leukoma:* A corneal cicatrix in which the iris tissue is incarcerated is known as adherent leukoma.

Following the perforation, there is a prolapse of iris through the ulcer. The ulcer heals with incarceration of the iris resulting in a condition known as adherent leukoma. Synechiotomy if needed.

d. *Anterior capsular cataract:* With perforation of a corneal ulcer, the aqueous escapes and the lens moves forward and the lens in the pupillary area comes in contact with the cornea. In a central corneal ulcer after perforation the lens in the pupillary area comes in contact with the ulcerated area. On coming in contact with inflamed cornea, the anterior capsular epithelium of the lens starts proliferating and laying the new fibers in an irregular manner which results in the opacity of the anterior capsule known as *anterior capsular cataract.*

e. *Corneal fistula:* In a case of a small perforation of corneal ulcer, the anterior chamber becomes shallow or absent. The ulcer is likely to heal faster with reformation of the anterior chamber. The healed ulcer is likely to rupture due to strain during cough, sneeze or at the stools. It again heals in a few days. *It is the frequent rupture and healing of a small perforated corneal ulcer results in formation of a permanent opening known as corneal fistula.* Advise patient to rest and avoid strain. Protect the eye by goggles or shield.

f. *Dislocation or subluxation of lens:* Sudden perforation of a large corneal ulcer allows the aqueous to escape suddenly and with force, therefore, the lens is likely to get subluxated.

If the perforation is large and centrally placed, then with sudden perforation, the lens may be dislocated out of the eye.

g. *Pseudocornea:* Sometimes the whole cornea sloughs and cast-off leaving a narrow rim of cornea in the periphery exposing the iris. In such a case, the iris gets covered with exudates which get organized forming a thin layer of connective tissue. The epithelium from the peripheral rim of the cornea grows to cover the iris completely resulting in formation of *pseudocornea*. This pseudocornea appears flat and whitish grey.

h. *Corneal anterior staphyloma:* Corneal anterior staphyloma is an ectatic cicatrix of the pseudocornea in which the iris tissue is incarcerated.

The pseudocornea cannot withstand the raised intraocular pressure, therefore, it bulges forward giving rise to a condition known as *corneal anterior staphyloma.*

i. *Intraocular or expulsive hemorrhage:* A sudden perforation of the corneal ulcer causes a sudden lowering of the intraocular pressure resulting in dilation of all the intraocular blood vessels. These blood vessels may rupture resulting in hemorrhage which may be choroidal, subchoroidal, subretinal or vitreal. The perforation of ulcer in an elderly wherein the vessels are arteriosclerotic, thereby their rupture may produce an expulsive hemorrhage. In an expulsive hemorrhage, the entire contents of the globe are extruded with the out-flowing blood.

j. *Purulent uveitis, endophthalmitis or panophthalmitis:* After perforation, the causative pyogenic organisms may gain entry into the eye. The vitreous being a very good culture medium, the organisms multiply fast and manifest as purulent iridocyclitis, endophthalmitis or panophthalmitis.

Microbiological Investigation

- Gram and Giemsa stained smear.
- 10% KOH wet preparation.
- Culture and sensitivity to identify the causative organism and fungal hyphae.

Management

Intensive broad-spectrum antibiotics
- Topical antibiotic eyedrops and ointment.
- Subconjunctivally.
- Systemic antibiotics, if needed.

Intensive supportive therapy
- Cycloplegic eyedrops to provide relief from ciliary spasm and to give rest to the eye.
- Systemic analgesics and anti-inflammatory drugs to relieve pain and edema.
- Carbonic anhydrase inhibitors, if required to keep the intraocular pressure low to prevent perforation.
- Cauterization of ulcer.
- Use of tissue adhesive such as N-butyl 2-ethyl cyanoacrylate monomer, if ulcer is threatening to perforate.
- Bandage soft contact lens.
- Good nourishing diet with vitamins.
- Cleanliness of the self, use goggles or shield and use sterile swab to clean the discharge from the angles of the eye.
- If no response in two days, then refer the case to ophthalmic center.

Hypopyon Corneal Ulcer (Fig. 13.1)

Patient presents with red eye, swollen lids, discharge, photophobia and blepharospasm with mild pain.

Slit-lamp shows a dull greyish white-yellowish disk-like ulcer, edema, infiltration and marked necrosis, conjunctival and circumciliary congestion along with pus in the anterior chamber.

The mild pain is the root cause for delay in presentation for treatment.

Diagnosis—hypopyon corneal ulcer.

A corneal ulcer with pus in the anterior chamber is known as a *hypopyon corneal ulcer.*

Etiology

Organisms Many pyogenic organisms like, *Staphylococcus, Streptococcus, Gonococcus, Moraxella,* may be a cause for a hypopyon ulcer, but the most common and virulent organisms are *Pseudomonas pyocyanea* and *Pneumococcus.*

Incidental factors
- Dacryocystitis
- Injury by a finger nail
- Infected foreign body of stone, coal, dust, etc.
- Weak resistance as in old age and debility
- Weak resistance following acute infectious diseases
- Diabetes
- Debilitated and alcoholic people.

Pathogenesis

The toxins liberated by bacteria can diffuse through the intact corneal lamellae and the base of the corneal ulcer.

The diffused toxins in the anterior chamber are irritant to the iris causing the anterior uveitis which may be so severe that there occurs an outpouring of leukocytes from the dilated capillaries of iris. It occurs to such an extent that these leukocytes settle at the bottom of the anterior chamber to form a *hypopyon.* It is important to remember that the leukocytosis is due to toxins and not due to actual invasion by bacteria, therefore, the hypopyon is sterile. The hypopyon consists of polymorphonuclear leukocytes. It has a tendency to appear and also disappear in a few hours. It may be small in amount or fill the chamber halfway or more. To begin with, hypopyon is fluid, shows a horizontal line and moves with the position of the head and settle to the lowest part of the anterior chamber.

Later the leukocytes become enmeshed in a network of fibrin.

The fibrinous hypopyon does not show a horizontal line and does not shift with the change in the position of the head rather the upper border is convex.

As the hypopyon is sterile, it is unnecessary to drain it. It absorbs with the healing of the ulcer. A large hypopyon covering more than half of the anterior chamber needs evacuation as the large hypopyon is usually fibrinous that does not absorb readily and leads to secondary glaucoma.

Symptoms

- In early stage, the symptoms consist of pain in the eye and brow with marked photophobia. *The pain reduces after the initial stage that is why the patient unduly delays the treatment.*

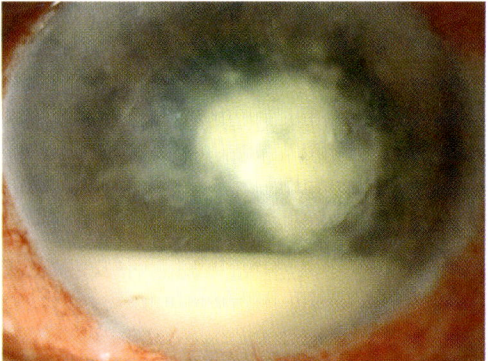

Fig. 13.1: Corneal ulcer with hypopyon

- Redness of the eye with lid swelling.
- Discharge from the eye.

Signs

- *Conjunctival and circumciliary congestion.*
- *Swelling of lid with blepharospasm.*

- *Greyish white or yellowish disk near the center of the cornea.*

The hypopyon corneal ulcer appears as disk-like area of greyish white or yellowish in color. The edges are well-marked in one particular direction. The ulcer has a tendency to progress towards this well marked edge. The ulcer increases in size and depth.

- *Lusterless:* Cornea appears dull, dry or misty.
- *Hypopyon* that may be fluid or organized

Management

Treatment of hypopyon ulcer is like that of any ulcer except that it needs early intensive and energetic management.

- Culture and sensitivity test.
- Curette the necrotic ulcer base before starting the antibiotic therapy.

Intensive broad-spectrum antibiotic therapy

Start a broad spectrum antibiotic therapy; locally, subconjunctivally and systemically as well. Instill eyedrops every 5 minutes for the first hour then every 15 minutes for next 2 hours and then every hourly until there is a good response. Change the antibiotic depending upon the report of the culture and sensitivity test.

Supportive therapy

- Atropine eyedrops 1% should be instilled three times a day until the pupil dilates well and maintains dilation at least for two weeks after healing of the ulcer.
- Systemic analgesics and anti-inflammatory drugs to relieve pain and edema.
- Carbonic anhydrase inhibitors, if required, to keep the intraocular pressure low to prevent perforation.
- Cauterization of ulcer.
- Use of tissue adhesive such as N-butyl 2-ethyl cyanoacrylate monomer, if ulcer is threatening to perforate.
- Bandage soft contact lens.
- Good nourishing diet with vitamins.
- Cleanliness of the self, use goggles or shield and use sterile swab to clean the discharge from the angles of the eye.

- If no response in two days, then refer the case to ophthalmic center.
- Paracentesis can be performed to prevent the perforation and its complications.
- Good nourishing diet with vitamins.
- Dacryocystorhinostomy, if associated with dacryocystitis.

Mycotic Corneal Ulcer

Farmer presents with history of mild injury while harvesting with red eye, dull grayish white-yellowish central ulcer and mild pain.

Slit-lamp shows a dry greyish white central corneal ulcer with elevated margin, multiple small satellite lesions, finger like projection in stroma under intact epithelium and large hypopyon yet no corneal vascularization.

The mild pain is the root cause for delay in presentation for treatment.

Diagnosis—mycotic corneal ulcer.

Etiology

A mycotic hypopyon corneal ulcer commonly occurs following infection with fungus such as *Aspergillus, Candida or Fusarium.*

Incidental factors

- Injury by vegetative material such as sharp leaf, thin branch of small tree, straw, hay or any kind of decaying vegetable material.
- Injury by animal tail.
- Patients with systemic or local immuno-supression.
- Excessive use of antibiotics and steroids predisposes the patient to fungal infection. Antibiotics disturb the symbiosis between bacteria and fungi. Steroids make the fungi facultative pathogens which are otherwise symbiotic saprophytes.

Clinical Features

- Symptoms are less marked than other corneal ulcers.
- Ulcer appears *dry, grey white* with elevated and rolled out margins.

- Ulcer is surrounded with *multiple small satellite lesions* and shows a yellow line of demarcation.
- Ulcer shows fine *feathery finger-like extension* in stroma under the intact epithelium.
- Ulcer is usually associated with large hypopyon which may not be sterile as fungi can penetrate into anterior chamber without perforation.
- Perforation is rare but can occur.
- Corneal vascularization is conspicuously absent.

Microbiological Investigation

- Gram's and Giemsa stained films for fungal hyphae
- 10% KOH wet preparation
- Calcofluor white
- Culture on Sabouraud's agar medium and sensitivity to identify the causative organism and fungal hyphae.

Management
Antifungal and antibiotic

- Topical antifungal eyedrops for 6–8 weeks:
  - Natamycin 5% eyedrops
  - Fluconazol 0.2% eyedrops
  - Nystatin 3.5% eye ointment
- Topical antibiotic eyedrops may be needed to control secondary bacterial infection.
- A few serious cases may require systemic antifungal drugs; fluconazole or keto-conazole for 2–3 weeks.

Supportive therapy

- Improve resistance by good diet and vitamins.
- Therapeutic keratoplasty have been considered as a treatment to save the eye and some vision.
- Do not use corticosteroids.
- Advise prophylaxis to the people working in agriculture field especially by use of plain glasses to avoid injury to cornea.

Marginal Catarrhal Corneal Ulcer
(Fig. 13.2)

Usually an elderly patient presents with mild pain, irritation, discomfort, photophobia and lacrimation.

Slit-lamp shows small, shallow and multiple marginal ulcers.

Diagnosis—marginal catarrhal corneal ulcer.

Etiology

The causative organisms are *Moraxella* or *Haemophilus aegyptius*. It is thought to be caused by a hypersensitive reaction to staphylococcal toxins.

Incidental Factors

- It is associated with chronic staphylococcal blepharoconjunctivitis.
- The marginal ulcers occur near the limbus especially in elderly people.
- Topical medication can induce hypersensitive reaction.

Clinical Features

- Mild ocular irritation, pain, photophobia and lacrimation.
- A few cases may present with neuralgic pain in the head and face.
- These marginal ulcers are shallow and multiple.
- Vascularization occurs followed by resolution and recurrences are common.
- Rare but serious form of deep marginal ulcer occurs in patients with polyarteritis nodosa caused by formation of antigen-antibody complexes at the limbus and turns into a *ring ulcer* which may lead to the necrosis of the whole cornea.

Management

Topical antibiotics and steroids Treat these ulcers with appropriate antibiotic. Steroids are helpful.

Supportive therapy Topical cyclosporin eye emulsion 0.05% twice a day to control limbal and eyelid inflammation.

Pay attention to associated blepharitis and chronic conjunctivitis.

Good nourishing diet with vitamins.

Herpes Simplex Keratitis (Fig. 13.2)

Patient presents with blurred vision along with mild irritation, discomfort, lacrimation, photophobia and blepharospasm following an attack of flu.

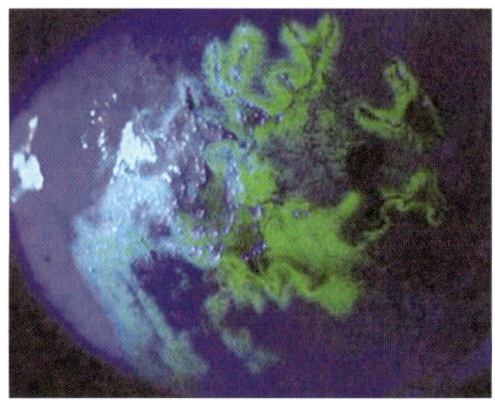

Fig. 13.2: Herpes simplex keratitis

Slit-lamp shows dendritic ulcer

Diagnosis—herpes simplex keratitis.

Etiology

- Herpes simplex virus is a DNA virus. The only natural host is human being. Herpes simplex virus is basically epitheliotropic but may become neurotropic.
- Herpes simplex keratitis is caused by herpes simplex virus-I (HSV-I) which causes infection above the waist involving skin, lips and eyes. HSV-1 infection is acquired by kissing and usually occurs in early years of life by transmission from parents, relatives and social visitors showering kisses on cheeks as expression of love.
- Herpes simplex virus-II (HSV-II) causes infection below the waist—herpes genitalis. It is transmitted to eyes of neonates through infected genitalia of the mother. HSV-2 infection is acquired by sexual contact and usually occurs in teenage or adult life. HSV-II also can cause ocular lesions.
- An attack does not confer immunity to the patient. A person once infected usually becomes a carrier and periodic attacks tend to occur on skin, lips and eyes. There is always a stress stimulus for attack and also for recurrence.

The stress stimulus can be:

- Low resistance following fever, flu, malaria, etc.

- Exposure to extreme heat, cold and wind.
- Psychiatric problems.
- Use of steroids locally and systemically.
- Use of immunosuppressive agents.
- Exposure to sunlight—ultraviolet rays.
- Emotional and physical stress.
- Minor unnoticeable trauma.

Symptoms

- Blurred vision associated with irritation, discomfort, lacrimation, photophobia and blepharospasm.
- History of fever or flu a few days before the onset of eye symptoms.

Signs

- *Follicular keratoconjunctivitis:* Follicles in the fornices with mild irritation and lacrimation.
- *Superficial punctate keratitis:* Numerous whitish plaques on cornea which are minute and often arranged in rows and groups. These desquamate quickly, form erosions, and heal rapidly leaving no opacity on the cornea. These are accompanied by irritation, lacrimation and blepharospasm. The cornea is insensitive and there is absence of corneal vascularization.
- *Dendritic or geographical ulcer:* More commonly, thin grey striae extend in all directions, increase in length and send out more lateral and linear branches classically ending as terminal end bulbs or knobs forming a figure known as *dendritic figure or dendritic ulcer* which is pathognomonic for herpes simplex. The surface over infiltrate breaks and a chronic type of ulcer is produced with swollen or raised border sending out fresh branches spreading over the cornea but not in depth. Sometimes infiltrates spread in all directions, coalesce with each other and form a large confluent shallow *geographical ulcer.*
  - *Staining:* Generally, one or two of the infiltrates stain with *fluorescein* at any one time and fresh spots are formed. The raised epithelial borders of the ulcer

does not stain with fluorescein, but are well stained with *rose bengal stain.*

- *Pathogenesis:* The pathogenesis of branching dendritic or geographical ulcer is believed to be related to the neuronal distribution and linear viral spread by contagious cell to cell movement.
- Sometimes stroma may be involved in the form of *disciform keratitis* associated with anterior uveitis.
- The cornea is insensitive.
- There is absence of vascularization.
- Recurrence is common.

Management
Topical antiviral eye ointment

- Topical antiviral acycloguanosine (acyclovir) is least toxic and most commonly used antiviral for herpes simplex keratitis.
- Acycloguanosine (acyclovir) 3% ointment to be applied five times a day for 7 to 14 days gives good response. Acyclovir gets in the viral infected cells. Acyclovir penetrates intact corneal epithelium and stroma achieving therapeutic levels in aqueous humor, therefore, it is effective for both the superficial epithelial and deep stromal lesions.

Supportive therapy

- Oral acyclovir 200 mg five times daily for 7 to 10 days, if needed.
- Topical cycloplegic in cases with photophobia and ciliary spasm.
- Antiglaucoma agents, if there is a rise of intraocular pressure.
- Good nourishing diet with vitamins.

Herpes Zoster Ophthalmicus (Fig. 13.3)

Patient presents with severe neuralgic pain even with the flow of fan air, combing or mild touch and limited to one side of head.

Examination shows red and warm skin on the affected side with a few minute vesicles.

Diagnosis—herpes zoster ophthalmicus.

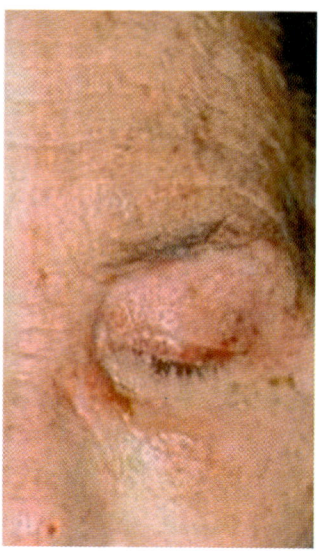

Fig. 13.3: Herpes zoster ophthalmicus

Etiopathogenesis

It is caused by *varicella-zoster virus* (VZV). It is a DNA virus. It produces acidophilic intranuclear inclusion bodies. It is neurotropic in nature affecting the first division of the trigeminal nerve.

After infection with virus in childhood which manifests as chickenpox, the virus lies dormant in the Gasserian ganglion of trigeminal nerve to manifest later particularly in the elderly age when there is low cellular immunity. The chief focus of infection is the Gasserian ganglion from where the infection travels down along one or more branches of the ophthalmic division of fifth nerve. The usual branches involved are supraorbital, supra- and infratrochlear and frequently the nasal branch. Lesions are unilateral strictly limited to one side of the midline of head.

Clinical features include general features, cutaneous lesions and ocular lesions. Ophthalmologist is primarily concerned with ocular features.

Symptoms

- *Severe neuralgic pain:* There is severe neuralgic pain along the course of the branches of ophthalmic division of fifth nerve. It is limited to one side. The neuralgic pain may be preceded by fever and malaise. A severe unilateral pain and limited to half side of the head should arouse suspicion before vesicles manifest.
- *Red and edematous skin of one side of head:* The part of the skin supplied by the ophthalmic division of fifth nerve appears red and edematous. It is tender to touch even on combing the hairs or even a strong wind initiates pain.
- *Vesicles on the skin:* The vesicles are limited to the area supplied by ophthalmic division of fifth nerve.

Signs

- *Edema and tenderness:* Skin of one side of head is red and edematous and tender to touch.
- *Intense pain and tenderness* even on touching the skin of the one side of middle line of head.
  - *Vesicles:* The vesicles have strict limitation to one side of the middle line of head. These vesicles suppurate, bleed and heal with permanent pitted scars. The eruptive stage lasts for about 3 weeks. There is anesthesia of the skin following subsidence of active stage.
  - *Cornea:* The cornea is definitely involved, if there is involvement of the nasociliary branch of the fifth nerve. On slit-lamp examination, one can observe numerous white spots in the epithelium and stroma as subepithelial punctate keratitis. The cornea is insensitive.
  - *Intraocular pressure:* It may be normal or high. Occurrence of secondary glaucoma is not unusual.
  - *Cranial nerve:* There is involvement of cranial nerves in some cases especially the third, fourth, sixth and seventh which recover within 6 weeks or so.
  - *Anterior uveitis:* Early sign being presence of keratic precipitates.

Complications

- Neuralgic pain may persist for years
- Insensitivity of cornea

- Anterior uveitis
- Cranial nerve palsies
- Secondary glaucoma
- Pitted and permanent scars.

Management

Antiviral, antibiotics and steroids therapy

Topical ocular

- *Topical antiviral:* Acyclovir 3% eye ointment five times daily for two weeks.
- Topical antibiotic eyedrops four times daily for two weeks.
- Topical steroids 2 to 4 times a day.

Systemic

- Acyclovir 200 mg five times daily for 10 days.
- Steroids, if there are neurological complications.

Local on skin lesions

Antibiotic, steroid and anesthetic skin ointment or cream three times daily to reduce pain and edema until skin lesions heal.

Supportive therapy

- *Topical cycloplegic:* Atropine eye ointment once a day so as to keep the pupil dilated for ensuing iridocyclitis.
- Good nourishing diet with vitamins.
- Topical timolol 0.5% eyedrops for raised intraocular pressure.
- Bandage soft contact lens, if needed.

It is advisable to refer the case to neurologist and skin specialist for general and skin lesions.

Mooren's Corneal Ulcer (Rodent Ulcer, Ulcer Serpens and Idiopathic Ulcer)

Usually an elderly patient presents with unilateral severe persistent neuralgic pain, lacrimation and photophobia in left eye since last two months or so.

Slit-lamp shows that the ulcer is undermining the epithelium with an advancing and overhanging edge which can be lifted easily. It is advancing circumferentially with heavy corneal vascularization.

Diagnosis—Mooren's corneal ulcer.

Mooren's ulcer is a chronic superficial peripheral ulcer of unknown etiology.

Etiology

- It is an idiopathic degenerative condition.
- It may be due to ischemic necrosis of limbal vessels.
- Erosion is initiated by autoimmunolysis of the epithelium with release of collagenolytic enzymes.
- It is an autoimmune disease.

Clinical Types

- *Benign form* of Mooren's ulcer is unilateral, usually affects elderly people and slow progressive in its character.
- *Virulent form* of Mooren's ulcer is bilateral, affects younger people and fast progressive in its character.

Clinical Features

- *Characteristic feature*: It spreads slowly with undermining the corneal epithelium at its *advancing and overhanging edge* which can be lifted up.
- Severe and persistent neuralgic pain and lacrimation, photophobia and diminished vision.
- Spread with intermissions until the whole cornea is involved with a nebular type of opacity and much loss of vision.
- Usually, both the eyes are involved but not always simultaneously.
- In early stage, the ulcer looks like a marginal ulcer with grey infiltration near the margin of the cornea.
- Ulcer tends to spread circumferentially or axially over whole of cornea.
- No tendency for perforation.
- Sclera remains uninvolved
- Healing takes place from the periphery with neovascularization. Healed areas are without superficial layers, heavily vascularized and remain permanently cloudy with very low vision.
- Prognosis is bad.

Management

- Treatment is uncertain, unsatisfactory and difficult.

- Topical antibiotics and steroids as initial therapy with poor response.
- Immunosuppressive therapy with systemic steroids may help.
- Classical treatment is the excision of the overhanging edge and free cauterization.
- Excision of 4–7 mm strip of conjunctiva adjacent to the ulcer margin may be helpful by eliminating conjunctival sources of collagenase and proteoglycogenase.
- Lamellar graft often melts or vascularizes.
- Try all the possible means to help the patient to alleviate his/her pain.

SUPERFICIAL KERATITIS

Exposure Keratitis

A male patient presents with incomplete closure of lids with mild discomfort and irritation in his left eye since 15 days.

Patient gives history of exposure to cold wave at his field.

Ocular examination shows Bell's palsy.

Slit-lamp shows superficial punctuate keratitis in the lower part of cornea.

Diagnosis—exposure keratitis due to Bell's palsy.

Etiology

Exposure keratitis occurs due to improper wetting or polishing of the corneal surface though there is normal secretion of tear fluid. This is due to inability of the lids to polish the cornea with each blink.

Causative Factors

- *Bell's phenomenon*: Absence of normal Bell's phenomenon.
- *Bell's palsy* or facial palsy due to any other factor.
- *Physiological lagophthalmos*: Exposure of cornea during sleep in healthy person.
- *Coma*: Exposure of cornea in state of coma.
- *Cicatricial ectropion*.
- *Symblepharon*
- *Proptosis—marked proptosis causes incomplete closure of lids.*

Pathogenesis

The epithelium of the exposed cornea dries up followed by desiccation. The epithelium is cast off and thereby falls prey to infective organisms. The initial desiccation occurs in the interpalpebral area or lower peripheral part of the cornea resulting in fine punctuate epithelial keratitis. It is followed by necrosis then ulcer with vascularization.

Clinical Features

- Diagnosis can be made easily by asking the patient to close the lids normally. Within a minute or two, one can observe a small opening between the lids exposing the conjunctiva and lower part of the cornea.
- The exposed conjunctiva and cornea loose the normal luster.
- Superficial vascularization of the cornea.
- Superficial erosions of cornea or even ulcer may be seen in the inferior part of cornea.
- Fluorescein staining may show punctate erosions or ulcer.

Management

- *Tarsorrhaphy*: If the process is likely to be permanent, then tarsorrhaphy is the ideal choice. This will save the eye and relieve the patient of his discomfort.
- If the process is likely to be of temporary nature, then use:
  - Artificial tear eyedrops—frequent instillation.
  - Bandage soft contact lens.
  - Air tight goggles.
  - At night, keep lids closed by a piece of tape from lid to cheek.
- Treat the causative factor.

Neuroparalytic Keratitis

Patient presents with red eye, blurred vision, discomfort with absence of pain and lacrimation.

Slit-lamp shows lusterless cornea with dull corneal reflex.

Corneal sensation is markedly diminished.

Diagnosis—neuroparalytic keratitis

Etiology

The neuroparalytic keratitis follows paralysis of the sensory nerve supply of cornea, i.e. the ophthalmic division of the trigeminal nerve. The corneal sensitivity is very important defensive mechanism of cornea against degeneration, ulceration and infection.

Causative Factors

- Inflammation of gasserian ganglion by herpes simplex virus or herpes zoster ophthalmicus.
- Alcohol-block or electrocoagulation of gasserian ganglion or section of the sensory root of trigeminal nerve for trigeminal neuralgia.
- Syphilitic or leprotic neuropathy.
- Traumatic injury to gasserian ganglion.
- Tumor pressing on gasserian ganglion.

Clinical Features

- Intense circumciliary congestion
- Cornea appears lusterless.
- Corneal reflex is dull.
- Conspicuous absence of pain and lacrimation.
- Corneal sensation test demonstrates diminished or absent corneal sensation.

Pathogenesis

Metabolic activity of corneal epithelium is disturbed due to paralysis of ophthalmic division of the fifth nerve. Corneal changes occur even with normal blink reflex and normal secretion of tear fluid. The characteristic corneal feature is presence of punctate epithelial erosions in the interpalpebral area followed by ulceration due to desquamation of the corneal epithelium. In early stage, it heals quickly and also breaks down rapidly, therefore, relapses are rule.

Management

The main fundamental of treatment is to keep the corneal surface moist. To achieve this:
- Shield to prevent exposure and evaporation of tear fluid.
- Closure of the lacrimal punctum.

- Artificial tears.
- Antibiotic eyedrops and ointment to prevent secondary infection.
- Soft contact lens.
- *Tarsorrhaphy is the best. If the lids are kept sutured for a year or so, then invariably tarsorrhaphy succeeds in stopping the process of desquamation of epithelium.*

Superficial Punctate Keratitis
(Recurrent Corneal Erosions)

A young professional presents with complain of blurred vision along with pain, watering, photophobia and foreign body sensation soon after waking up in the morning.

Slit-lamp with fluorescein staining shows a few minute dots in the central cornea.

Diagnosis—superficial punctate keratitis

Superficial punctate keratitis is characterized by multiple raised gray dots-like lesions in the superficial epithelial layers of cornea. Slit-lamp shows multiple epithelial opacities appear as superficial slightly raised gray dots mainly over the central area of the cornea.

It may manifest as:
- Punctate epithelial erosions
- Punctate epithelial keratitis
- Punctate subepithelial keratitis
- Filamentary keratitis.

Recurrence is common.

Etiopathogenesis

- *Viral infection* such as herpes simplex, herpes zoster, adenovirus, epidemic keratoconjunctivitis and so on.
- *Chlamydial infection* covers trachoma and inclusion conjunctivitis.
- *Toxic lesions* due to staphylococcal toxin associated with blepharoconjunctivitis.
- *Trophic lesions* as in exposure and neuroparalytic keratitis.
- *Allergic lesions, e.g. vernal and phlyctenular keratoconjunctivitis.*
- *Dry eye syndrome—keratoconjunctivitis sicca.*

Clinical Features

- These dots do not stain easily with fluorescein but turns deep red with rose bengal.
- Patient presents with blurred vision, foreign body sensation, mild photophobia and lacrimation with discomfort.
- It is usually associated with mild conjunctivitis.
- Cornea appears dull and the corneal reflex is not bright.
- Slit-lamp shows multiple minute dots.

Management

- *Topical steroids* show early and marked symptomatic relief.
- *Artificial tear* provides soothing effect.
- *Antiviral and antibiotic*—topical instillation as per need.
- *Supportive therapy*—good nourishing diet with vitamins.

Phlyctenular Keratitis

Young mother enters the clinic holding the hand of her female child and complains that she keeps her left eye closed almost all the time with watering and discharge since 10 days.

General inspection shows rhagades at left canthus and nostril with free flow of nasal discharge. Mother and daughter both are malnourished.

Slit-lamp shows fascicular ulcer.

Diagnosis—phlyctenular keratitis.

Etiology

Phlyctenular keratitis is believed to be a delayed hypersensitivity (type IV—cell mediated) response to endogenous microbial proteins; such as *tuberculous proteins* and now more commonly to *Staphylococcus proteins*.

Types

1. *Ulcerative phlyctenular keratitis:* It manifests in three forms:
   a. *Sacrofulous phlyctenular keratitis* manifests as a shallow marginal ulcer due to break-off of superficial epithelium from the apex of the phlycten. It heals without scar.
   b. *Fascicular phlyctenular keratitis* manifests as progressive ulcer followed by prominent leash of blood vessels. It heals with band-shaped scar.
   c. *Miliary phlyctenular keratitis* manifests as multiple phlyctenular ulcers around the limbus.
2. *Diffuse infiltrative phlyctenular keratitis:* Diffuse infiltrative phlyctenulr keratitis manifests as diffuse central infiltration with rich vascularization of the cornea from the limbus.

Symptoms

- *Corneal phlycten:* Corneal phlycten astrides the limbus. The symptoms are minimal until the corneal epithelium is cast-off. There may be one or more phlycten around the limbus.
- *Pain, lacrimation and photophobia:* These symptoms manifest due to reflex irritation of fifth nerve ending of cornea after the corneal epithelium is cast off from the apex of the phlycten.
- *Congestion:* Usually localized around the phlycten.
- *Nasal discharge:* Free flow of nasal discharge.

Signs

- *Corneal phlycten:* A corneal phlycten is a gray nodule slightly raised from surface and looks yellow ulcer, when epithelium is cast-off. The corneal phlyctens are localized infiltration may be one or more around the limbus. Some may be astriding the limbus the other may be on the cornea and may be involving the conjunctiva alone.
- *Congestion* is localized around the phlycten. In some cases, there may be associated conjunctivitis then the whole conjunctiva is congested.
- *Fascicular ulcer:* In a long-standing untreated case, the phlycten advances towards the center of cornea followed by a leash of blood vessels. This type of ulcer is

known as *fascicular ulcer*. The peripheral part of the ulcer heals while the half moon like progressive central margin of the ulcer remains active eating away its way across the cornea preceded by gray infiltration and followed by a leash of vessels from limbus. The fascicular ulcer is a superficial ulcer and never perforates. On healing, it leaves a band shape superficial opacity which is dense at the advancing edge. The vascularization gradually diminishes. It affects the vision.

- *Skin rash or eczema* around the nose and lids.
- *General malnutrition:* Patient is usually a child and looks ill-nourished and sick.

Complications

- *Fascicular ulcer:* An occurrence of fascicular ulcer indicates that the case has not been treated for a long time. Steroids topically in the form of eyedrops and ointment improve the condition remarkably.
- *Corneal opacity:* A corneal phlycten always leaves a triangular scar with base towards the limbus.

A triangular opaque scar with base towards the limbus is diagnostic for phlyctenular keratitis.

Management

Antibiotics and steroids
- Topical steroids eyedrops four to six times a day and ointment at bedtime until there is good response and thereafter gradually reduce the instillation.
- Topical antibiotic eyedrops and ointment to cover any secondary infection of conjunctiva.

Supportive therapy
- Cycloplegic atropine 1% eye drops 1% twice a day to keep the pupil well dilated as preventive measure for iritis.
- Treat rhagades at the canthi and skin eczema with antibiotic and steroid eye ointment three times daily.
- Good nourishing diet with vitamins.

DEEP KERATITIS

Interstitial Keratitis (Fig. 13.4)

Interstitial keratitis is broad term that denotes a non-ulcerative, non-suppurative inflammation of corneal stroma characterized by cellular infiltration. It is often associated with vascularization of stroma without primary involvement of the epithelium and endothelium.

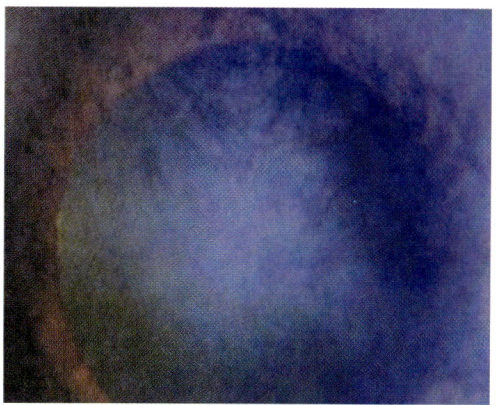

Fig. 13.4: Interstitial keratitis

Interstitial keratitis is an immune-mediated process thought to be caused by cellular and humoral response against antigens in the corneal stroma, residual infectious antigens or both. Although syphilis is the leading cause of interstitial keratitis, it can be caused due to bacteria, viral, parasitic and autoimmune factors. Now herpes simplex virus is one of the leading causes for interstitial keratitis.

It is associated with:
- Congenital syphilis
- Herpes simplex virus
- Herpes zoster virus
- Tuberculosis
- Acquired syphilis
- Leprosy
- Sarcoidosis
- Cogan's syndrome
- Onchocerciasis

Syphilitic Interstitial Keratitis

Etiology It manifests due to local antigen-antibody reaction.

It is a late manifestation of congenital syphilis affecting mostly children between the age of five and fifteen. An injury acts as an exciting factor. Indeed the disease is primarily anterior uveitis but the keratitis masks the picture. It is essential that energetic treatment is directed towards uveitis and keratitis both.

It is bilateral in congenital syphilis and unilateral in acquired syphilis.

Symptoms

- *Circumciliary congestion:* It is marked in the florid stage of the disease.
- *Pain, lacrimation, photophobia and blepharospasm:* These symptoms are marked in the florid stage of the disease.
- *Diminution of vision:* Vision is reduced to hand movements.

Signs

- *Opaque cornea (ground glass appearance):* To begin with one or more hazy patches appear in deep layers of the cornea near the corneal margin or at the center of cornea. These hazy patches spread from margin to the center, or from center towards the periphery, until they cover the whole cornea. The cornea appears like a ground glass.
- *Deep vascularization (salmon patch appearance):* There is deep vascularization which consists of radial bundles of brush-like vessels. As these vessels are covered by an opaque cornea, these appear like a patch of dull reddish pink color rather than individual vessels of bright color. Because of their dull reddish pink color like the color of salmon fish; these are known as *"salmon patch appearance"*.
- *Superficial vascularization:* Minimal only in the periphery of the cornea.
- *Heaping of the conjunctiva at limbus:* At the limbus, the conjunctiva may be heaped up like an *epaulette*.
- *Keratic precipitates*: Easily seen by slit-lamp.
- *Visual acuity:* Vision is reduced to just hand movements.

Course

The clinical features can be classified in three stages:

1. *Progressive stage:* The malady starts with edema of the endothelium and deeper stroma secondary to anterior uveitis with mild symptoms and signs of uveitis and keratitis.
2. *Florid stage:* The malady shows deep vascularization with acute symptoms and signs of uveitis and keratitis.
3. *Regressive stage*: After the disease has reached its height of *florid stage*, the cornea starts clearing slowly from the margin towards the center and ultimately the whole cornea is clear except in some worst cases. The vessels get obliterated and appear as *ghost vessels* seen as radial opaque lines. The acute stage lasts for 6 weeks or more. It takes months for the cornea to become clear. Do not expect much improvement after 18 months.

Diagnosis

- Typical clinical picture of cornea with deep vascularization.
- Other clinical evidences of congenital syphilis are as follows:
  - Prominence of frontal eminences
  - Flatness of the bridge of the nose.
  - Hutchinson's teeth notching of the two upper central incisors in the permanent dentition.
  - Rhagades at the angle of mouth
  - Shotty cervical nodes
  - Periosteal nodules on the tibia.
- Positive VDRL or *Treponema pallidum* immobilization test confirms the diagnosis.

Management

Systemic anti-syphilitic and steroids

- Course of anti-syphilitic treatment. It will shorten the course of the disease.
- Topical steroid eyedrops during day and ointment at bedtime. Topical steroids should be continued for at least a year as maintenance dose to prevent relapse.

Supportive therapy

- Cycloplegic-atropine 1% eyedrops twice a day to control anterior uveitis.
- Dark goggles for photophobia.
- Penetrating keratoplasty for cases with left over central corneal opacity.

Disciform Keratitis

Disciform keratitis is most common type of endothelitis. It presents as stromal edema with overlying keratic precipitates on the endothelium.

Etiopathogenesis

- It manifests due to delayed hypersensitivity reaction to the HSV antigen.
- There is low grade stromal infiltration with involvement of endothelium resulting in corneal edema.
- It is probably a tissue response between antigen liberated by virus in the epithelium and antibodies produced in the stroma.

Clinical Features

- Mild irritation which lasts for months.
- Vision is markedly reduced.
- Cornea is insensitive.
- No ulceration.
- Characterized by appearance of a central gray disk in the middle layers of stroma which is dense in the central part.
- Slit-lamp shows thickening of the cornea, fold in Descemet's membrane and keratic precipitates.
- Intraocular pressure may be raised.

Management

Topical steroids with antiviral cover Topical steroid eyedrops 4 times a day with antiviral cover acyclovir 3% twice daily. Dilute and taper the steroids over a period of several weeks.

Supportive therapy Tarsorrhaphy may be needed in some worst cases due to insensitive cornea.

DEGENERATIVE AND DYSTROPHIC CONDITIONS

Arcus Senilis

- Arcus senilis is an age-related malady of lipid infiltration of the cornea usually in elderly people.
- Lipid infiltration commences as crescentic grayish white line concentric with the upper and lower margins of the cornea which finally meet to form a circle round the cornea.
- About 1 mm broad sharply defined on the peripheral side and fading off on the central side.
- Typically characterized by a clear rim of cornea (*lucid interval of Vogt*) between the arcus senilis and the margin of the cornea.
- Does not affect the vision or the vitality of the cornea.

Arcus Juvenilis

- Arcus juvenilis is a rare condition which affects the people under the age of 40 years.
- Lipid profile is indicated in a case that shows arcus in the younger age to exclude a heritable anomaly with serious prognosis for life.
- Characterized by a clear rim of cornea between the arcus and the limbus.

Band Shape Keratopathy (Fig. 13.5)

An elderly malnourished patient presents with marked loss of vision and mild discomfort since years.

Slit-lamp shows gray white band shape opacity with dots, holes and chalk-like crusts covering the entire length of cornea in the midline leaving a small clear cornea at both the ends.

Diagnosis—band shape keratopathy.

Band shape keratopathy denotes a condition in which calcium salts are precipitated on the surface of the cornea either due to local or systemic factors.

Band shape keratopathy is characterized by the development of a gray-white band of opacity in the exposed part of the cornea in the palpebral aperture slightly below the middle of the pupil.

Band shape keratopathy is a degenerative condition of the cornea associated with varied ocular condition. The most common are the following four types of cases:

1. Primary band shape keratopathy.
2. Constitutional factors with systemic maladies.
3. Secondary to ocular malady such as glaucoma, uveitis, keratitis.
4. Following ocular trauma.

Usually band shape keratopathy manifests in the following cases:

- Elderly people with malnourishment.
- Elderly people with degeneration of cornea.
- Old and untreated cases of glaucoma, uveitis and keratitis.

Clinical Features

- First change is appearance of slight opacity at the level of Bowman's membrane in which dark round holes are seen by slit-lamp examination. This change occurs initially near the periphery with a clear zone between the opacity and the limbus.
- Gradually, the opacity spreads towards the center resulting in an unbroken band across the cornea in the palpebral aperture.
- To begin with, the opacity is situated below the epithelium. Later there are changes in the epithelium giving an appearance with many *grey dots, holes and chalk-like white crusts.*
- Deposition of calcium salts in the subepithelial space and on Bowman's membrane and superficial stroma as seen by slit-lamp. The overlying epithelium is usually intact though it is irregular.
- No symptoms till the epithelium is intact except mild irritation with dim vision.
- Fluorescein stain shows staining of epithelium in a punctate manner.
- If no ocular etiological factor, then rule out systemic factors.

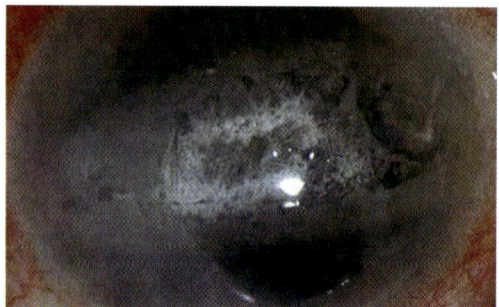

Fig. 13.5: Band shape keratopathy

Management

Chemical chelation of deposited calcium salts is the mainstay of management. The epithelium overlying the lesion is mechanically debrided using a spatula. EDTA (*ethylene-diamine-tetra-acet*ic *acid)*, neutral solution 1% or 2% (0.05 mol) is applied over the lesion using soaked tipped applicator for about 5 minutes. Scrap the calcium particles with blade edge. Repeat the procedure till visual axis is cleared. Bandage soft contact lens or pressure bandage till the epithelium heals.

Supportive therapy

- Treat ocular and or systemic malady.
- *Phototherapeutic keratectomy* with excimer laser in cases wherein the corneal surface is very irregular.
- *Keratoplasty* is effective providing good vision in cases with primary keratopathy.

Salzmann's Nodular Degeneration

- Seen in cases with old phlyctenular keratitis, trachoma or interstitial keratitis.
- Characterized by multiple bluish white elevated subepithelial nodules in an opaque cornea or at the edge of the transparent cornea.
- Bowman's layer is replaced by scar tissue and the epithelium is irregular.
Keratoplasty is effective.

Reis-Bücklers Corneal Dystrophy

- Presents in early childhood.
- Autosomal dominant inheritance.
- Characterized by superficial ring-shaped opacities which appear like a honeycomb.

- Opacities lie at the level of Bowman's membrane.
- Most cases develop recurrent erosions.
- Vision is markedly affected.
- Keratoplasty is needed to improve the vision.

Fuch's Endothelial Dystrophy

- Fuch's endothelial dystrophy affects elderly females in 5th and 6th decades of life.
- Usually, bilateral and slowly progressive.
- Mostly, autosomal dominant inheritance. Family history is present in 30% of cases.
- Commonly associated with primary open-angle glaucoma.

Etiopathogenesis

- An increased apoptosis of the corneal endothelium with changes in the Descemet's membrane.
- In early stage, the changes consist of cornea guttata which become numerous and spread to periphery giving *'beaten metal'* appearance.
- Later endothelial decompensation causes *edema of stroma*.
- Later there is epithelial edema which results in *bullous keratopathy* causing pain.
- Edema and vascularization of stroma lead to *opaque and vascularized cornea* that causes marked loss of vision.

Symptoms

- Patient presents with glare, blurred vision that is worse on awakening in the morning.
- Vision gets blurred with epithelial and stromal edema.
- Pain and photophobia with recurrent erosions of the cornea due to ruptured bullae.

Signs

Slit-lamp shows:
- Cornea guttata
- Central edema of the stroma
- Epithelial edema
- Bullae

- Folds in Descemet's membrane
- Subepithelial stromal scarring and vascularization

Investigations

- Intraocular pressure
- Pachymetry
- Specular microscopy
- Confocal microscopy

Management

Sodium chloride 5% eyedrops in daytime and eye ointment at bedtime.

Supportive therapy

- Control intraocular pressure, if more than 20 mm Hg.
- Bandage soft contact lenses provide some relief during bullous keratopathy.
- Follow-up every month and later every 3 months.
- Keratoplasty for stromal scarring provides relief and vision.
- Take care to preserve endothelium during surgical interference.

ECTATIC CONDITIONS

Keratoconus (Fig. 13.6)

Teenager girl presents with gradual loss of vision since about 1 year or so more in her left eye. She finds difficulty in coping with her studies.

Slit-lamp shows mild keratoconus

Diagnosis—keratoconus.

Keratoconus denotes—a non-inflammatory, bilateral, asymmetric ectasia of the cornea characterized by thining of the apical cornea and corneal scarring of obscure etiology.

Usually, it is bilateral though one eye may be more affected. It manifests at puberty.

It may be associated with numerous other ocular abnormalities such as retinitis pigmentosa, Leber's optic atrophy, vernal conjunctivitis, ectopia lentis, congenital cataract, aniridia, Down's syndrome and Marfan's syndrome.

Clinical Features

- Gradual loss of vision, photophobia and monocular diplopia.

- Almost invariably bilateral.
- Usually, manifests at the puberty and more common in females.
- Most of the cases do not have a positive family history.
- Visual acuity is markedly reduced with distorted vision.
- Dim vision with myopic astigmatism.
- Corneal sensation is diminished.
- Retinoscopy will reveal a scissor reflex or yawning reflex.
- Refraction shows a high degree of irregular myopic astigmatism.
- Photokeratoscopy shows distortion of circles.
- Keratometry will give high cylinders with oblique axis.
- Peculiar unusual glistening and luster in the central area of the cornea.
- *Munson's sign*, is an angular curve of the lower lid margin when the patient looks down.

Slit-lamp shows:

- Thinning of the cornea at the apex even to the extent that the pulse beat of the intraocular pressure may be clearly seen.
- An endothelial reflex in the central portion of the cornea due to increased concavity of the posterior surface.

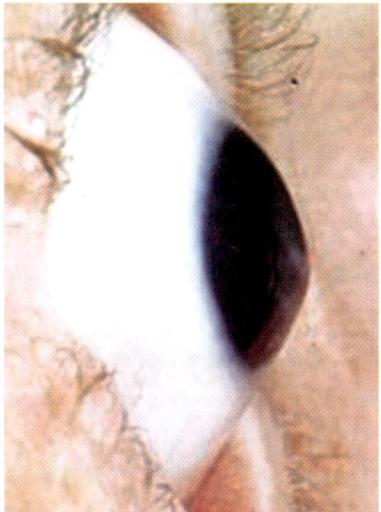

Fig. 13.6: Keratoconus

- Increased visibility of the nerve fibers.
- Ruptures in the Descemet's and Bowman's membranes.
- *Vogt's striae*: Fine vertical lines in the deeper layers of the stroma due to stretching phenomenon.
- *Fleischer's ring*—iron ring scarring at the base of the cone.

Management

- *Corneal collagen cross-linking:* It is a new technique of corneal collagen cross-linking (CXL or C3R) by the photosensitizer riboflavin and ultraviolet type rays (UVA). It increases biomechanical strength of cornea and thereby arrests the progression of keratoconus. This is used only in cases wherein progression of keratoconus has been well documented.
- *Phakic IOLs:* Phakic implants can be used to correct or reduce the refractive error.
- *Contact lens:* Contact lens improves the vision. The optimal correction can be provided by plain rigid gas permeable lenses.
- *Intacs:* Intracorneal ring segments can be used to decrease astigmatism.
- *Full thickness keratoplasty:* Once it is concluded that the condition is progressive, then it is better to put a graft early rather than wait and allow the cornea to get damaged.

Keratoglobus

Keratoglobus is a hemispherical protrusion of the whole cornea occurring bilaterally as a congenital anomaly. It is non-progressive and inherited as an autosomal recessive trait. It is a familial and hereditary condition.

Differentiated from the *buphthalmos* by the following points:

1. No rise of intraocular pressure
2. Cornea is clear
3. Normal angle of anterior chamber
4. No cupping of the disk on fundus examination.

CORNEAL PIGMENTATION

Blood Staining of Cornea (Fig. 13.7)

A young adult presents with his son with complain of complete loss of vision in his son's left eye following an incident of stone pelting while plucking mangos.

Slit-lamp shows red rusty brown cornea with clear ring in periphery.

Diagnosis—blood staining of cornea.

Blood-stained cornea gives a classical clinical picture. If seen once, then one can never forget and miss the diagnosis later throughout life.

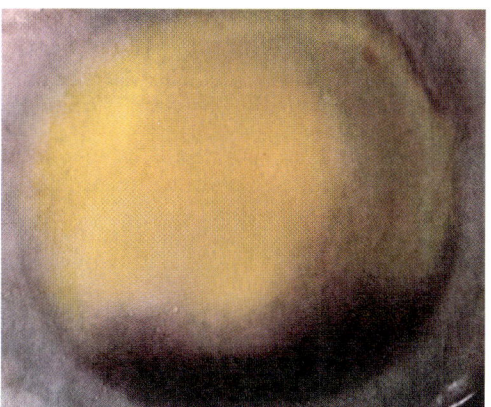

Fig. 13.7: Blood staining of cornea

Etiology

The most common cause of blood staining of cornea is a contusion injury to the eyeball and stone pelting is most common cause for contusional injury.

Pathogenesis

Blood staining of the cornea is due to absorption of the disintegrated products of the erythrocytes which have broken down in the anterior chamber in a case of total hyphema typically associated with a raised intraocular pressure.

Most likely, the blood products enter the cornea through the damaged endothelium. Thus two factors, *raised intraocular pressure and damage to endothelium*, play the important role in blood staining of the cornea.

Clinically, blood staining of cornea starts in the central part of the corneal stroma. It spreads to periphery covering the entire cornea leaving only a small clear ring round the periphery. To begin with, the *cornea appears red rusty brown which later changes to greenish yellow or grey in color.* Eyeball ultimately ends up as *atrophic bulbi.* Patient is able to perceive the light for long time. Eye is usually lost and needs artificial eye for cosmetic and social uplift.

Management

There is no treatment for blood-stained cornea.

Supportive preventive therapy

Blood staining of the cornea can be completely prevented, if the total hyphema is treated early and energetically. If the hyphema is fluid, then just control the intraocular pressure by medical therapy. If the hyphema though fluid does not show signs of absorption in a few hours, then plan to evacuate the blood from the anterior chamber by surgical procedure. If the hyphema is organized, then the only choice is to evacuate the organized blood from the anterior chamber under medical therapy to lower the high ocular pressure. A simple surgical procedure to evacuate the hyphema from the anterior chamber can save the eye and vision.

Krukenberg's Spindle

- *Krukenberg's spindle is a condition in which the pigment derived from the uveal tract is deposited on the endothelium of the cornea in a shape of a vertical small or large spindle.*
- Usually, diagnosed in routine by slit-lamp biomicroscopy.
- Usually seen in the aged and mostly in myopes and females.
- Acquired in nature and pigment is derived from the uvea.
- Associated with development of pigmentary glaucoma in later years and with diabetes also.

A case with Krukenberg's spindle must be watched for glaucoma, diabetes and myopia.

Wilson's Disease (Hepatolenticular Degeneration, Kayser-Fleischer Ring)

It is due to deficiency of the alpha-2 globulin ceruloplasmin and is characterized by deposition of copper in the tissue.

Classical ocular manifestation is Kayser-Fleischer ring in the peripheral part of the cornea in the Descemet's membrane and may show a green 'sunflower' cataract.

SYMPTOMATIC CONDITIONS

Corneal Opacity

A student of 12th standard presents with eye ache followed by headache after a few hours of study.

Slit-lamp shows central nebular opacity of cornea.

Diagnosis nebular opacity of cornea.

Corneal opacity denotes loss of transparency of cornea due to scar on healing of corneal ulcer. The density of the scar depends on the depth of the corneal thickness involved.

The corneal opacity can be of three types:

- Nebular corneal opacity
- Macular corneal opacity
- Leukomatous corneal opacity.

Nebular corneal opacity: A thin scar of the cornea is known as nebula. In this condition there is destruction of epithelium, Bowman's membrane and superficial layers of the substantia propria. It is easily diagnosed by slit-lamp examination. It affects the vision considerably if situated in the pupillary area. The vision can be improved by the use of contact lenses after complete healing.

Macular corneal opacity: A slightly denser scar than the nebular scar is known as macular opacity of the cornea. In this condition, there is destruction of epithelium, Bowman's membrane and about one-third thickness of the substantia propria. It affects the vision if situated in the pupillary area. In such case, the only treatment is lamellar keratoplasty.

Leukomatous corneal opacity: A dense, thick and white scar of the cornea is known as leukoma of the cornea. In this condition, there is destruction of epithelium, Bowman's membrane and more than one-third thickness of the substantia propria. It also affects the vision if situated in the pupillary area. The only treatment available is penetrating keratoplasty.

Management

- *Optical iridectomy* in central macular and leukomatous corneal opacity.
- *Phototherapeutic keratectomy* is indicated in nebular corneal opacity.
- *Keratoplasty* provides good vision in macular and leukomatous corneal opacity.
- *Cosmetic-colored contact lens* relieves the patient from his social embarrassment.

Xerophthalmia

Xerophthalmia covers all the ocular manifestation of vitamin A deficiency including changes affecting conjunctiva, cornea and retina along with biophysical functional disorders of retinal rods and cones.

Etiology

It occurs due to dietary deficiency of vitamin A or its defective absorption along with protein-energy malnutrition.

Vitamin A

Vitamin A is available in two forms:

1. Retinol, a preformed vitamin A
2. Beta carotene, which is converted to retinol in the intestinal mucosa.

One international unit of vitamin A is equivalent to 0.3 µm of retinol.

Daily Requirement

- Daily requirement of vitamin A is 3000 units for an adult.
- Lactating mother needs about 5000 units daily.
- Children need from 1000 to 3000 units depending on the age.

Natural Sources

- Animal food in the form of milk and milk products such as ghee, butter, paneer, and egg yolk, fish, fish liver oil of cod, halibut and shark fish.

- Vegetable food in form of green leafy vegetables such as spinach and amaranth, both available in abundance and throughout the year, and in form of yellow vegetables or fruits such as ripe mango, pumpkin, papaya, cabbage, tomato, orange, and green leaves.
- Liver has an enormous capacity to store the vitamin A in form of retinol palmitate. A healthy person has a store of vitamin A in his liver to supply him for about 6 months.

Functions of Vitamin A

- It is required for night vision. Its deficiency leads to night blindness.
- To maintain the normal functioning of the glandular and epithelial tissues.
- It is essential for normal skeletal and body growth.
- It offers good resistance to infection.

Deficiency Causes

Systemic manifestations include hyperkeratosis, anorexia, growth retardation and a general low resistance to the infection.

Ocular manifestation results in xerophthalmia.

Deficiency symptoms manifest, if the serum level is lower than 10 μg/dl, i.e. about 30 units per 100 cc of serum.

WHO Classification of Xerophthalmia

- *XN—night blindness:* It is the earliest symptom in children.
- *XIA—conjunctival xerosis:* There are thickening, wrinkling and pigmentation of conjunctiva.
- *XIB—Bitot's spot:* It is usually bilateral, raised white foamy triangular patch of keratinized epithelium on temporal side of the bulbar conjunctiva in the interpalpebral aperture.
- *X2—corneal xerosis:* Cornea appears dry and lusterless usually in the lower nasal quadrant.
- *X3A—keratomalacia:* Less than one-third of cornea surface.
- *X3B—keratomalacia:* More than one-third of cornea surface.

- *XS—corneal scar:* Thick scar in form of leukomatous opacity.
- *XF—fundus changes:* Fundus shows seed-like raised white lesions scattered uniformally.

XN—Night Blindness

Mother presents her child with complain that my baby girl is unable to pick up even her food to eat and cannot find her way home after sunset.

Diagnosis—night blindness
Usually night blindness is the first symptom to appear in a child who is deficient of vitamin A and proteins.

Deficiency symptom of night blindness manifests, if the serum level is lower than 10 μg/dl, i.e. about 30 units per 100 cc of serum.

Often the mother brings the child with a complaint that the child is not able to see after sunset or in dim light. At this stage, a single high dose of vitamin A orally with advice to give him egg or milk daily cures him of his night blindness. If the child is not taken care of at this stage and happens to suffer from an attack of acute diarrhea, then most often, the child is brought with corneal xerosis or even keratomalacia.

XIA—Conjunctival Xerosis

- Clinically, an early visible sign is the appearance of dry, lusterless conjunctiva.
- Conjunctiva appears dry and wrinkled in the palpebral area usually adjacent to the limbus.
- Chronic case may show brown pigmentation of the conjunctiva followed by appearance of Bitot's spots.

XIB—Bitot's Spots (Fig. 13.8)

Teenage girl presents with white foamy patches at limbus slightly away from and on temporal side of cornea in her both the eyes since her early child hood. She complains that these patches get stained with 'kajal' resulting in cosmetic embarrassment for me.

Slit-lamp shows slightly raised white foamy triangular patches on temporal side of both the cornea in both eyes.

Diagnosis—Bitot's spots.

- Bitot's spots appear as a triangular pearly white foamy spots on bulbar conjunctiva on either side of the cornea.
- Usually bilateral.
- Presence of Bitot's spot indicates low vitamin A and protein energy malnutrition in early childhood. These spots have been observed in pellagra and other nutritional deficiency also. These spots do not disappear even after giving a high dose of vitamin A and proteins. These spots are otherwise harmless except as cosmetic embarrassment.
- Remove surgically, if the patient desires.

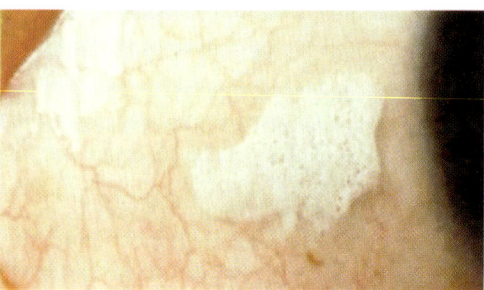

Fig. 13.8: Bitot's spot

X2—Corneal Xerosis

- Cornea appears dry and lusterless with a few white spots also. Even at this stage, if the child is brought to an ophthalmologist, then high dose of vitamin A in form of injection followed by oral therapy with diet rich in proteins can cure him/her.
- Even delay for a day or two may result in keratomalacia.
- An attack of diarrhea at this stage certainly leads to keratomalacia.

X3A and X3B—Keratomalacia (Fig. 13.9)

An elderly debilited person presents with his grandson in his lap. The child is extremely malnourished and apathetic.

Inspection shows; malnourished child with open eyes, dry luster less conjunctiva and hazy necrosed cornea with absence of any inflammatory signs.

Diagnosis—keratomalacia

Keratomalacia (xerophthalmia, xerotic keratitis) is defined as dry, cloudy and melting of cornea due to extreme deficiency of vitamin A, proteins and diet.

Clinical Features

- Keratomalacia is a condition in which there is necrosis of the cornea and cornea seems to melt away within a few hours.
- It is due to marked deficiency of vitamin A.
- It affects extremely malnourished infants who have recently suffered from acute infectious illness or acute diarrhea and look extremely ill and frequently die.

On examination of the eyes:

- Conjunctiva looks dry, lusterless with xerotic spots.
- Cornea appears dull, insensitive and hazy with necrosis. Soon the whole cornea gets necrosed and melts away.
- *Characteristic feature is the absence of any inflammatory reaction in the eyes.*
- Infant is in apathetic condition to the extent that he cannot close the lids exposing the cornea.
- If the patient has been brought in the early stage, when there are only a few spots of haze in the cornea, then probably the eyes can be saved by intensive treatment. Admission in the hospital is essential to keep a watch and treat intensively and energetically.

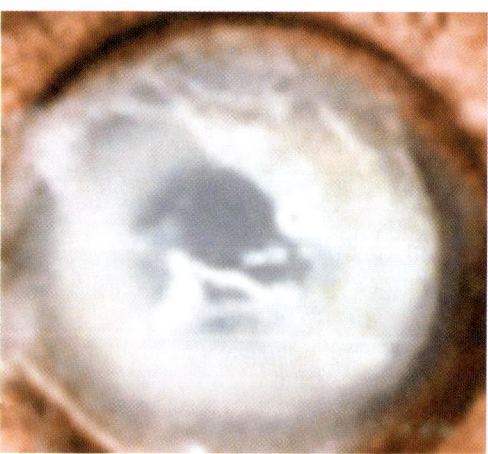

Fig. 13.9: Keratomalacia

XS—Corneal Scar

Thick scar in form of leukomatous opacity.

XF—Fundus Changes

Fundus shows seed-like raised white lesions scattered evenly.

Treatment of Xerophthalmia

Therapeutic therapy with vitamin A

- Inject vitamin A (aqueous) intramuscular; two lac units immediately followed with one lac units for four days. Thereafter daily dose of vitamin A tablets of 10,000 units daily for a month and maintenance dose of 5000 units for long time.
- Take care of protein-energy malnutrition.

Supportive therapy

- Topical broad-spectrum antibiotic eye-drops and ointment as required.
- Artificial tear eyedrops in case of conjunctival xerosis.
- Replace body fluids by intravenous route and orally as well in cases with diarrhea and dehydration.
- Feed the infant with mother's milk.
- Supplement with vitamins, minerals, high protein with good nourishing diet.

Preventive or prophylactic therapy

Under 'child survival and safe motherhood' as follows:

- As a national program to prevent blindness due to vitamin A deficiency.
- Vitamin A in concentrated form in oil base is available at all the primary health centers. It is given orally.
- Strategy is to administer a single massive dose of 200,000 lac units of vitamin A in oil (retinol palmitate) orally every 6 months to pre-school children of 1–6 years of age and 100,000 lac units of vitamin A to children between the age of 6 months and 1 year. In this way, infant and child are covered against xerophthalmia.
- Along with this the staff at the health center advises the mother about the intake of diet rich in vitamins and proteins using egg, milk, spinach, amaranth, etc. in daily diet.

Toxic Effect of High Intake of Vitamin A

Toxic effects can be nausea, vomiting, anorexia, disturbance of sleep, liver enlargement and edema of papilla.

It is rare for a person to take such high doses of vitamin A so as to cause toxic effects.

Photophthalmia

An industrial worker presents usually at mid-night with severe neuralgic unbearable pain, feeling of extreme burning, lacrimation, reflex blepharospasm and marked swelling of the lids following exposure to arc light while welding.

Slit-lamp shows marked conjunctival congestion with chemosis. Fluorescein stain is covering entire cornea.

Diagnosis—industrial photophthalmia.

Etiology

The most common cause for photophthalmia is an exposure of the eye to a source of light rich in short waves used in many occupation such as:

- Flash light in cinematography
- Photograph
- Arc welding
- Tending in arc-furnaces
- Ultraviolet lamps and lights used in medical profession.
- The main factor responsible for photophthalmia is not wearing protective goggles or not using protective screens while on job.
- Repeated small exposures over a period of 12–16 hours of working period are additive in effect. A cumulative few minutes of exposure at intervals would result in acute photophthalmia.
- Photophthalmic symptoms are produced by exposure to about 150 lumen/sq.ft measured in terms of visible light.
- Yet, a cumulative few minutes exposure from an arc light at intervals even from a distance at which the intensity of light is only 10 lumen/sq ft will manifest as an acute photophthalmia.

The photophthalmia is caused by ultraviolet rays especially from 311 to 290nm. It is commonly caused by:

- Bright flash of short circuit
- Exposure to naked arc light during welding or in studios.
- Reflection of ultraviolet rays from snow in *snow blindness*.

Solar Photophthalmia (Snow Blindness)

The solar photophthalmia is the result of solar energy reflected from these extensive areas of high reflectivity. Solar photophthalmia is encountered more on snow, therefore, it is popularly known as 'snow blindness'. Usually, it is an amature mountaineer at high altitudes suffers from this uninvited malady by sheer negligence of not using protective goggles.

Any person who happens to look at the dazzling reflection of sufficient intensity from a surface of large extensity such as sea, desert, snow or ice fields or snow mountains for long hours is likely to develop the symptoms and signs of photophthalmia.

Symptoms and Signs

The symptoms and signs may be *mild, moderate or severe*.

- Latent period of 6 to 10 hours between exposure and onset of symptoms and signs. Therefore, the patient presents at ophthalmic clinic in late hours usually at midnight. Patient wakes up because of acute symptoms of foreign body sensation, pain, burning and swelling of lids.
- Symptoms vary in intensity depending upon the time and the intensity of the exposure. With extreme intensity of exposure, the symptoms manifest even in half an hour.
- With less time and low intensity the latent period may be long even 24 hours but never more than that as the natural factor of physiological repair counteracts the abiotic effect of the radiation.
- With weak intensity and short time of exposure, the patients have mild symptoms of burning and irritation.

- Patient cannot bear even home light and feels distressed with slightest attempt to open the eyes.
- Examination can only be carried out only after proper local anesthesia of the cornea. The whole cornea may stain with fluorescein.

A typical case presents with the following·

Symptoms
- Sensation of foreign body as if the eye is full of sand particles.
- Neuralgia—severe pain, lacrimation, photophobia, reflex blepharospasm and extreme burning of the eyes.
- Marked swelling of the lids.

Signs
- Marked edema of lids.
- Edema of the corneal epithelium. Thereafter the epithelium is desquamated to form epithelial erosions usually involving the whole corneal epithelium.
- Fluorescein stain covers almost entire cornea.
- Congestion and chemosis of the conjunctiva.
- Pupil is miotic due to cyclitis.

Management

Normally, the symptoms subside after 2 days with repair of corneal epithelium. Mild symptoms of congestion and irritation persist for a few days even after complete healing of corneal epithelium.

Topical broad-spectrum antibiotic eyedrops during day and ointment at night for a week even after healing of corneal erosions.

Supportive therapy
- Cycloplegic 1% atropine eyedrops once daily to keep the pupil dilated.
- Ask the patient to sleep over. Give him/her good dose of analgesics and sedative orally or intramuscularly to make him/her sleep over to provide relief from pain and burning of the eyes.
- Assure him/her that he will get the complete vision in 2 to 3 days time, when the corneal epithelium regenerates and cover the cornea.

- Advise him/her to use protective goggles in future all the time, when he/she is exposing himself/herself to arc light or solar light.

Corneal Vascularization (Fig. 13.10)

Daily wage earner presents with irritation, photophobia, lacrimation, dim vision and difficulty in carrying out his normal work in fields or construction sites.

Slit-lamp shows corneal vascularization.

Diagnosis—corneal vascularization.

Corneal vascularization is a malady wherein cornea is invaded by blood vessels in a pathological state primarily as a defense mechanism against the disease or injury.

Corneal vascularization has a beneficial effect in resolving an inflammatory lesion. The invasion of cornea by blood vessels results in some loss of transparency and is the cause of opacification of graft due to development of antigen-antibody reaction by providing antibodies.

Clinical Types

Superficial vascularization In superficial vascularization of cornea, the vessels originate from the superficial limbal plexus by budding or loop formation and pass without interruption. The superficial vascularization can be pannus, fascicular and equalet.

Pannus An extensive superficial vascularization of cornea has been termed as a *pannus*.

Pannus can be of four types:
 a. Pannus trachomatous
 b. Pannus leprosus
 c. Pannus phlyctenulosus
 d. Pannus degenerativus

Interstitial vascularization It is derived from the anterior ciliary arteries. The new vessels are straight and do not anastomose. Slit-lamp shows that the vessels appear to disappear from the view as they traverse the boundary between the cornea and the sclera. It can be of the following types:

- *Terminal loops:* There is growth of small loops which grow out from the limbus in a deeper plane.
- *Brush form:* The vessels run in the substantia propria parallel and without any anastomosis giving an appearance of a brush.
- *Umbel form:* A large vessel runs far into the cornea and then breaks up into a star-shaped branches.
- *Network form:* There is a free communication of loops to give an appearance of a network.
- *Interstitial arcades:* These are derived from episcleral vessels and seen in the anterior portion of the cornea typically in the sclerosing lesions due to tuberculosis and leprosy.
- *Aberrant vessels:* The vessels arise from episcleral vessels and traverse the stroma of the cornea in an irregular fashion.

Deep vascularization It is a rare phenomenon, occurring in interstitial keratitis of syphilitic origin, when associated with uveitis. The vessels invade along the deepest layers of the stroma in front of Descemet's membrane.

Management

An early treatment results in reducing the opacification of cornea. An infective lesion should be treated by suitable antibiotic. Other treatments available are:

- Use of steroids locally and subconjunctivally
- Peritomy
- Superficial keratectomy.

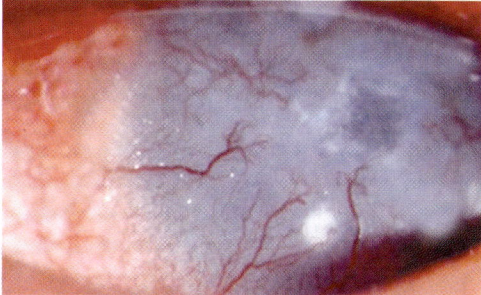

Fig. 13.10: Corneal vascularization

- Lamellar corneal graft.
- Irradiation.

Corneal Staphyloma (Fig. 13.11)

An elderly person holding the hand of his grand-daughter aged about 8 years or so presents with a straight question. Can her vision be restored by a donor eye. She lost her eye and vision following an attack of 'choti-mata'—measles, when she was 4 years of age.

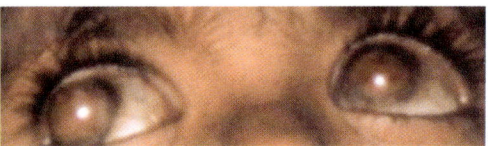

Fig. 13.11: Corneal staphyloma

Slit-lamp shows the cornea of the left eye is bulging forward like a small grape with a slight rim of healthy cornea in the upper periphery.

Diagnosis—corneal staphyloma.

Corneal staphyloma is an ectatic condition of the extensive corneal defect in which the iris gets incarcerated.

Pathogenesis

- It usually follows extensive corneal ulcer which has sloughed and cast off leaving an extensive corneal wound with normal peripheral rim of cornea and complete iris exposed. At this stage, the epithelium from the intact and healthy peripheral rim of the cornea proliferates and grows over the entire iris filling all the cervices. The cicatrization consisting of epithelium, iris stroma and exudation may be rapid and dense so that it can withstand the intra-ocular pressure and the cornea becomes flat resulting in *applanatio cornea.*

- In some cases, there is degeneration and shrinkage of the corneal scar tissue resulting in a contracted and shrunken scar *phthisis cornea.*

- If the pseudo-cornea is thin, then the iris tissue provides it with deep blue black color. Most often the thin pseudo-cornea gives way to the raised intraocular pressure and bulges as *corneal staphyloma* resulting in an embarrassing cosmetic appearance.

Management

- It is advisable to excise the eye and give an artificial eye to free the patient from his cosmetic embarrassment.
- It shall help to rebuild confidence within.

Cystoid Cicatrix and Fistula

Cystoid cicatrix and fistula result due to improper healing of the corneal scar.

- Minimal scar tissue which is loosely arranged with spaces in between. The anterior wall may be formed by epithelium and the posterior wall by the pigment layer of the iris. Thin scar gives way to the normal intraocular pressure resulting in an *ectatic cicatrix of cornea.*

- In some cases the aqueous percolates the iridic tissue and fill up the cystoid spaces in the scar forming *bullae* underneath *ectatic cystoid cicatrix.*

- In some cases, the cicatrix may burst through the epithelium to form a *corneal fistula.* Fistula favors the down growth of the epithelium making the track permanent and may also line the inner surface of the cornea, angle of the anterior chamber and the anterior surface of the iris resulting in *secondary glaucoma.*

14

Maladies of Sclera

- Episcleritis
- Anterior scleritis
- Necrotizing scleritis
- Scleromalacia perforans
- Posterior scleritis
- Scleral staphylomas
- Blue sclera

The sclera is the outer fibrous layer of the eyeball. It is covered by a thin layer of elastic tissue. The sclera is supplied by ciliary nerves. It is pierced by the optic nerve, long and short posterior ciliary arteries and nerves, four vortex veins and short anterior ciliary arteries and veins. All the six extrinsic muscles of the eyes are inserted in the sclera. The disease processes of the sclera are chronic and show poor and delayed response to treatment due to its comparative avascularity.

Episcleritis

Patient presents with localized diffuse congestion near limbus with mild pain and discomfort and pain on pressure along with joint pains.

Slit-lamp shows diffuse localized congestion near limbus.

Diagnosis—episcleritis.

Episcleritis is mild, self-limiting and recurrent inflammation of the episcleral tissue.

Etiopathogenesis

- Episcleritis is common in females.
- Hypersensitivity reaction to an endogenous toxin from any septic focus in the body especially to tubercular and streptococcal toxins.
- Most of the cases are idiopathic.
- Affects people between fourth and fifth decade.
- Many cases show associated rheumatoid arthritis or chronic systemic disease.

Symptoms

- Localized diffuse or nodular redness in the sclera with mild discomfort, photophobia and lacrimation.
- Localized diffused or nodular swelling is tender to touch and pressure.

Signs

- *Localized congestion around the diffuse swelling or nodule* is due to involvement of scleral vessels. The congestion appears purple and not bright in color as the vessels are covered by the conjunctiva.
- *Nodules near the limbus:* One or more small nodules of dense leukocytic infiltration are seen near the limbus. The nodules are hard, immovable and tender to touch. The conjunctiva moves freely over the nodules.
- The diffuse swelling or nodule never ulcerates and on healing it leaves a slate color scar to which the conjunctiva is adherent.

Complications

- Scleritis and uveitis.
- It heals with scar formation.
- Recurrence is common.

Management

- Topical steroid eyedrops and ointment is rewarding.
- Systemic administration of aspirin and salicylates is helpful in the case with a history of rheumatism.
- Investigate the case to find any septic focus or any chronic systemic disease and treat accordingly.

Anterior Scleritis (Fig. 14.1)

Patient presents with localized diffuse or nodular congestion near limbus with severe boring (piercing) ocular pain which is worse at night and awaken the patient from sleep. On asking, patient gives history of long-standing associated joint pains.

Slit-lamp shows localized deep nodular congestion which is extremely tender to touch and pressure.

Diagnosis—anterior scleritis.

Scleritis is much more severe inflammation than episcleritis. Majority of cases show association with underlying systemic immunological disease. It manifests in the second to sixth decades of life. It is more common in females and bilateral in more than half cases.

Etiology

1. *Autoimmune collagen disorders* are associated with more than 50% of cases of scleritis. It is most commonly associated with *rheumatoid arthritis*. Other common collagen disorders associated with scleritis are polyarteritis nodosa, systemic lupus erythematosus, non-specific arteritis, Wegener's granulomatosis, dermatomyositis and polychondritis.
2. *Granulomatous disorders* like tuberculosis, sarcoidosis, syphilis, and leprosy can cause scleritis.
3. *Metabolic disorders:* Gout, psoriasis and thyrotoxicosis are common metabolic diseases which can cause scleritis.

Clinical Types of Anterior Scleritis

1. Anterior diffuse non-necrotizing scleritis (brawny scleritis).
2. Anterior nodular non-necrotizing scleritis.

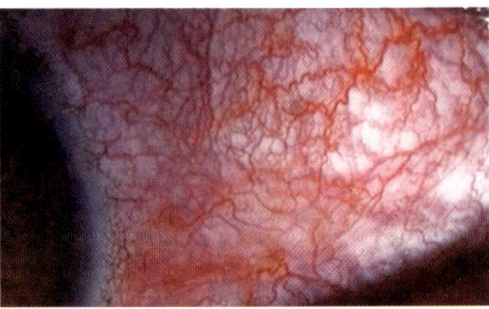

Fig. 14.1: Anterior nodular scleritis

3. Anterior necrotising scleritis with inflammation.
4. Anterior necrotizing scleritis without inflammation (scleromalacia perforans).

Symptoms

- Localized congestion with watering and discomfort.
- Mild to severe pain.
- Tenderness on touch or pressure.

Signs

- Nodule slightly away from the limbus which is hard, immovable and tender to touch.
- Localized congestion over and around the nodule.
- Conjunctiva over the nodule moves freely.

Complications

1. *Sclerosing keratitis:* Cornea adjacent to the affected sclera becomes opaque. The opacity near the corneal margin is triangular in shape with its apex towards the center of the cornea. There is no vascularization and it never ulcerates.
2. *Annular scleritis:* Involvement of the sclera all around the cornea. There is a diffuse type of nodules and congestion which appears purple and not bright red.
3. *Uveitis:* Involvement of the uveal tissue manifesting as iritis, cyclitis or anterior choroiditis.
4. *Ciliary staphyloma:* Scleritis heals leaving a thin sclera through which the uveal tissue is seen as purple cicatrix. The weak

sclera is unable to withstand even the normal intraocular pressure resulting in formation of a raised cicatrix known as ciliary staphyloma.

5. *Secondary glaucoma:* Occurrence of secondary glaucoma is common squeal due to uveitis.

6. *Scar:* Heals with gray color scar.

Investigations

- Complete blood picture with hemoglobin and ESR.
- Serum uric acid for gout.
- FTA-ABS,VDRL for syphilis.
- Tests for immunological survey; serum levels of complement (C3), immune complexes, rheumatoid factor, antinuclear antibodies, and LE
- Montoux test
- X-rays of sacroiliac joint and chest are helpful in diagnosis.
- Scleral biopsy for infective organism can be done.

Management

Steroids systemic and topical

- Systemic steroid therapy is necessary. Start steroids with a high dose and gradually reduce it to maintenance dose and withdraw soon, if there is a good response.
- Topical steroid eyedrops and ointment.
- Topical antibiotic to cover secondary infection.

Supportive therapy

- Aspirin and salicylates are helpful in resolving the nodules.
- Systemic non-steroid anti-inflammatory drugs (NSAIDs) such as indomethacin, oxyphenbutazone or flurbiprofen.
- Treat causative factor.
- Systemic antibiotics in infective scleritis.

Necrotizing Scleritis

Patient presents with severe pain out of proportion to inflammatory signs.

- Necrotizing scleritis is characterized by a localized area of congestion and necrosis which ultimately results in thinning and destruction of the sclera.
- Medical therapy in form of steroids is beneficial and effective in its early stage prior to advent of necrosis.
- Due to thinning of the sclera, a ciliary staphyloma develops in course of time.
- Use of steroid is contraindicated in later stage. Refer the case to rheumatologist also.

Scleromalacia Perforans

Scleromalacia perforans is a rare disease characterized by thinning and melting of the scleral tissue without any signs of inflammation and pain because of destruction of nerves.

- Scleromalacia perforens is usually associated with severe form of long-standing *rheumatoid arthritis.*
- Treatment consists in treating the underlying cause if detected on investigations.
- Repair the thin area of sclera with a segment of homologous preserved sclera.

Posterior Scleritis

The posterior scleritis is difficult to diagnose as the clinical signs are not visible.

Symptoms of pain, proptosis of the eyeball, limitation of the ocular movements and no obvious pathology in the anterior segment should arouse suspicion of posterior scleritis.

Treat like a case of anterior scleritis.

Ultrasound B Scans

Presence of T sign on ultrasound B scan, i.e. fluid in Tenon's sheath around optic nerve is one of the pathognomonic sign of posterior scleritis

Scleral Staphyloma

Scleral staphyloma is an ectatic condition of the sclera in which the uveal tissue is incarcerated.

Clinically, there are *five types* of scleral staphyloma:

1. *Anterior staphyloma:* The anterior staphyloma is obvious which is usually heavily pigmented. Due to uneven thinning of the sclera, the anterior staphyloma appears as lobulated dark blue color protrusions.

2. *Intercalary staphyloma:* It occurs between the anterior extremity of the ciliary body and the limbus where the sclera is weak due to presence of the anterior ciliary veins and the canal of Schlemn.
3. *Ciliary staphyloma* (Fig. 14.2): It occurs in the region of the ciliary body where the anterior ciliary arteries penetrate.
- It is difficult to differentiate the ciliary staphyloma from the intercalary staphyloma even than the location of anterior ciliary arteries is helpful to differentiate.

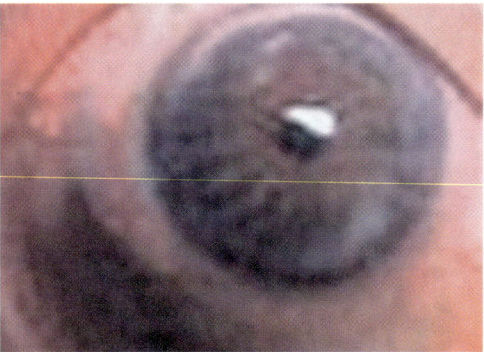

Fig. 14.2: Ciliary staphyloma

- In the ciliary staphyloma, the anterior ciliary arteries emerge at the anterior border of the bulge and the dark striae of the ciliary processes can be seen on transillumination.
- In the intercalary staphyloma, the anterior ciliary arteries emerge posterior.
4. *Equatorial staphyloma:* It occurs due to weakness of the sclera at the site where the vortex veins penetrate the sclera. It is diagnosed during surgery undertaken for retinal detachment wherein the equatorial region of the sclera is exposed. There are no symptoms of any kind.
5. *Posterior staphyloma:* Posterior staphyloma is seen in a case of high myopia. It can be diagnosed only by ophthalmoscopy. The posterior pole bulges backwards giving rise to kinking of retinal vessels. In fact it is only ectasia of the sclera.

Complications of Staphyloma

- *Glaucoma:* Common complication of anterior staphyloma.
- *Retinal detachment:* Retinal detachment is common in a case of equatorial staphyloma.

Management

Glaucoma surgery in a case of anterior staphyloma is enough to retard or even stop the progress of staphyloma.

An equatorial staphyloma can be managed by scleral resection, buckling operation, or scleroplasty.

Blue Sclera

The normal sclera is white and opaque. Thinning of the sclera allows the underlying uveal tissue to be seen through, therefore, the sclera appears blue in color. Blue sclera is seen in normal infants, in keratoconus and in keratoglobus. Blue sclera is seen in osteogenesis imperfecta, pseudoxanthoma elasticum and Marfan's syndrome. The treatment is not required.

15

Maladies of Uveal Tract

Congenital Anomalies

- Persistent pupillary membrane
- Coloboma
- Albinism
- Heterochromia iridium
- Heterochromia iridis
- Aniridia (irideremia)
- Polycoria
- Corectopia (ectopia pupillae)

Uveitis—Inflammation of Uveal Tract

- Anterior uveitis
- Posterior uveitis
- Detachment of the choroid
- Sympathetic uveitis

Lens Induced Uveitis

Phacoanaphylactic uveitis

Viral Uveitis

- Herpes simplex uveitis
- Herpes zoster uveitis

Fungal Uveitis

Candiasis

Uveitis due to Chronic Systemic Maladies

- Tubercular uveitis
- Syphilitic uveitis
- Leprotic uveitis
- Uveitis with sarcoidosis
- Uveitis with toxoplasmosis
- Uveitis with onchocerciasis
- Uveitis with brucellosis
- Uveitis with arthritis (ankylosing spondylitis)

Syndromes Associated with Uveitis

- Posner-Schlossman syndrome (glaucomato-cyclitic crisis)
- Fuch's uveitis syndrome
- Ocular histoplasma syndrome
- Uveoparotitis (Heerfordt's) syndrome
- Behçet's syndrome (recurrent iridocyclitis with hypopyon)
- Reiter's syndrome and uveitis
- Vogt-Koyanagi-Harada's syndrome (uveo-meningitis syndrome)

Degeneration—Dystrophy

- Essential atrophy of iris
- Gyrate atrophy of choroid
- Choroideremia
- Senile central choroidal atrophy

Purulent Uveitis

- Endophthalmitis
- Panophthalmitis

CONGENITAL ANOMALIES

Persistent Pupillary Membrane (Fig. 15.1)

Persistent pupillary membrane is due to persistence of the part of the anterior vascular sheath of the lens which normally disappears before birth. It is common in babies and disappears with age but may persist permanently.

- Slit-lamp shows fine threads of iris tissue stretching across the pupil to be anchored on the opposite side or on the lens.
- Persistent pupillary membrane either in form of fine threads or pigment on the lens does not affect the visual acuity.

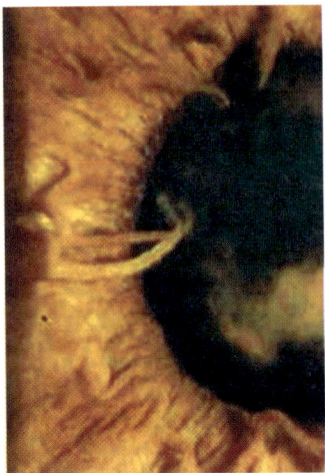

Fig. 15.1: Persistent pupillary membrane

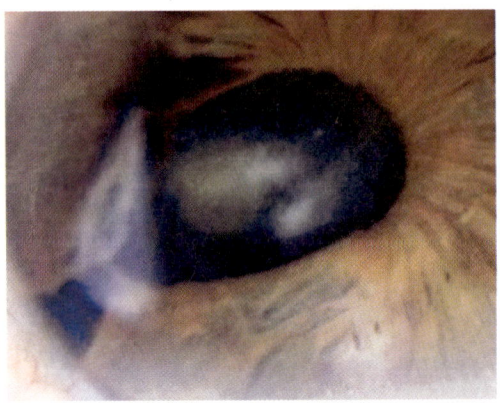

Fig. 15.2: Iris coloboma

- In some cases, the pigment is seen on the lens surface as fine brown spots, small in size, stellate in shape, numerous and regularly arranged with no signs of iridocyclitis.
- These spots are to be differentiated from the pigment spots left on the lens in iridocyclitis after the synechia has broken. These spots are thick, much less in number, irregularly arranged and with all the signs of iridocyclitis.

Coloboma (Fig. 15.2)

As a rule, the coloboma is due to defective closure of the embryonic cleft, therefore, the coloboma occurs in the lower part of the eye.

One of the commonest congenital defects of the eye is coloboma in which the tissues of the uvea and associated retinal tissues are deficient.

Typical coloboma of iris is pear-shaped, runs downwards and slightly inwards and extends from the pupil towards the ciliary body but not always up to it.

Atypical coloboma of iris occurs in other direction.

Coloboma of retina and choroid is oval in shape with rounded apex towards the optic disk which may or may not be included. A few retinal vessels may crossover the surface. The choroidal vessels are at the edges. The vision is affected and there is a scotoma in the field corresponding to the coloboma.

Albinism

Albinism is a hereditary disorder of defective development of pigment throughout the body.

The albinism may be ocular, oculocutaneous and cutaneous in form.

The ocular albinism has the following features:
- The iris looks pink
- There is photophobia
- Nystagmus
- Diminution of vision
- Occasionally strabismus
- Fundus shows the retinal and choroidal vessels against white ground of sclera.
- Partial albinism is common wherein the absence of pigment is limited to choroid and retina and the iris appears blue. These cases have fair hair as children.

There is no treatment except that the patient can be advised to use dark glasses to avoid photophobia.

Heterochromia Iridium

In this condition, the color of iris in right eye differs from the color of iris in the left eye.

Heterochromia Iridis

In this condition, usually a sector of iris in one eye may differ in color from the rest of the iris in the same eye.

Aniridia (Irideremia)

Aniridia is a rare condition in which the iris is extremely rudimentary.

It has the following features:

- The pupil appears very large.
- On focal illumination and slit-lamp examination, the margin of the lens, the zonules and even ciliary process can be seen.
- Diminution of vision.
- Marked photophobia.
- Nystagmus.
- The patient is prone to glaucoma due to anomaly at the angle of anterior chamber.

Polycoria

Polycoria is a condition in which there is more than one pupil.

It is rare to have more than one pupil with a sphincter. Thus the other pupil is a hole in the iris and falls in the category of coloboma.

Corectopia (Ectopia Pupillae)

Corectopia is a condition in which the pupil is not at its normal position.

The normal position of the pupil is slightly down and in from the center of the iris. In corectopia, the most common position of the pupil is up and out. It is usually bilateral. The eyes are myopic with poor vision.

UVEITIS—INFLAMMATION OF UVEAL TRACT

*The term **uveitis** covers inflammation of the uveal tract, the iris, ciliary body and choroid as a whole.*

Anatomical Classification

- Anterior uveitis—iridocyclitis
- Posterior uveitis—choroiditis

Clinical Classification

- Acute uveitis
- Chronic uveitis

Pathological Classification

- Exudative uveitis
- Granulomatous uveitis

Etiology of Uveitis

1. *Endogenous infection:* The endogenous infection results due to the organisms lodged in other organs of the body reaching the uveal tissue or the eyeball through the bloodstream. It can be bacterial, viral, fungal, parasitic and rickettsial infection.

2. *Secondary to infection of other ocular tissues:* The structures in close relation to the uveal tract are the cornea, sclera and the retina. The infection from these tissues can easily spread to the associated uveal tissues— iris, ciliary body and choroid.

3. *Exogenous infection:* The exogenous infection is usually suppurative resulting in an acute uveitis—iridocyclitis, endophthalmitis or even panophthalmitis. It is due to entry of organisms into the eye through a perforating injury or a perforating corneal ulcer.

4. *Allergic inflammation:* An allergic reaction of the uveal tissue is common. There is a primary source of infection present in some organs of the body. When the organisms from these sources enter the bloodstream and while circulating in the system make the ocular tissues sensitive to them with formation of antibodies. Later after months or years the original primary focus of infection becomes active again and causes fresh dissemination of organisms or their proteins into the bloodstream which on coming in contact with the already sensitized ocular tissue excites an allergic inflammatory response. The most common source of infection is teeth, paranasal sinuses, tonsils, prostate, genitourinary tract.

5. *Autoimmune uveitis:* It is seen in association with autoimmune maladies such as; rheumatoid arthritis, ankylosing spondylitis, Reiter's disease, systemic lupus erythematosus and Wegener's granulomatosis.

6. *HLA- associated uveitis*: Human leukocytic antigens denote histocompatibility antigens such as:
    i. *HLA-B27*-associated with ankylosing spondylitis and Reiter's disease.

ii. *HLA-B5*-associated in Behçet's syndrome.

iii. *HLA-DR4* and *DW15*-associated in Vogt-Koyanagi-Harada syndrome.

7. *Toxic uveitis:* The toxins can be endotoxins, endocular or exogenous.

8. *Traumatic uveitis:* Any kind of trauma can induce uveitis.

Pathogenesis

Granulomatous uveitis occurs due to invasion of the eye by living organisms. The inflammation tends to be insidious in onset and chronic in nature with minimal reaction of the tissue.

Such inflammations are characterized by dense nodular infiltration of the tissue rather than the diffuse exudative reaction. If immunity develops, the infiltration becomes circumscribed and relapse occurs, if the resistance is low. If hypersensitivity develops, then the further invasion by organisms leads to necrosis and caseation.

Clinically, such an inflammation is characterized by formation of dense synechia and large mutton fat keratic precipitates are seen on the back of the cornea. The clinical picture varies with the type of organism concerned.

Exudative uveitis

Exudative type of reaction tends to be of acute onset, short duration, diffuse in nature and without focal lesions in the iris.

There is a flare in the aqueous and keratic precipitates.

Relapses are common and each attack of uveitis causes further impairment of vision and the iris shows patches of atrophy.

Anterior Uveitis

Patient presents with his left eye covered by hanky and palm of his left hand and complains of acute intense pin pricking pain, red eye, photophobia and watering of the left eye since yesterday evening.

Ocular examination shows circumciliary congestion, pin point pupil and hazy cornea.

Topical atropine 1% eyedrops until the pupil dilate. The dilation of pupil provides immediate relief from *intense pin pricking pain in the eyes and slit-lamp biomicroscopy shows pigment on the lens, synechia, cells and aqueous flare.*

Diagnosis—acute anterior uveitis—iridocyclitis.

Anterior uveitis *refers to* **iridocyclitis**—*an inflammation of iris and ciliary body as a whole; as iritis is always associated with some cyclitis and cyclitis with some iritis.*

Pathogenesis

To understand the pathogenesis of *anterior uveitis or iridocyclitis*, it is essential to keep in mind the anatomy of the iris and ciliary body and the pathological changes which occur in these due to inflammatory process.

The iris is a diaphragm of radially arranged blood vessels, unstripped muscle fibers, and loose spongy stroma. The pupillary margin slides freely upon the lens capsule.

The ciliary body consists of ciliary muscle which slackens the suspensory ligaments of the lens in the act of accommodation and ciliary processes which secrete the aqueous humor.

The iris and ciliary body respond to inflammation as all the connective tissue in the body showing the same characteristics, i.e. dilation of blood vessels with impairment of capillary walls and therefore, exudation of protein rich fluid into the spongy connective tissue of the iris and ciliary body with production of protein rich aqueous humor (plasmoid aqueous) into the anterior chamber.

The rich blood supply of the iris, the radial arrangement of blood vessels of the iris, the loose spongy stroma of iris, the unstripped muscles the dilator and sphincter papillae, plasmoid aqueous and the nerves the parasympathetic, the sympathetic and sensory; all of which result in a special generic features in form of symptoms and signs of inflammation which vary with the intensity of causative factor and tissue response.

Symptoms

1. *Redness around the limbus:* It is due to hyperemia of anterior ciliary vessels which supply the iris.

2. *Intense pain in the eye:* It is due to irritation of the sensory nerve supply of the iris by the toxic substances in the exudation which collects in the spongy iris tissue. The patient complains of severe pin pricking pain in the eye. It is more at night and on exposure to the bright light. It may be referred to forehead, cheeks, nose and teeth.

3. *Photophobia:* It is due to irritation of sensory nerve supply of the iris, when the pupil constricts, when exposed to bright light.

4. *Lacrimation:* It is due to hyperemia and reflex irritation.

5. *Floating black spots:* It is due to vitreous opacities. It is a positive sign of cyclitis.

6. *Dim vision:* It is due to aqueous flare, keratic precipitates, constriction of pupil with exudates in the pupillary area and vitreous.

7. *Tenderness to touch:* It is a typical symptom of cyclitis.

Signs

Slit-lamp is mandatory to elicit most of the early signs for diagnosis and treatment.

1. *Circumciliary congestion:* It is due to dilated anterior ciliary vessels which supply the iris.

2. *Muddy iris (waterlogged iris or loss of the pattern of iris):* As the iris stroma is a spongy connective tissue, it can withhold the exudation from the impairment of the capillary walls of the iris capillaries. This waterlogging of the iris results in:
   - *Muddy iris*—loss of the pattern of iris.
   - *Sluggish pupillary reaction* due to impairment of the free movement of the pupil.
   - *Change in the color of the iris* due to atrophy.

3. *Constriction of the pupil:* The constriction of the pupil is one of the most important signs of iridocyclitis. It occurs due to the following three factors:
   a. Due to hyperemia, the radially arranged vessels of the iris become full and straight thereby result in constriction of the pupil.
   b. The waterlogged iris is unable to move freely, therefore, the pupillary reaction

becomes sluggish and later the pupil constricts with no reaction.

   c. The toxin in the iris stroma causes irritation of the nerve supply of the iris. The pupil constricts since the sphincter muscle overcomes the dilator muscle, i.e. the third nerve the parasympathetic nerve supply overpowers the sympathetic nerve supply.

4. *Aqueous cells:* It is an early sign. The cells in the aqueous can be counted in an oblique beam with intense light and magnification.

5. *Aqueous flare:* The aqueous flare is due to presence of protein-rich aqueous humor— the *plasmoid aqueous* into the anterior chamber. It is due to exudation of fluid from the impaired capillary walls of the iris. The aqueous flare can be seen only by a short 2 mm beam of light from a slit-lamp directed obliquely. The light beam appears empty, if the aqueous is clear. *The aqueous flare is visible, only when the aqueous is plasmoid in character.*

6. *Keratic precipitates* (Fig. 15.3): Keratic precipitates are typically seen in a triangular form in the lower part of the corneal endothelium.

   This peculiar distribution is due to convection current in the aqueous humor. The keratic precipitates are composed of chronic inflammatory cells such as macrophages, lymphocytes and plasma cells. The corneal endothelium gets covered by hundreds of keratic precipitates.

   - *Micro or medium size keratic precipitates* are pathognomonic for *exudative uveitis*. These are small or medium size, discrete, dirty

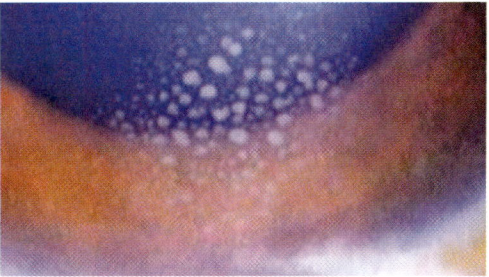

Fig. 15.3: Keratic precipitates

white, numerous and composed of lymphocytes.
- *Large size keratic precipitates* are pathognomonic for *granulomatous uveitis*. These are few large, thick, fluffy keratic precipitates giving waxy in appearance, therefore, known as *'mutton fat'* keratic precipitates. These are composed of epitheloid cells and mononuclear macrophages.
- *Fresh keratic precipitates* are white in color and round in shape.
- *Old keratic precipitates* are shrunken and pigmented.
  Presence of keratic precipitates is diagnostic for cyclitis.
  Keratic precipitates are best examined by retroillumination method of slit-lamp biomicroscopy. In the retroillumination, the cornea is illuminated by the light reflected from the iris and fundus.

7. *Vitreous opacities:* The vitreous may show opacities due to inflammatory cells and exudates poured in the vitreous humor usually in patients with predominant cyclitis.

8. *Retinal phlebitis:* There may be inflammation of the retinal vessels which may leak to result in vitreous hemorrhage.

Complications

All the complications of anterior uveitis or iridocyclitis are due to exudation which is being poured out from the impaired capillary walls of uveal tissue—the iris and ciliary body. The complications depend on the type and the amount of exudation and where it collects and gets organized.

1. **In relation to cornea**: Keratic precipitates.
2. **In relation to anterior chamber**
   - Aqueous cells
   - Aqueous flare.
3. **In relation to iris**: Synechia—adhesion of the iris to other tissue of the eye is synechia.
   - *Anterior synechia:* The iris gets adherent to the posterior surface of the cornea. It usually follows perforating injury or perforating corneal ulcer.
   - *Peripheral anterior synechia:* The adherence of the peripheral iris to the back of the cornea at the angle of the anterior chamber is known as the peripheral anterior synechia. It causes block of the angle, therefore, leads to secondary glaucoma. A filtering operation is needed to treat the secondary glaucoma.
   - *Annular or ring synechia or seclusio pupil:* In this condition, the whole pupillary margin is adherent to the lens capsule. As there is no passage for the aqueous to enter the anterior chamber, the aqueous collects behind the iris which becomes bowed forwards like a sail of a yacht. This condition of bowing forward of the iris is known as *'iris bombe'*. In this condition, the anterior chamber appears funnel-shaped, i.e. the chamber is shallow in the periphery and deep in the center. It leads to secondary glaucoma due to block at the angle and at the pupil. In early stage, before the peripheral anterior synechia becomes organized a simple iridotomy or four dot iridotomy may relieve the block by providing a passage to the aqueous from the posterior chamber to the anterior chamber. A laser iridotomy is preferable.
   - *Posterior synechia* (Fig. 15.4)*:* The adhesion of the iris to the anterior lens capsule is known as posterior synechia. It is better appreciated, when the pupil is dilated by mydriatic and cycloplegic. The pupil appears irregular, free at certain part of the pupillary margin and adherent at certain part of the pupillary margin.
   - *Total posterior synechia:* The complete adherence of the posterior surface of the iris to the underlying lens is known as total posterior synechia. In this condition the chamber appears deep throughout especially in the periphery due to retraction of the iris.

4. **In relation to pupil**
   - *Festooned (irregular) appearance of the pupil:* In the late stage of posterior

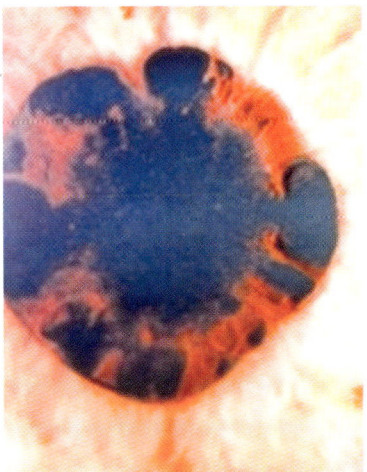

Fig. 15.4: Posterior synechia

synechia the adhesion between the iris and the lens capsule gets organized. Cycloplegic causes dilation of the part of the pupil which is not firmly adherent, thereby the pupil assumes a festooned (irregular) appearance.

An irregular pupil is pathognomonic and diagnostic sign of present or past iridocyclitis.

- *Ectropion of the uveal pigment at the pupillary margin:* It occurs due to contraction of organizing exudates upon the iris, thereby the pigment epithelium on the posterior surface of the iris is pulled around the pupillary margin so that the patches of the pigment on the posterior surface of iris at the pupil are visible as an ectropion of the uveal pigment.
- *Occlusio-pupil or blocked pupil:* The exudates organize across the entire pupillary area giving an appearance of formation of an opaque film. The pupil is not visible as the margin is covered by the organized film of exudates.

5. In relation to lens
- *Pigment deposits on anterior lens capsule:* In an early stage of posterior, synechia if the pupil is dilated by mydriatic and cycloplegic, then the synechia may break leaving the pupil dilated and circular in shape. In such a case spots of pigment derived from the posterior layer of the iris are left permanently upon the anterior capsule of the lens due to breaking of synechia by mydriatic and cycloplegic. These spots are thick, a few in number and irregularly arranged. These pigment spots are a valuable evidence of previous anterior uveitis or iridocyclitis.

However, these spots need to be differentiated from the congenital spots of pigment due to *persistent pupillary membrane.* The congenital spots are much smaller in size, stellate in shape, much more in number and regularly arranged with absence of any signs of iridocyclitis.

There is no treatment by which these spots of pigment can be removed whether due to iridocyclitis or congenital. They do not interfere with vision.

- *Complicated cataract:* Typical features of complicated cataract in early stage are 'Polychromatic luster' and 'bread-crumb' appearance in the posterior capsule.
- *Cyclitic membrane or pseudoglioma:* The exudates may form a membrane behind the lens which gives a white reflex from the pupil, when examined with the ophthalmoscope or slit-lamp or even by a simple torch. Patient with glioma also gives a white reflex from the pupil.

Differentiate the white reflex of glioma from white reflex due to cyclitic membrane.

6. In relation to vitreous
- *Vitreous opacities:* The vitreous opacities occur most commonly in patient with predominant cyclitis. The opacities are wandering leukocytes, coagulated fibrin and albuminous particles. The free mobility of these opacities shows that the vitreous gel has become fluid in nature. The exudates may organize in the vitreous as fibrous strands which become anchored to the retina at various places. These strands on contraction lead to retinal detachment. The vitreous opacities cause dim vision.

7. In relation to intraocular pressure

- *Hypertensive iridocyclitis: A* rise in the intraocular pressure during iridocyclitis is labeled as hypertensive iridocyclitis. The rise in the intraocular pressure can occur due to following factors:
  a. By the height of the pressure in the dilated capillaries.
  b. Difficulty in drainage of plasmoid aqueous through the filtration channels at the angle of the anterior chamber.
  c. Block to the drainage of aqueous at the pupil due to ring synechia or at the angle due to peripheral anterior synechia.

- *Pthisis bulbi or soft shrunken eyeball with low tension:* Phthisis bulbi occurs in the later stage of iridocyclitis due to atrophy of ciliary processes, thereby there is less or no secretion of aqueous humor. It affects the nutrition of the eyeball. The vitreous becomes fluid and the lens gets opaque.

The eyeball appears shrunken and soft which is an *ominous sign.*

Diagnosis

With all the symptoms and signs as described above, there should be no difficulty in the diagnosis of iridocyclitis.

In the early stage, the presence of cells in the aqueous, aqueous flare or keratic precipitates is pathognomonic and diagnostic.

Investigations

- Complete blood picture with ESR and smear.
- Blood sugar-fasting and postprandial to exclude diabetes.
- Complete urine examination. Culture if pus cells.
- Stool examination for cyst and ova.
- X-ray chest, paranasal sinuses.

Management

1. *Topical mydriatic and cycloplegic drugs*: Mydriasis and cycloplegia is usually achieved by topical use of atropine 1% eye-drops three times a day. The aim is to break the synechia and achieve full mydriasis and cycloplegia and maintain it for at least 2 to 3 weeks after the subsidence of acute phase of anterior uveitis.

These act in the three ways:

a. It provides relief from pain by *dilation of pupil and paralysis of ciliary muscle,* thereby putting the iris and ciliary muscle to rest. As there is no movement of the iris and no action of the ciliary muscle, there is no irritation of sensory nerve endings, therefore pain is markedly reduced.

b. It reduces hyperemia there by the exudation is reduced and thus all the signs, symptoms and complications associated with exudation are reduced.

c. It prevents formation of synechia and breaks down the synechia already formed, if not firmly organized. With the prevention of formation of synechia or breaking down the synechia, many complications associated with synechia formation are avoided.

2. *Systemic and topical steroids:* Steroids should be used topically, subconjunctivally and in some cases even systemic. The results are dramatic. Steroids reduce exudation, therefore, the eye becomes normal rapidly with almost no complications.

3. *Systemic and topical broad-spectrum antibiotic:* A course of systemic and topical antibiotic to cover up any focus of infection.

4. *Supportive therapy:*

- *Anti-inflammatory and analgesics* such as aspirin, paracetamol, salicylates, brufen, phenylbutazone, oxyphenbutazone.

- *Systemic antibiotics* should be given depending upon the investigation reports or finding any focus of infection which may be presumed as the etiological factor.

- Good nourishing diet with vitamins.

- Rest to the patient for few days until he/she shows signs of recovery from acute phase.

Posterior Uveitis

Patient presents with complain of dim vision, objects appear smaller than normal, one black spot in the field of vision and many black floaters.

Ophthalmoscopy shows a patch of choroiditis close to macula and many scattered spots.

Diagnosis—posterior uveitis choroiditis.

Posterior uveitis *refers to* **choroiditis**—*an inflammation of choroid.*

Pathogenesis

The pathogenesis of choroditis can be easily and clearly observed by ophthalmoscopy and slit-lamp.

A recent focus of choroiditis appears as a yellowish area which lies deeper to retinal vessels, when close to it.

In early stage of disease process, the membrane of Bruch is intact, therefore, only fluid can pass through it. This passage of fluid makes the overlying retina cloudy and grey with ill-defined edges. The fluid passes into the retina and vitreous giving rise to fine punctate or diffuse vitreous opacities.

Though the membrane of Bruch offers a good resistance but later it is destroyed by the inflammatory process, thereby allowing the leukocytes to pass in the retina and through it in the vitreous showing a whitish yellow patch in the retina and marked haze of the vitreous.

Later due to fibroblastic activity of the choroidal stroma, the spots of exudation become organized, thereby fusing the retina and the choroid.

The color of the spots gradually changes to white partly due to fibrous tissue and partly by the reflex from the sclera. The pigment of the destroyed retinal pigmentary epithelium tends to become heaped up into masses usually at the edges of the healed spots of choroiditis. The pigment cells also proliferate to form masses of black pigment in the white opaque spots.

Thus the ultimate picture of a spot of healed choroiditis is a white spot of scar tissue surrounded by black pigment at the edges or in the opaque areas lying deep to retinal vessels. This remains unaltered permanently.

Symptoms

1. *Diminution of vision:* If the lesions are located at the macula or near about it and due to vitreous opacities.

2. *Photopsia:* The patient complains of seeing flashes of light usually in dark and on movement of the eyeball. The flashes occur due to the irritation of the retina as the fluid vitreous affects it during the movement of the eyeball.

3. *Metamorphopsia:* The patient complains of seeing a straight line as a wavy line. This is due to edema at the macula or near about thereby the contour of the retina is altered so the line appears wavy instead of a straight line.

4. *Micropsia and macropsia:* The image of an object is formed at the macula. The size of the image so formed depends on the distance of rods and cones from each other. In macular or central choroiditis due to exudation at the macula, the rods and cones may either get separated or crowded together.
   If there is separation of rods and cones, then the objects appear smaller—the condition known as *'micropsia'*.
   If there is crowding together of rods and cones then the objects appear larger—the condition known as *'macropsia'*.

5. *Positive and negative scotoma:* Any active and fresh lesion of the retina and choroid excites a visual sensation. This lesion of retina and choroid gives rise to a feeling of seeing *a black spot in the field of vision* corresponding to the lesion. This area perceived by the patient as a black spot in his/her field of vision is referred to as a *'positive scotoma'*. This feeling persists until the retina is viable and can excite visual sensation.
   Later due to fibrosis and healing the retina is destroyed and cannot excite a visual sensation. The patient no more complains of seeing a black spot in his field of vision corresponding to the lesion. Though the patient does not complain but the area of the lesion can be charted on charting the visual field and this area so charted is referred to as *'negative scotoma'*.

6. *Floating black spots:* In choroiditis, the exudation enters the vitreous giving rise to vitreous opacities. These vitreous opacities appear as black spots moving freely before the eye in patient's field of vision. These opacities can be easily seen by an ophthalmoscope. These appear as black spots in the red reflex from the fundus. Ask the patient to move his/her eyes and then look straight forward. The vitreous opacities are seen moving freely in the vitreous though the eye is stationary.

Signs

- Yellowish spot deeper to retinal vessels is pathognomonic.
- White grey spot with ill-defined edges.
- White grey spot with black pigments heaped up along its edges and in the opaque area also.
- Vitreous shows numerous fine or course floating opacities.

Types of Choroiditis

Choroiditis has been classified in various types depending on the number and location of lesions.

Disseminated choroiditis The lesions are scattered over large part of the fundus usually behind the equator. Every lesion undergoes all the stages and heals leaving a scar, i.e. a white area with black pigments at the edges. Fresh lesions occur and pass through the same process. So, one can see almost all the stages. *Ultimately almost whole of the posterior fundus is covered with atrophic areas.*

Anterior choroiditis The lesions are located in the periphery of the fundus thereby they can pass unnoticed by the patient as there are no symptoms observed by him/her. They are usually noticed on a routine examination of fundus. They should be differentiated from the lesions due to myopic degeneration and senile degeneration. There is mild cyclitis. Slit-lamp biomicroscopy may show a few keratic precipitates.

Central choroiditis The lesions involve macula only or macula may be involved in association with disseminated choroiditis. There is marked loss of vision.

Juxtapapillary choroiditis The lesions are located close to the optic disk. There may be an isolated single lesion or the lesions may surround the optic disk. The lesions are oval-shaped and about same size as of the optic disk.

It leaves a sector-shaped defect in the field of vision. It may also be the cause of the enlargement of the blind spot.

Management

Systemic broad-spectrum antibiotic and steroid

- *Start a course of systemic broad-spectrum antibiotics.*
- Start a course of systemic steroids 80-100 mg prednisolone daily for 5 days and taper it off in about 30 days to the minimum maintenance dose for long time.
- Topical broad-spectrum antibiotic and steroid if there are signs of cyclitis.

Supportive therapy

- *Rest to the patient for few days until he/she shows signs of recovery from acute phase.*
- Good nourishing diet with vitamins.

Detachment of the Choroid

Clinical Features

- The most common condition in which there occurs a detachment of the choroid is following an intraocular operation usually cataract operation.
- Due to low intraocular pressure, there is vasodilation and exudation in the outer lamellae of the choroid.
- Slit-lamp shows very shallow anterior chamber.
- Ophthalmoscopy, a dark mass is visible in the upper quadrant. The prognosis is good as usually the choroid is replaced and the chamber is formed in course of few days.
- In a case wherein the intraocular pressure remains low for a longer period, then there are chances for development of secondary obstructive glaucoma due to formation of

peripheral anterior synechia at the angle of anterior chamber due to shallow or absent chamber.

Management

- Sometimes wait and watch with systemic administration of acctazolamide proves useful.
- It is essential that every case is thoroughly examined for any leak of the wound and treat it.

Sympathetic Uveitis

Patient presents with history of severely injured right eye with no useful vision, with mild symptoms of discomfort, photophobia, lacrimation and difficulty in near work.

Slit-lamp examination shows few cells and mild aqueous flare.

Diagnosis—sympathetic uveitis ophthalmitis.

Sympathetic uveitis (ophthalmitis) is a condition in which the normal eye (sound eye) gets inflamed after an injury to the other eye.

The malady is rare now because of better and early management of the injured eye and use of steroids.

Etiology

The etiology is unknown but two views postulated:

- *Infective:* As no organism has been demonstrated, a hypothetical virus infection has been thought of.
- *Allergic:* On the other hand, purely allergic origin to uveal pigment has been postulated. The uveal pigment can act as an allergen.

The viral infection may be the initiating factor by modifying uveal proteins to the extent that they become unusually antigenic or by damaging the cells directly uncover intracellular antigens.

Predisposing Factors

1. Sympathetic uveitis always occurs after perforating wounds, especially when the area involved is the ciliary zone, the "dangerous zone" involving the ciliary body and leading to its incarceration in the wound.
2. Sympathetic uveitis is more common in the cases with wounds in which there is incarceration of iris, ciliary body and lens capsule.
3. Children are more susceptible to it.
4. Sympathetic uveitis usually sets in after 4 to 8 weeks of the injury. The earliest reported case is 9 days and it may be delayed for many months or years.

Pathology

The microscopic features are same in both the exciting and sympathising eyes. The microscopic examination shows nodular aggregations of lymphocytes, plasma cells scattered throughout the uveal tract. The pigment epithelium of the iris, ciliary body and choroid proliferates to form nodular aggregations known as *Dalen-Fuch's nodules* and the tissues become invaded by lymphocytes and epithelioid cells. Later the giant cells appear. The picture is almost like that in tuberculosis of the uveal tract although caseation is never present.

Symptoms and Signs in Injured—Exciting Eye

There are always some symptoms and signs of iridocyclitis in the injured eye even though it may have remained quiescent for months.

Symptoms in the Uninjured-Sympathizing Sound Eye

Prodromal symptoms

- Mild discomfort
- Photophobia
- Transient blurring of near vision due to weak accommodation.
- Mild lacrimation.
- Tenderness of the eyeball
- Dim vision
- Circumciliary congestion.

Signs in the Uninjured—Sympathizing Sound Eye

- Circumciliary congestion
- Cells and aqueous flare
- Keratic precipitates
- Vitreous opacities
- Edema of the disk on fundus examination **showing** occurrence of neuroretinitis
- Lesions of posterior uveitis—choroiditis
- All the signs of iridocyclitis.

Treatment

Prophylactic treatment

- It should be kept in mind that sympathetic ophthalmitis never occurs after the excision of the injured eye unless it has already commenced at the time of excision. *Therefore, an early excision of the injured eye is a safeguard against the malady.* Thus, it is advisable to excise any eye in which it is impossible to save useful vision.
- In case of doubt, take utmost care to free the uveal tissue and lens material from the wound to reduce the chances of constant irritation.

If the sympathetic ophthalmitis has already set in, then it is wise to wait and treat the case with the entire care using steroid and decide later. It is probable that the injured eye may retain more useful vision than the uninjured eye.

Curative treatment Use steroid topically and systemically in high dose.

- Steroid—systemic, subconjunctival and topical.
- Steroids are used for long period and taper gradually.
- Treat sympathetic uveitis as a case of acute iridocyclitis.

LENS-INDUCED UVEITIS

Phacoanaphylactic Uveitis

Patient presents with pain, redness and dim vision after cataract surgery.

- An autoimmune response to lens protein in the sensitized eye.
- Type of severe granulomatous anterior uveitis.

- Lens-induced uveitis can occur following a trauma to lens, after extracapsular cataract surgery and in cases with hypermature cataract.
- In hypermature cataract, lens capsule leaks and the lens material passes into the anterior chamber causing an inflammatory reaction characterized by accumulation of plasma cells, mononuclear phagocytes and a few polymorphonuclear cells.
- Eye is painful with intense circumciliary congestion and small pupil.
- Management lies mainly in removal of the lens and lens material with free use of systemic and topical steroids.

VIRAL UVEITIS

Herpes Simplex Uveitis

Patient presents with deep keratitis with symptoms and signs of anterior uveitis.

- Patient presents with superficial dendritic ulcer associated with mild symptoms and signs of anterior uveitis.
- Severe uveitis has been observed with deep herpetic keratitis.
- Topical steroids give a good response which favours an immune nature of the uveitis.
- Look for hyphema, iris atrophy and some corneal signs in a case of herpes simplex.
- Slit-lamp may reveal nebular opacities and iris atrophy.
- Iris atrophy tends to affect small areas nearer to the pupil in herpes simplex. than in herpes zoster wherein the iris atrophy tends to affect large areas close to root of the iris in herpes zoster.

Manage by topical antibiotic, antiviral and cycloplegic eyedrops and ointment.

Herpes Zoster Uveitis

Patient presents with vesicles limited to one side of head with pain, redness, photophobia and blurred vision.

Herpes zoster uveitis soon follows the involvement of nasociliary nerve that supplies cornea.

Symptoms and Signs

- Severe pain in the eye
- Marked circumciliary congestion
- Diminished corneal sensation
- Corneal opacities
- Iris atrophy
- Some case may show hyphema and raised intraocular pressure.

Management

- Topical antibiotic, antiviral, steroid and cycloplegic eyedrops and ointment.
- Control raised pressure with carbonic anhydrase inhibitor.
- Refer the case to neurologist.

FUNGAL UVEITIS

Candidiasis Uveitis

Patient presents with symptoms and signs of chronic uveitis.

The fungal uveitis is caused by *Candida albicans.* It is yeast-like fungus. It is frequently present in the human skin, mouth, gastrointestinal tract and vagina.

It can acquire pathogenic properties in the following three conditions:

1. Through the use of non-sterile needles and syringes.
2. Patients with long-term indwelling catheters.
3. Patients with decreased immunity; AIDS, malignancy, long-term use of steroids, antibiotics, cytotoxic drugs and drug addicts.

Ocular Features

- Anterior uveitis
- Posterior uveitis—chorioretinitis
- Endophthalmitis
- Retinal detachment

Management

- Topical antifungal and cycloplegic eyedrops.
- Systemic antifungal drugs.
- Vitrectomy, if needed in cases with endophthalmitis.

UVEITIS DUE TO CHRONIC SYSTEMIC MALADIES

Tubercular Uveitis

Patient presents with symptoms and signs of chronic uveitis.

Clinical Features

- Exudative uveitis is probably allergic in nature.
- Clinical picture is like any other exudative type of uveitis.
- Mutton fat keratic precipitate
- Translucent nodules '*Koeppe's nodules*' on the iris near the pupillary border.
- Metastatic granulomatous uveitis may occur in solitary or miliary form. There are one or more yellowish white nodules surrounded by many smaller nodules usually near the pupillary or ciliary margin of the iris.
- Choroiditis occurs in acute or chronic form.
- Ophthalmoscopy shows one or more pale yellow spots of exudation near the disk or any part of the fundus.

Management

- Systemic antitubercular drugs.
- Topical cycloplegic and steroid eyedrops.
- Refer the case to tuberculosis specialist.

Syphilitic Uveitis

Patient presents with symptoms and signs of chronic uveitis.

Clinical Features

- Simple plastic uveitis occurs in the secondary stage of syphilis in a congenital syphilis as an accompaniment of interstitial keratitis and as a *Herxheimer reaction.* Herxheimer reaction occurs 24 to 48 hours after the first therapeutic dose of penicillin probably due to the flooding of the system with treponemal toxins.
- Gummatous uveitis occurs late in the secondary stage of syphilis. It is characterized by formation of yellowish red vascularized nodules near the pupillary and ciliary margins of the iris.

- Uveitis is usually bilateral and associated with much exudation and thick broad synechia.
- Pain is not the important symptom.
- Choroiditis may manifest as disseminated, peripheral or diffuse lesions.

Management

- Topical antibiotic, cycloplegic and steroid therapy.
- Systemic penicillin or other antisyphilitic drugs.
- Refer the case to physician.

Leprotic Uveitis

Patient presents with lepromatous cutaneous form or tuberculoid neural form. Once seen, one can diagnose a leprotic patient as he enters the clinic.

Clinical Features

Leprosy (Hansen's disease) is caused by *Mycobacterium leprae*, acid-fast bacilli.

Leprosy manifests in two forms:

1. *Lepromatous (cutaneous) form* is associated with depressed cellular immunity and frequent eye involvement.
2. *Tuberculoid (neural) form* is associated with good systemic resistance and the eye complications are due to *neuroparalytic keratopathy*.

Eyes are involved late in the course of lepromatous leprosy.

Ocular Manifestation

- Conjunctivitis
- Episcleritis
- Keratitis
- Lens opacities
- Visual loss
- Non-reacting pupil
- Iridocyclitis and iris atrophy

Management

- Dapsone is the drug of choice and the usual dose is 50–100 mg.
- Topical antibiotic, cycloplegic and steroids eyedrops and ointment as required.

- Refer to leprosy center for free supply of drugs as leprotics need a long-term therapy and consistent follow-up.

Uveitis with Sarcoidosis

Patient presents with multiple cutaneous and sub-cutneous nodules with symptoms and signs of uveitis.

Clinical Features

- Sarcoidosis is a chronic granulomatous disease of unknown etiology.
- Characterized by multiple cutaneous and subcutaneous nodules with similar invasion in the viscera and bones.
- Periodic remissions and relapses.
- No caseation.
- Chronic bilateral anterior uveitis of granulomatous type with nodules on the iris and keratic precipitates in 30% cases.
- Posterior uveitis is characterized by multiple lesions in choroid and peri-vasculitis.

Diagnosis

- Typical clinical picture.
- X-ray chest
- Raised levels of serum angiotensin converting enzyme (ACE).
- Rarefaction in bones.
- Positive biopsy of cutaneous nodules.
- *Kveim test:* It shows a localized granuloma following an injection of *suspension of sarcoid tissue* in the skin of the patient.

Management: The malady responds well to steroids.

Uveitis with Toxoplasmosis

Patient presents with blurred vision. Ophthalmoscopy shows a clear cut punched out scar with heavy pigmentation usually at the macula.

Clinical Feature

Toxoplasmosis is caused by a protozoan 'Toxoplasma gondii'. Toxoplasmosis affects eye in form of chorioretinitis.

- *In infants:* Infection occurs in fetal life. Infants are acutely ill with history of convulsions. If the infant survives, they show the following diseased conditions: hydrocephalus, calcification in the brain, mental retardation and posterior uveitis—choroiditis.

- *Ophthalmoscopy* shows a clear cut punched out scar with heavy pigmentation usually at the macula.
- *In adults:* Diffuse choroiditis with recurrent attacks often at the edge of the previous scar associated with exudation in the vitreous.

Diagnosis

- Typical lesions of choroiditis in fundus.
- Sabin-Feldman test with a titer greater than 1:16.
- Complement fixation test.
- ELISA test
- Indirect fluorescein antibody test

Management

- Systemic antitoxoplasmic drugs such as sulphadiazine, clindamycin, pyremethamine, spiramycin.
- Topical and systemic broad-spectrum antibiotic and steroid.

Uveitis with Onchocerciasis

Patient presents with conjunctivitis and keratitis.

It is endemic in tropical Africa and central and South America. The usual ocular infection results in conjunctivitis and keratitis causing blindness in millions in that region.

The onchocerciasis is caused by *Onchocerca volvulus*, a filarial nematode worm. It is transmitted to humans by the bite of black fly (sand fly) *Simulium damnosum.*

Microfilaria can pass into the anterior chamber and cause chronic iridocyclitis.

Microfilaria can be seen swimming in the anterior chamber and vitreous.

Severe inflammation follows after the death of the organism.

Clinical Features

- Low grade iridocyclitis
- Microfilaria in the anterior chamber

- Localized atrophy of the iris
- Chorioretinitis with pigmentation
- Skin nodules
- Eosinophilia.

Management

- Systemic administration of hetrazan (diethylcarbamazine citrate) 100 mg four times a day for 10–14 days. In endemic zone, 50 mg of hetrazan daily provides a good cover.
- Antihistamines and steroids to reduce the side effects caused by the death of the organisms.
- The skin nodule should be excised to avoid further dissemination of microfilaria.

Uveitis with Brucellosis
(Undulant Fever, Malta Fever, Melitensis)

Patient presents with chronic granulomatous uveitis.

Brucellosis is caused by infection with *Brucella* and is widespread throughout the world. Relapses are common.

Clinical Features

- Chronic granulomatous uveitis is common.
- Keratitis, choroiditis and optic neuritis are rare.

Investigations

- Agglutination test
- Cutaneous test
- Opsonocytophagic test.

Management

- Systemic sulfonamides or chlortetracycline.
- Topical antibiotic, cycloplegic and steroid eyedrops and ointment as required.

Uveitis with Arthritis
(Ankylosing Spondylitis)

Patient presents with complains of low backache, morning stiffness of joints, blurred vision, redness and pain in the eyes.

- It is a chronic inflammatory arthritis of unknown etiology.

- Acute recurrent exudative anterior uveitis—iridocyclitis.
- Slit-lamp shows keratic precipitates, aqueous flare, cells, posterior synechia and even hypopyon.
- Usual complications are cataract, chronic cystoid macular edema and glaucoma.

Management: Topical antibiotic, cycloplegic and steroid are helpful.

SYNDROMES ASSOCIATED WITH UVEITIS

Posner-Schlossman Syndrome
(Glaucomatocyclitic Crisis)

Patient presents with history of halos and complains of blurring of vision but no pain.

Clinical Features

- Recurrent attacks of secondary open angle glaucoma with mild anterior uveitis.
- During attack, there may be aqueous flare, few pigmented keratic precipitates, epithelial edema of cornea, heterochromia, but no posterior synechia.
- It affects young adults 40% of whom are positive for HLA-BW54.
- During the attack, the intraocular pressure may rise to 40–60 mm Hg.
- In between the attacks, the eye is normal with normal intraocular pressure, normal visual fields and normal optic disc.
- Usually, unilateral but 50% patients have bilateral involvement.

Management

- High incidence of associated diabetes so check for blood sugar.
- During attack, control the intraocular pressure by medical therapy—topical timolol maleate and systemic carbonic anhydrase inhibitors.
- Topical steroids with care as many of these patients may be steroid responders. Most of these cases have open angle glaucoma.

Fuch's Uveitis Syndrome
(Fuch's Heterochromic Cyclitis)

*Patient presents with **triad** of ocular symptoms: Heterochromia iris, keratic precipitates, cataract.*

Clinical Features

- Iris stromal atrophy
- Diffusely scattered small white keratic precipitates
- Mild aqueous flare and cells
- Anterior vitreous shows cells
- Normal fundus.

Pathogenesis

Syndrome is said to be associated with some disturbance of the sympathetic nerve supply as this nerve controls the chromatophores accounting for the depigmentation as well as the tone of blood vessels so that in their dilated condition the white cells escape and get deposited on the posterior surface of the cornea as precipitates.

Management

Malady responds well to steroids.

Ocular Histoplasma Syndrome

Patient presents with triad of ocular symptoms: Multifocal atrophic choroidal spots, peripapillary atrophy, hemorrhagic disciform maculopathy.

- It is common among the age group of 20–50 years.
- It is 20 times more common in whites than in blacks.
- Patient complains of metamorphopsia and blurred vision due to involvement of the macula.
- Steroids have been found to be useful in aborting the attack of macular disease.

Uveoparotitis (Heerfordt's) Syndrome

Patient presents with malaise and fever accompanied by either granulomatous anterior uveitis or painful swelling of the parotid glands followed later by diplopia due to palsy of ocular nerves.

It is bilateral and characterized by involvement of:

- Entire uveal tract
- Parotid glands
- Cranial nerves.
- Affects young people between the age group of 10 and 30 years of age.
- Malady is self-limiting.

Behcet's Syndrome
(Recurrent Iridocyclitis with Hypopyon)

Patient presents with hypopyon due to uveitis and is associated with ulcers in mouth, on tongue and genitals.

Etiology is unknown but the viral and immunologic factors have been proposed.

Ocular Manifestations

- Acute anterior uveitis
- Hypopyon
- Vitreous haze
- Macular edema
- Retinal phlebitis and obliterative arteritis.

Management

Steroid and immune-suppressive under supervision of physician.

Reiter's Syndrome and Uveitis

Patient presents with **triad** *of symptoms: Urethritis, arthritis, conjunctivitis often with anterior uveitis.*

Acute anterior uveitis occurs independently of the conjunctivitis and features are like that seen in ankylosing spondylitis.

It is of unknown etiology.

Serologic evidence has confirmed its relationship with ankylosing spondylitis.

Treat anterior uveitis with cycloplegic and steroid.

Vogt-Koyanagi-Harada Syndrome
(Uveomeningitic Syndrome)

Patient presents with uveitis, meningeal signs, vitiligo, poliosis alopecia and auditory signs.

Clinical Features

- Exudative detachment of retina which settles and leaves the characteristic mottled fundus appearance of Harada's disease.
- Common complications are macular pathology, cataract, posterior synechia and glaucoma.
- Syndrome resembles clinically and immunologically with sympathetic ophthalmia.

DEGENERATION—DYSTROPHY

Essential Atrophy of Iris

Patient presents with unilateral slowly progressive atrophy of the iris—a malady of unknown etiology.

- Starts insidiously in early adult age.
- Areas of iris atrophy coalesce and progress to form lacuna.
- Vision is ultimately lost due to glaucoma which develops due to down-growth of an endothelial membrane at the angle of the anterior chamber.
- Prognosis is poor.

Gyrate Atrophy of Choroid

Patient presents with progressive atrophy of choroid, the pigment epithelium and the retina.

To begin with, atrophy is patchy and distributed irregularly.

These coalesce in the final stage thereby the fundus disappears leaving only macula.

Choroideremia

Patient presents with fundus picture that resembles the terminal stage of gyrate atrophy of choroid.

It is a hereditary degeneration and the prominent symptoms are night blindness and extreme concentric contraction of visual fields.

Senile Central Choroidal Atrophy

It occurs in two forms

1. *Central guttate choroidal atrophy (Tay's choroiditis):*
   - *Patient presents with numerous minute yellowish white spots round or with crenated edges in the macular region.*
   - These spots are due to peculiar hyaline excrescences on the surface of choroid commonly known as *drusen* or *colloid bodies.*
   - Malady is bilateral with minimal loss of vision.
2. *Central areolar choroidal atrophy (sclerosis):*
   - Patient presents with large circular or oval patch of degeneration in the macular region.
   - Sclera shines through it and the patch appears white with large choroidal vessels traversing it.
   - Absolute central scotoma.

PURULENT UVEITIS

Endophthalmitis (Fig. 15.5)

Endophthalmitis is severe usually unilateral inflammation of the vitreous and the adjacent structures. The inflammation does not extend beyond the sclera.

The incidence is rare due to awareness in the mind, availability of good hospital with specialist and improved socioeconomic status with better environmental living conditions.

Etiology

- Causative organisms are Gram-positive cocci, *i.e. Staphylococcus, streptococci, Pseudomonas, Bacillus subtilis.*
- *Exogenous infection* following penetrating injury. The common causative organism is *Bacillus subtilis*, a common containment. It gets entry either by a penetrating injury or during surgery.
- *Complication* of post-cataract or filtration surgery.
- *Uveitis* is a common cause.
- *Endogenous* metastatic infection.
- *Fungal* infection by *Candida albicans.*

Pathogenesis

The vitreous is a very good culture media for organisms to grow and multiply rapidly as the vitreous is avsacular with no natural defense mechanism. The organisms grow without any hindrance from antibiotics as these are not able to reach the vitreous whether administered topically or systemically.

Clinical Features

- Pain in the eye.
- Intense circumciliary congestion.
- Dim and blurred vision.
- Cornea appears dull due to edema of corneal endothelium.
- Ophthalmoscopy shows white yellow reflex from the fundus.
- Indirect ophthalmoscopy may show choroiditis or retinochoroiditis.
- Slit-lamp shows hazy vitreous with cells.
- Raised intraocular pressure.

Management

Prognosis depends on early diagnosis and intensive treatment.
Systemic and topical broad-spectrum antibiotics and steroids:
- Intravitreal
- Subconjunctival
- Systemic and topical antibiotics and steroids.

Supportive therapy:
- Topical cycloplegics
- Topical and systemic antiglaucoma drugs.

Early surgery if no or slow response
Vitrectomy to save the vision and the eye.

Panophthalmitis

Panophthalmitis is a severe and unilateral purulent inflammation of the whole eyeball. *The incidence is rare due to awareness in the mind, availability of good hospital with specialist and improved socioeconomic status with better environmental living conditions.*

Etiology

- *Exogenous:* It is caused by an infected wound, usually due to a perforating injury, or following an intraocular operation, or an infected corneal ulcer. The infection may spread from anterior to the posterior part of the eyeball or the whole eyeball gets

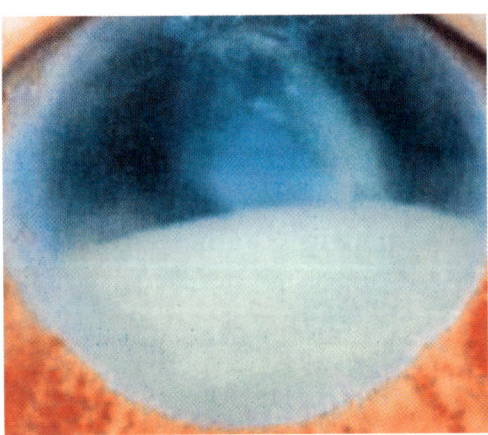

Fig. 15.5: Endophthalmitis with hypopyon

involved following infection of the vitreous which acts as a good culture medium.

- Causative organisms: *Pneumococcus, Staphylococcus, Streptococcus, Escherichia coli, Pseudomonas pyocyanea, Bacillus subtilis,* etc.
- *Endogenous* metastatic infection.

Symptoms

- General symptoms of malaise and fever.
- Severe pain in the eye and around it.
- Marked purulent discharge from the eye
- Complete loss of vision.

Signs

- Eyeball appears swollen and proptosed.
- Lids are swollen and red.
- Marked congestion of the whole conjunctiva with chemosis.
- Intense circumciliary congestion
- Corneal wound appears yellow and necrotic with hypopyon.
- Marked purulent discharge.

- In endogenous cases, there is a yellow reflex from the pupil with great loss of vision may be to perception of light.
- In very severe cases of panophthalmitis, the pus may burst through the walls of the globe usually at the limbus.

Complications

- Orbital cellulitis
- Cavernous sinus thrombophlebitis

Management

Systemic and topical broad-spectrum antibiotics and steroids: Intravenous antibiotics along with steroids.

Supportive therapy: Analgesics and anti-inflammatory drugs to provide relief from general symptoms and intense pain.

Surgery

- Vitrectomy in endogenous panophthalmitis may save the eye.
- Evisceration with frill excision of sclera.

16

Maladies of Lens

Developmental Cataract

- Zonular cataract
- Rubella cataract
- Coronary cataract
- Blue dot cataract
- Fusiform cataract
- Embryonal nuclear cataract
- Anterior capsular (polar) cataract
- Posterior capsular (polar) cataract

Acquired Cataract

- Senile cataract
- Senile cortical (soft) cataract
- Senile nuclear (hard) cataract
- After cataract
- Complicated cataract

Cataract Associated with Systemic Diseases

- Diabetes
- Parathyroid
- Myotonic dystrophy
- Syndermatotic cataract

Cataract due to other Causes

- Infrared cataract
- Irradiation cataract
- Electric cataract
- Ultrasonic cataract
- Chlorpromazine cataract
- Steroid cataract

Traumatic or Concussion Cataract

- Vossius's ring
- Rosette-shaped cataract
- Opacification of lens

Cataract due to Deficiency of Enzyme

- Galactokinase deficiency cataract
- Fabry's disease
- Wilson's disease (hepatolenticular degeneration)
- Mannosidosis
- Galactosemia

Congenital Abnormalities of the Lens

- Ectopia lentis
- Coloboma of lens
- Lenticonus

Syndromes Associated with Cataract

- Down's syndrome (mongolism)
- Werner's syndrome
- Rothmund's syndrome
- Lowe's syndrome

Displacement of the Lens

- Dislocation of lens (luxation of lens)
- Subluxation of lens (partial dislocation)

Any opacity in the lens or its capsule is called cataract.

The lens is a biconvex, avascular, colorless and transparent structure with permeable capsule. Anterior capsule is lined with sub-capsular epithelium. The lens with its capsule is suspended behind the iris by suspensory ligaments which connect it with ciliary body. Lens focus the light rays coming from a distant object on the retina without use of any accommodation. The divergent light rays coming from near objects are brought to focus on the retina by virtue of the act of accommodation by which the refractive power of the lens is increased with an increase in its anterior curvature. Maladies of a lens are cataract, subluxation and dislocation. Management of these disorders is either IOLs implant or prescription of suitable glasses.

DEVELOPMENTAL CATARACT

Most people show some kind of minute opacity of the lens, if examined by slit-lamp under full mydriasis. The developmental cataract is seen in many forms, shapes, sizes and at varied locations. The lens is formed in layers and the central nucleus is the earliest formation around which concentric zones are laid down. Therefore, the developmental cataract has a tendency to affect a particular zone which got disturbed during its formation. The lens fibers laid down prior to the disturbance and subsequently are normal. Thus the opacity of the lens due to developmental defect follows the architectural pattern of the lens. The location of the lens opacity gives a fair idea of the stage at which it developed during formation of lens.

The factors which play part are not yet clear. A developmental cataract usually remains stationary although these cases develop senile cataract earlier than usual. Most of the developmental cataracts do not interfere with vision unless large in size and centrally placed.

Zonular Cataract

Young mother with her child presents with complain of white opacity in left eye of her child.

Slit-lamp under full mydriasis shows zonular cataract.

Diagnosis—zonular cataract.

Clinical Features

Patient presents with white opacity in one or both the eyes and may be associated with squint or nystagmus due to low vision which does not allow the proper development of macula.

- Zonular cataract is usually bilateral.
- Frequently, the zonular cataract is formed just before the birth or shortly after birth and in these cases the opacity is large to fill the pupillary aperture affecting vision.
- There is an opaque zone in the lens around the embryonic nucleus in one or both the eyes.
- The opaque zonal area is sharply demarcated and the lens within and around the opaque zone is clear.
- In some cases, there may be linear opacities from the opaque zone running towards the equator.
- Some cases may even show two zones of lens opacity.

Etiology

- Deficiency of vitamin D appears as a potent factor as evidence of rickets has been observed in these cases especially affecting the teeth. The incisors and canines show erosion and transverse lines.

Symptoms

- White opacity in the eyes.
- Dim vision with abnormal position and movement of the eyes.

Signs

- Low visual acuity
- Zonular cataract
- Squint or nystagmus due to mal-development of macula due to low vision.
- Ophthalmoscopy shows black opacity in the red background.

Management

- If the opacity is small and does not interfere with vision, then the child does not need any treatment. Follow periodically for any increase in the size of cataract.
- If the lens opacity is placed centrally and large enough to cover the pupil and there is a tendency for development of squint or nystagmus then the surgical interference is essential without any further delay.
- IOLs implant is the ideal choice of surgery.

Rubella Cataract

Young mother presents with her newborn infant and complains of white opacity in the eyes of her newborn infant.

Consultant could elicit the history of rubella during her second month of pregnancy.

Diagnosis— rubella cataract.

Rubella or German measles is a mild contagious disease which manifests with fever, pharyngitis, and eruptions on the skin. To begin with the eruptions appear on face, neck and then spread to the trunk and extremities which fade in three days.

Progressive type of developmental cataract is associated with the occurrence of Rubella in the mother during her second or sometimes in the third month of pregnancy.

Rubella virus reaches the fetus before it has developed an immunological defence mechanism.

- Slit-lamp shows cataract.
- Ophthalmoscopy shows fine pigmentary deposit (*salt-and-pepper retinopathy*) at the posterior pole of the fundus.
- Systemic manifestation may show other congenital anomalies such as patent ductus arteriosus, microphthalmos, microencephaly, mental retardation, deafness and dental defects.
- IOLs implant is the ideal choice.

Coronary Cataract

Coronary cataract is diagnosed accidentally only by slit-lamp under full mydriasis as routine examination.

- Coronary cataract manifests as corona of *club-shaped opacities* in the periphery of the lens.
- The axial region of the lens and extreme periphery is clear.
- The coronary cataract manifests at puberty. Therefore, it is situated in the deeper layers of the cortex and superficial layers of nucleus.
- It is a non-progressive type of cataract.

Blue Dot Cataract

Blue dot cataract is diagnosed accidently only by slit-lamp under full mydriasis as routine examination.

The blue dot cataract is the most common manifestation of developmental cataract and is seen in large number of cases.

- The spots are multiple and scattered all over the lens. Under slit-lamp beam, these appear as tiny blue dots, therefore, it is known as *'blue dot cataract'*.
- Sometimes, these dots get crowded in the Y sutures then it is known as sutural cataract or anterior axial embryonic cataract.
- These do not disturb the vision and are of no significance.

Fusiform Cataract

Fusiform cataract is diagnosed accidently only by slit-lamp under full mydriasis as routine examination.

Fusiform cataract manifests as an anteroposterior spindle shape, axial or coraliform cataract.

It has a genetic origin and occurs in families.

Embryonal Nuclear Cataract

Embryonal nuclear cataract is diagnosed accidently only by slit-lamp under full mydriasis as routine examination.

Embryonal nuclear cataract manifests as opaque central nucleus due to inhibition of the development of the lens at a very early stage of development.

Small dot does not disturb the vision and is of no significance.

Anterior Capsular (Polar) Cataract

Congenital anterior capsular (polar) cataract occurs due to delayed formation of the anterior chamber.

Acquired anterior capsular (polar) cataract is more common and it manifests as white plaque due to contact of the lens capsule with the cornea most commonly after the perforation of a corneal ulcer in ophthalmia neonatorum in early infancy. In some cases, it may project in the anterior chamber as '*anterior pyramidal cataract'* or underlying cortex becomes opaque as *'anterior cortical cataract'* or as a*nterior reduplicated cataract'* an imprint of the superficial opacity.

Small dot does not disturb the vision and is of no significance.

Posterior Capsular (Polar) Cataract

Posterior capsular (polar) cataract occurs due to persistence of dot-like posterior part of the vascular sheath of the lens.

Small dot does not interfere with vision and is of no significance

ACQUIRED CATARACT

Any factor which disturbs the critical intra- and extracellular equilibrium of water and electrolytes, or deranges the colloid system within the lens fibers can be a cause for the acquired cataract.

Biochemically, *hydration* and *sclerosis* are the two factors which play an important role in the process of degeneration of lens fibers resulting in acquired cataract.

Clinically, when the process of *hydration* is predominant then it results in formation of *cortical soft cataract* and when the process of *sclerosis* is dominant then it results in formation of *nuclear hard cataract.*

Process of *hydration i*s seen relatively in early age while the process of *sclerosis* is seen in later years of life.

The following factors may lead to the changes which results in formation of acquired cataract.

- *Impaired semipermeability of the lens capsule* results in an increase in inactive and insoluble proteins and the oxidation system becomes less effective.
- *Deficiency of amino acids* such as tryptophane or vitamin riboflavine can lead to formation of cataract.
- *Systemic use of toxic substances* such as naphthalene, thallium, dinitrophenol produce lens opacity in the posterior cortex.
- *Any toxic product* in the aqueous humor due to ocular disease results in posterior cortical cataract.

- *Hypocalcemia* is known to cause lens opacity by altering the ionic balance.
- *Steroids–systemic or topical* for long period lead to cataract.
- *Osmotic imbalance* due to diabetes causes cataract.
- *Trauma* of any kind results in cataract formation.

SENILE CATARACT

The occurrence of senile cataract is universal over the age of seventy and affects both the sexes equally. It is bilateral but often one eye shows lens opacity earlier than the other.

Patient presents with dim vision, polyopia, halos, black spot, improved near vision and change in his/her color perception.

Ocular examination shows white opaque lens, grey pupil, and iris shadow.

Slit-lamp examination after full mydriasis shows cataract in its various stages.

Ophthalmoscopy further informs about the etiology and visual outcome after surgery.

IOLs implant is the ideal choice to restore the vision.

Diagnosis—senile cataract.

Senile Cortical (Soft) Cataract

In senile cortical soft cataract, the signs of hydration followed by coagulation of proteins appear primarily in the cortex.

Clinical Features and Treatment at Various Stages

1. Stage of lamellar separation

- Lamellar separation can only be seen by slit-lamp. There is demarcation of the cortical fibers due to their separation by hydration seen only by slit-lamp. If the *lamellar separation* is due to diabetes, then control of diabetes may reverse the process or at least arrest the further progress of hydration.
- Once the opacity has developed, then the changes are irreversible.

- Pupil appears grey due to increase in reflection and scattering of light entering the pupil.
- No treatment for this stage.

2. *Stage of incipient cataract* (Fig. 16.1)

a. **Cuneiform cataract:** Slit-lamp shows wedge-shape spokes of lens opacity with clear areas in between the periphery of lens cortex mostly in the lower nasal quadrant. The base of the wedge-shape opacity is peripheral and apex towards the pupil. These are preceded by sectorial alteration in the refractive index of the lens fibers giving rise to symptoms of dim vision and polyopia.

Clinically:

- Ophthalmoscopy under full mydriasis shows black spokes against a red back ground.
- Slit-lamp under full mydriasis shows grey spokes of lens opacity in the anterior and posterior cortex usually in the lower nasal quadrant.
- Symptoms of dim vision and polyopia manifest in dim light as the pupil gets dilated and spokes of opacities come in the visual line.
- *Polyopia* occurs due to break up of the image by the spokes of lens opacity.

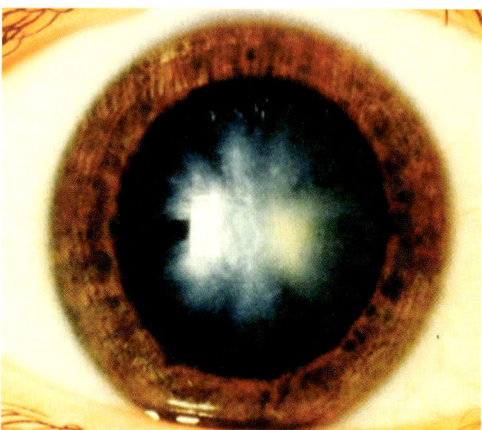

Fig. 16.1: Incipient cataract

- *Dim vision* occurs due to sectorial alteration in the refractive index of the lens fibers.
- Correct the refractive error by prescribing suitable lens.
- Bright illumination improves the vision.

b. **Cupuliform cataract:** Slit lamp shows aggregation of opacities in the posterior cortex close to capsule.

Clinically:

- Visual acuity is very low.
- Lens appears grey.
- Iris shadow is present.
- No polyopia or halos.
- Dark spot in his/her line of vision.
- Ophthalmoscopy shows slightly dark area in the field against the red back-ground at the posterior pole.
- Slit-lamp examination shows dense yellowish layer at the posterior pole of the lens.
- IOLs implant is the ideal choice to restore full vision.

3. *Stage of intumescent cataract:* Opacity of lens becomes more diffuse and progressive hydration of cortical fibers result in swelling of the lens leading to shallow anterior chamber.

Clinically:

- Vision is markedly reduced.
- Lens appears cloudy and eventually white and opaque.
- Ophthalmoscopy shows no red glow.
- Anterior chamber is shallow and it may induce secondary glaucoma.
- IOLs implant is the ideal choice.

4. *Immature cataract* (Fig. 16.2): As long as there is any clear lens substance between the pupillary margin of the iris and the opacity in the lens the iris throws a shadow upon the grey opacity of the lens.

Presence of iris shadow is a sure sign of an immature cataract.

Clinically:

- Visual acuity is very low.
- Pupil appears grey white.

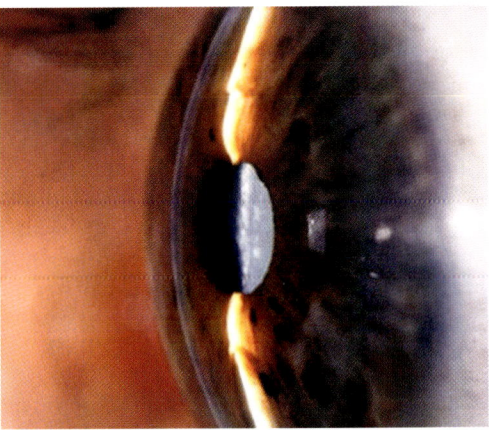

Fig. 16.2: Immature cataract

- Iris shadow is present.
- Ophthalmoscopy—no red glow.
- IOLs implant is the ideal choice.

5. *Mature cataract (Fig. 1.6.3):* Entire cortex is opaque and the swelling of the lens subsides. Lens nucleus shows only progressive sclerosis.

Clinically:
- Visual acuity is reduced to hand movements or even to perception and projection of light.
- White reflex from the pupil.
- Lens appears white and opaque.
- No iris shadow.
- Ophthalmoscopy—no red glow.
- IOLs implant is the ideal choice.

6. *Hypermature cataract:* Cortex of the lens becomes disintegrated and turns into a soft mass.

Clinically:
- Visual acuity is reduced to perception and projection of light.
- No iris shadow.
- Lens appears shrunken and yellowish in color.
- Anterior capsule is thick and dense at the anterior pole.
- Anterior chamber is deep.
- Iris is tremulous.
- Lens may subluxate.
- IOLs implant is the ideal choice.

7. *Morgagnian cataract (Fig. 16.4):* Sometimes the cortex of the lens becomes fluid and the lens nucleus sinks to the lower end of the lens capsule.

Clinically:
- Lens appears milky white.
- Lens nucleus sinks to bottom of capsule and give rise to an appearance of a semicircular yellowish brown line in the pupillary area.
- IOLs implant is the ideal choice.

Senile Nuclear (Hard) Cataract

Sclerosis of the lens nucleus and the cortical fibers remains transparent. With the passage of time, the nucleus of the lens becomes

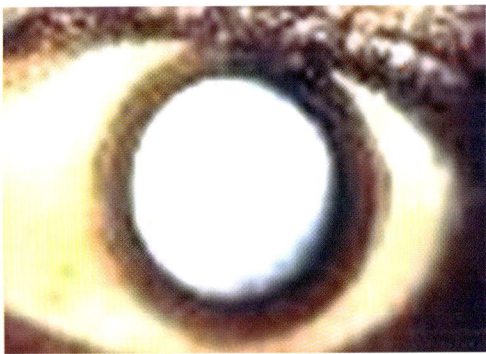

Fig. 16.3: Mature cataract

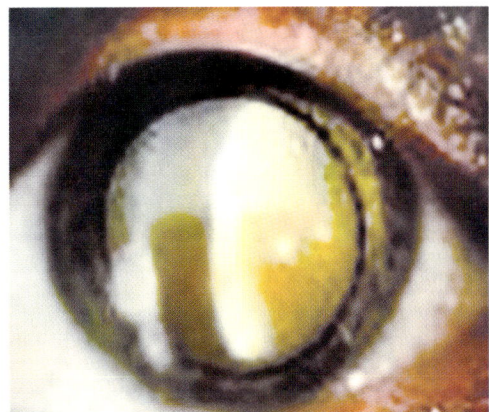

Fig. 16.4: Morgagnian cataract

diffusely cloudy extending almost to the capsule thereby reaching its maturity.

Occasionally, the lens nucleus becomes dark brown or dusky red or even black in appearance. This change in the color of the lens nucleus is due to deposition of melanin derived from the amino acids in the lens. This colored nuclear cataract is known as *cataracta brunescens*, or *black cataract*.

Symptoms of Senile Cataract

1. *Diminution in visual acuity* In *senile cortical cataract*, the lens opacities are in periphery of the lens, thereby a good vision is maintained for a long time. In fact, the vision improves in bright light due to contraction of pupil and there is some deterioration of vision in dim light due to exposure of spokes of lens opacities and irregular refraction. These patients feel comfortable in bright light.

In *senile nuclear cataract*, the lens is opaque in the central and posterior part of the lens, therefore, the central vision is affected early and much more due to its location at the nodal point of the eye. The vision improves in dim light due to dilation of the pupil. These patients are comfortable in evening and dim illumination. The vision is diminished in bright light due to contraction of the pupil.

2. *Uniocular polyopia* Uniocular polyopia is another early symptom of senile cortical cataract. Polyopia denotes doubling or trebling of the objects seen by the eye. The polyopia is due to sectorial alteration in the refractive index of the lens fibers and spokes of lens opacity which breaks the image in the *stage of incipient cataract*. The patient from a rural area usually complains of seeing two, three or more images of the moon. The patient from an urban area usually complains of seeing two, three or more images of a bulb in the home or head light of vehicles.

3. *Color halos* Patient complains of seeing colored rings around the lights, therefore, usually seen after dark, when the lights are put on in the home. The colors are distributed as in the spectrum, the red color is the outer most and the blue color is the inner most. The halos are seen due to hydration of the lens during the *stage of intumescent cataract*.

The only other condition in which the halos are seen is glaucoma. In glaucoma, the halos are seen due to accumulation of fluid in the corneal epithelium. The halos seen are due to cataract or glaucoma can be differentiated by Fincham's test. In this test, a stenopic slit is passed before the eye across the line of vision. As the slit passes in front of the eye, the halos due to glaucoma remain intact while the halos due to cataract are broken up into segments which revolve as the slit is moved. The patient becomes able to appreciate the halos better, if he/she can be demonstrated the appearance of halos by his/her looking through a thin layer of lycopodium powder enclosed between two glass plates making it as a trial lens.

4. *Black spot in front of eye* Seeing a black spot before the eye is an early complaint from the patient. The spot is stationary and retains its relative position in the field of vision in different position of the eye. It is to be differentiated from black spots seen due to muscae volitantes, which are found due to degeneration of the vitreous and appear like cotton wool, and moves continually even though the eye is stationary. The black spot is due to a tiny dense spot at the posterior pole of the lens in nuclear cataract.

5. *Change in color perception* The change in color perception affects mostly the blue end of the spectrum. In nuclear cataract, there is some diminution in acuity of perception of the blue color due to its physical absorption by increase of amber pigment in the lens nucleus. It is much more in a black cataract. It is also known as *blue blindness*. The blue end of the spectrum is also affected in the diseases of the retina and choroid. This change in color perception usually affects the pictures of artists in their late years of life, when the sclerosis of the lens nucleus increases. The red color value is accentuated.

6. *Second sight of aged* The persons in whom the nuclear sclerosis is prominent, there is an increase in the refractive index of the lens causing progressive myopia. Therefore, a

previously presbyopic person is able to read again without the use of his/her near vision spectacles. This gain in the near sight is known as *'second sight'*. Patient improves in his/her distance visua l acuity with myopic correction.

Signs of Senile Cataract

Slit-lamp under full mydriasis shows:
- Central or diffuse dense lens opacity.
- Lens opacity in various form, shape, size and location.
- Spokes of lens opacity in periphery.
- Hydration of lens or shrunken lens.
- Anterior chamber normal, shallow or deep
- Lens—milky white, grey, brown or even black in color.
- Ophthalmoscopy—hazy fundus or black spots in red background.

Management of Senile Cataract

- Refractive error may be corrected from time to time to improve the visual acuity of the patient.
- Surgical treatment for removal of cataract is indicated, when the visual acuity falls below 6/18 or when the visual acuity is low to the extent that the person is not able to earn his/her living.
- It is essential to exclude any systemic or ocular disease which may affect the surgical results.

General and Systemic Examination

Examine the patient for any systemic disease and any septic focus, especially in the upper respiratory tract and genitourinary tract.

Diabetes is one of the most common malady that should be excluded or controlled.

Ocular Examination

A thorough examination of the eye is necessary as a routine to exclude any ocular disease which may be causative factor for complications or affect the ultimate surgical results.

Surgical Management

The best management of cataract is phaco-emulsification with intraocular lens implant.

Types of Intraocular Lenses

1. *Anterior chamber lenses* Anterior chamber lens lies entirely in the anterior chamber in front of iris. The lens gets fixed by its haptics supported against the scleral spur in the angle of anterior chamber. There are many designs of anterior chamber lens available. Each surgeon has his own choice. The most popular anterior chamber lens is the mark VIII and IX of Choyce.

2. *Iris supported lenses* The iris supports the lens. It is important that the iris has a good structural integrity. There are many designs but the basic principal is same.

3. *Posterior chamber lens—in ciliary-sulcus fixation* These lenses lie behind the iris. The flexible haptics are inserted into the ciliary sulcus a groove between the root of the iris and the ciliary body.

4. *Posterior chamber lens—in capsular bag fixation* The intraocular lens is fixed in the lens capsule of the patient. A planned extracapsular cataract extraction is performed. The lens is placed in the capsular bag with haptic of lens between the anterior and posterior capsuleS in periphery. It provides good capsular fixation. It is the most widely accepted mode of management of cataract.

Posterior chamber lens are available as rigid IOLs, foldable IOLs and rollable IOLs (Fig. 16.5).

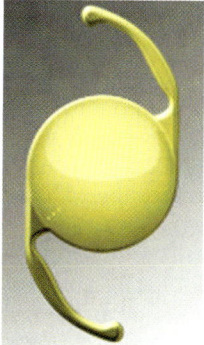

Fig. 16.5: IOLs

After Cataract

The incidence of posterior capsule opacification has markedly by reduced due to advances in surgical techniques, IOL designs and bio-materials. Patient may also complain of increase in glare day by day.

Slit lamp shows opacification of the posterior capsule.

Management

The choicest treatment is a capsulotomy with Neodymium YAG laser. It is safe, painless and can be performed as an out-door procedure.

Complicated Cataract

Aqueous humor provides nutrition to the lens. Therefore, any condition that disturbs the circulation, formation and constituents of aqueous humor shall lead to development of lens opacities.

Complicated cataract may remain stationary for a long time or in some cases the opacity spreads to cover the entire lens.

Thorough examination of the eye involved and the other eye is essential to know the causative factor.

Etiology

- Uveitis is one of the most common factor.
- Degenerative disease of retina such as retinitis pigmentosa and myopic chorio-retinal degeneration.
- Retinal detachment of long-standing.
- Intraocular tumor.

Pathogenesis

Anterior capsule of the lens is lined with epithelium. The inflammation of the anterior segment of the eye such as anterior uveitis disturbs the subcapsular epithelium which results in opacification of lens cortex.

Posterior capsule of the lens is semipermeable allowing toxins to pass through it in any inflammatory or degenerative disease of the eye. This results in a characteristic opacification of the posterior cortex at the posterior pole of the lens.

Clinical Features

- Low visual acuity due to the location of opacity at the nodal point of the eye.
- Slit-lamp shows opacity in the posterior cortex with irregular border and extends diffusely towards the equator and nucleus of the lens. In the beam of the slit-lamp, the opacity gives *'bread-crumb appearance'* and characteristic rainbow colors known as *'polychromatic lustre'* of red, green and blue.
- Ophthalmoscopy shows ill-defined dark area in the center with red background.

Management

- If the posterior opacity is stationary with reasonably good vision, then leave it alone and take care of the disease of the eye energetically and consistently with regular follow-up.
- IOLs implant, if the patient demands good visual acuity to earn living.

CATARACT ASSOCIATED WITH SYSTEMIC DISEASES

Diabetes

- Typical diabetic cataract occurs bilaterally.
- *Slit-lamp shows white punctate or snowflake-like opacities in the anterior and posterior capsules.*
- These occur due to osmotic overhydration of the lens.
- Senile cataract develops at an early age and progresses rapidly than usual in diabetics.
- Control diabetes energetically and consis-tently.

Parathyroid

- Atrophy of the parathyroid gland or its removal during a thyroidectomy can lead to opacity of the lens.
- *Slit-lamp shows large number of small discrete opacities in the cortex separated from the capsule by a clear zone.*
- Prevented by administration of para-thyroid hormone and calcium.

Myotonic Dystrophy

Slit-lamp shows fine dust-like opacities interspersed with tiny iridescent spots in a sharply defined zone of cortex under the anterior and posterior capsules.

Usually, it remains stationary.

Syndermatotic Cataract

- Cataract can develop in the skin diseases such as atopic eczema, poikiloderma, scleroderma, keratosis follicularis.
- Such cataracts are bilateral, fast progressive and affect young people.
- Essential to control the allergy to have good prognosis for surgery.
- IOLs implant is the ideal choice.

CATARACT DUE TO OTHER CAUSES

Infrared Cataract

- Cataract occurs due to absorption of heat by the pigment of the iris and the ciliary body which influences the fibers of the lens indirectly.
- Clinically, this type of cataract is seen in glass blowers, tin plate mill-men and chain makers.
- In early stage, there is a small disk of lens opacity in the posterior cortex.

  IOLs implant is the choice to restore vision.

Irradiation Cataract

- Irradiation cataract is caused by X-rays, Y-rays, and neutrons.
- Usually seen in the patients undergoing radiation therapy for malignant tumor near the eye and unprotected technicians and workers in atomic energy plants. It was seen in survivors of atomic bomb attack over Japan.
- Clinically, there is a thin opacity at the posterior pole of the cortex alike the infrared cataract.
- IOLs implant is the ideal choice.

Electric Cataract

- Cataract develops rapidly after an electric current passes through the body.
- Usually seen after a flash of lightening or short-circuiting of high voltage current passing through the body.
- Lens opacity starts as subcapsular punctate opacities and rapidly progresses to involve the entire cortex.
- IOLs implant is the ideal choice.

Ultrasonic Cataract

Ultrasonic waves cause cataract due to heat and concussion effect on the lens fibers.

Chlorpromazine Cataract

Intake of chlorpromazine for a long period may cause deposition of fine yellow brown granules under the anterior lens capsule in the pupillary area. The drug also gets deposited in the retina causing its atrophy.

Steroid Cataract

- Long-term therapy with steroids whether systemic or topical leads to formation of posterior subcapsular cataract.
- An alternate day therapy for systemic intake is safe for long-term use of steroids.
- Gradually, taper and keep the patient on the minimum maintenance dose.
- Safe to record the intraocular pressure before and at periodical intervals during steroid therapy whether local or systemic.
- Early withdrawal of steroids may arrest the progress of opacity of lens.
- Open angle glaucoma due to steroid is reversible on withdrawing the drug. Topical timolol maleate eyedrops help to reduce the intraocular pressure.

TRAUMATIC OR CONCUSSION CATARACT

A concussion cataract is due to a contusion injury to the eyeball. Clinically, it can appear in the following forms.

Vossius's Ring

- Slit-lamp shows small circular ring of faint or stippled opacity on the anterior surface of the lens due to multitudes of brown granules of pigment lying on the capsule and derived from the iris.

- It is due to impression of the iris on the lens produced by the force of the contusion injury pushing the cornea and iris backwards to hit the lens.
- It needs no treatment and usually the granules disappear in course of time. Minute subcapsular opacities may persist.

Rosette-shaped Cataract

- Slit-lamp shows rosette-shaped cataract in the posterior cortex.
- There is an accumulation of fluid which marks out the architectural arrangement of the lens. It results in showing the star-shaped cortical sutures and from these feathery lines of opacities radiate outlining the lens fibers.
- It may remain stationary or may progress to complete opacification of the lens.
- IOLs implant is gratifying.

Opacification of Lens

- Complete opacification of the lens may occur due to mechanical effect of injury or more commonly due to entrance of the aqueous in the lens due to tear of the capsule or change in the semipermeability of the capsule.
- IOLs implant is the choice.

CATARACT DUE TO DEFICIENCY OF ENZYME

Galactokinase Deficiency Cataract

This is due to deficiency of galactokinase (GK), which is the first enzyme in the metabolic pathway of galactose utilization. The children are at risk to develop lens opacity early in life. It is presumed that some presenile cataracts are due to mild deficiency of galactokinase.

Fabry's Disease

This is due to deficiency in the enzyme, α galactosidase A. The ocular features are cornea verticillata and spokes of lens opacities.

Wilson's Disease
(Hepatolenticular Degeneration)

It is due to the deficiency of the α-2-globulin ceruloplasmin which leads to widespread deposition of copper in the tissues. It can be treated with D-penicillamine. The ocular features include, Kayser-Fleischer ring in the peripheral parts of the Descemet's membrane of the cornea and sunflower cataract.

Mannosidosis

This is due to deficiency of the enzyme α-mannosidase. The patient develops spoke or wheel-like opacities in the posterior capsule. The absence of the corneal changes helps to differentiate it from Hurler's disease.

Galactosemia

This is due to severe impairment of galactose utilization due to absence or deficiency of galactose-1-phosphate uridyltransferase (GPUT). The malady is fatal unless galactose in the form of milk and milk products is completely withdrawn from the diet of the infant. The infant develops bilateral cataract in first few days or weeks of the life. The cataract appears as oil droplets-like central lens opacities. The lens opacities are reversible, if diagnosed early and milk is withdrawn from the diet.

CONGENITAL ABNORMALITIES OF THE LENS

Ectopia Lentis (Fig. 16.6)

Ectopia lentis is a congenital condition of subluxation of the lens. The displacement is

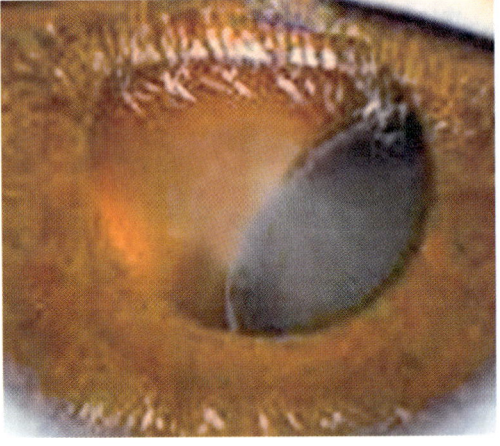

Fig. 16.6: Ectopia lentis

upwards, or upwards and inwards. It is a bilateral condition. It is often hereditary.

Lens is small and usually the edge of the lens is visible, when the pupil is dilated.

Signs of subluxation such as deep or irregular anterior chamber with tremulous iris are seen.

Sometimes associated with Marfan's syndrome or homocystinuria.

Coloboma of Lens

Coloboma of lens appears as a notched-shaped defect usually in its inferior margin. It is due to defective development of part of the suspensory ligament. It does not interfere with vision.

Lenticonus

Lenticonus is a rare congenital defect at the posterior pole of lens which has an abnormal curvature in the form of a cone towards the vitreous. It causes myopia and irregular astigmatism.

Ophthalmoscopy shows it as an oil globule in the center of the red reflex.

IOLs implant is the ideal choice.

SYNDROMES ASSOCIATED WITH CATARACT

Down's Syndrome (Mongolism)

Ocular features include lens opacity, strabismus, nystagmus, keratoconus and myopia.

Systemic features are mental retardation, stunted growth, mongoloid facies and congenital heart defect.

Werner's Syndrome

Ocular feature is bilateral cataract manifesting between the age 20 and 40 years.

Systemic features are premature senility, diabetes, hypogonadism and arrested growth.

Rothmund's Syndrome

Ocular feature consists of bilateral cataract which develops during second to fourth decades of life predominantly in females.

Systemic manifestations are as follows:

- Skin changes in form of atrophy, pigmentation and telangiectasis usually manifesting in early infancy
- Bony defects
- Disturbance in hair growth
- Hypogonadism
- Saddle-shaped nose.

It is a rare hereditary syndrome which affects predominantly females.

Lowe's Syndrome
(Oculocerebrorenal Syndrome)

- It is a rare disease with inborn error of amino acid matabolism which predominantly affects boys.
- Lens is small and thin with lens opacities which may be capsular, lamellar, nuclear or total.
- Glaucoma is associated in 50% of the cases.
- Mother of the child may show multiple punctate lens opacities.
- Systemic features of syndrome include mental retardation, dwarfism, osteomalacia, muscular hypotonia and frontal prominence.

DISPLACEMENT OF THE LENS

Dislocation of the lens occurs, when the fibers of suspensory ligament are torn.

When all the fibers of suspensory ligament are torn, then it gives rise to complete dislocation of the lens known as *luxation of lens.*

When only few fibers in a sector of suspensory ligament are torn, then it gives rise to partial dislocation of the lens known as *subluxation of lens.*

Dislocation of Lens (Luxation of Lens)

Etiology

It can be either congenital or traumatic. Congenital luxation is rare. Luxation of the lens due to trauma is not uncommon.

Usually, a subluxated lens gets luxated even with a trivial trauma to the eyeball.

Clinical Features

The clinical features vary depending on the location of the luxated lens. Lens can be dislocated posteriorly in the vitreous, anteriorly in the anterior chamber, outside the eye under the conjunctiva or may be expelled out of the eyeball.

Posterior Dislocation of the Lens in the Vitreous

Posterior dislocation of the lens in the vitreous is the most common result of a trauma. A clear lens may remain clear in the vitreous for a long time, or may become opaque soon, if there has been some rupture of capsule. A clear lens is seen with difficulty but an opaque lens is visible as a yellow globular mass usually close to ciliary body.

Clear and intact lens does not give rise to any symptoms other than an aphakic eye.

Opaque lens may give rise to all the signs and symptoms of chronic cyclitis.

Better to leave the quiet lens alone.

If there are signs of cyclitis or phacolytic glaucoma, then treat medically and plan for IOLs implant.

Anterior Dislocation of the Lens

Anterior dislocation of the lens occurs usually after a blow to the eye from the side, i.e. a slanting blow to the eye. A trivial injury to a hypermature shrunken lens or a subluxated lens results in anterior dislocation.

Clear lens in the anterior chamber looks like a globule of oil in anterior chamber. With oblique illumination, it shows a golden rim due to total reflection of the light. The lens in the anterior chamber causes spasm of the sphincter muscle of the pupil. The lens is more globular and refraction of the eye is myopic due to increased curvature and anterior placement of the lens.

Delay in extraction causes iridocyclitis and secondary glaucoma. IOLs implant shall restore good vision.

Subconjunctival Dislocation of the Lens

Subconjunctival dislocation of the lens follows a severe contusion to eyeball causing rupture of the sclera. Treat the injury, repair the sclera and remove the lens.

Expulsion of the Lens from the Eyeball

Complete expulsion of the lens from the eyeball also follows a contusion injury which results in rupture of the sclera.

Subluxation of Lens (Partial Dislocation)
Marfan's Syndrome

It is an inherited connective tissue disorder characterized by the following features.

Ocular Features

- Subluxation of the lens upwards in 80% of the cases
- Angle anomaly
- Hypoplasia of dilator muscle of pupil.
- Glaucoma
- Cornea may show flattening
- Axial myopia
- Lattice degeneration of retina.

Systemic Features

- Cardiac anomalies such as aneurysm and aortic regurgitation.
- Skeletal anomalies—long limbs, spider-like long fingers (arachnodactyly), laxity of joints and high arched palate.
- Muscular under development.
- Patient is long in height but of thin built.

Clinical Features

- Features vary depending on the displacement of the lens, the direction of the displacement, and whether the subluxated lens is clear or opaque.
- No symptoms in an opaque subluxated lens.
- Annoying symptoms with a clear subluxated lens.

Symptoms

Uniocular diplopia Patient complains of seeing double image of the objects. It occurs, when the lens has been displaced to uncover only half of the pupillary area. In this condition, the half pupil is phakic and half of the pupil is aphakic, therefore, forming two images of the object, seen through two different refractive media.

Dim vision Dim vision for distance is due to change in the refraction to myopia. The lens becomes more globular. There is an associated astigmatism also.

Near vision There is difficulty in near vision due to disturbance of accommodation.

Signs

Irregular anterior chamber It is deep where the lens is absent and normal or shallow in the area where the lens has been displaced.

Iridodonesis *Dark edge of the lens* in the pupillary area by distant direct ophthalmoscopy.

Indirect ophthalmoscopy Optic disk appears double. One image of the disc being seen through the phakic area and the other image through the aphakic area.

Refraction Phakic area is myopic and astigmatic. Refraction through the aphakic area is hypermetropic.

Color of pupil Half of the pupil is normal grey and half of the pupil is jet black.

Complications

- Secondary glaucoma
- Uveitis
- Cataractous changes

Management

- Subluxated lens may remain quiet for a long time.
- IOLs implant is the ideal choice.

17

Maladies of Glaucoma

GLAUCOMA

Congenital Glaucoma

- Infantile glaucoma (buphthalmos, hydro-phthalmos, congenital glaucoma, juvenile glaucoma)

Primary Glaucoma

- Primary open angle glaucoma
- Primary angle-closure glaucoma

Specific Types of Glaucoma

- Normal (low) tension glaucoma
- Ocular hypertension
- Ciliary block glaucoma (malignant glaucoma)
- Aphakic/pseudophakic glaucoma

Secondary Glaucoma

- Lens induced glaucoma
- Hypertensive uveitis
- Hemogenic glaucoma
- Pigmentary glaucoma
- Neovascular glaucoma
- Glaucoma capsulare
- Steroid glaucoma
- Angle recession glaucoma

Glaucoma Associated with Syndromes

- Posner-Schlossman syndrome (glaucomato-cyclitic crisis)
- Sturge-Weber syndrome
- Von-Recklinghausen's neurofibromatosis
- Plateau iris syndrome
- Iridocorneal endothelial syndrome

GLAUCOMA

Glaucoma is a symptomatic complex in which there is raised intraocular pressure essentially due to obstruction to the drainage of aqueous humor at the pupil and/or at the angle of the anterior chamber or beyond the angle of anterior chamber in the drainage channels.

Glaucoma causes gradual loss of vision and visual field.

Malady is bilateral and must be genetically determined probably by multifactorial or polygenic inheritance. Specific glaucoma syndromes are transmitted as autosomal dominant disease.

Incidence of glaucoma over the age of 40 years is about 2%. Primary open angle affects more than 80% of cases. Primary angle close glaucoma affects less than 5% of primary glaucoma cases.

Ophthalmoscopy shows cupping of the optic disk and later glaucomatous optic atrophy.

Topical miotics *facilitate the outflow of aqueous* through the drainage channels.

Topical epinephrine and timolol maleate and systemic acetazolamide *inhibit the secretion of aqueous* by the ciliary epithelium and processes. Object of surgery is to create new subconjunctival filtration channel to drain the aqueous out of the anterior chamber.

Glaucoma leads to blindness, if not treated.

An early diagnosis and regular treatment can maintain a good visual acuity and visual fields for the life.

CONGENITAL GLAUCOMA

Congenital glaucoma refers to developmental anomaly of the angle with abnormally high ocular pressure but without any other associated ocular or systemic anomaly.

It has been classified according to the age of onset of rise in ocular pressure:

- *True congenital glaucoma:* Infant is born with ocular enlargement and high intraocular pressure. It affects 40% of cases.
- *Infantile glaucoma:* Glaucoma manifests prior to child's third birthday. It manifests in 50% of cases.
- *Juvenile glaucoma:* Glaucoma manifests between 3–16 years of age. It occurs in 10% cases.

Infantile Glaucoma (Buphthalmos, Hydrophthalmos, Congenital Glaucoma, Juvenile glaucoma)

Young mother presents with complains of large eyes with watering and photophobia in her infant's eyes.

Ocular examination shows enlarged eyeball with mild corneal haze.

Diagnosis—infantile glaucoma.

Etiology

- It is a rare disease.
- It is inherited as an autosomal recessive trait.
- It is caused by the developmental defect of the angle of the anterior chamber.

Symptoms

Parents bring the child, when they observe an abnormally large eye with associated symptoms of corneal haze, epiphora, photophobia and blepharospasm.

Signs

- Increased corneal diameter above 11.5 mm.
- Edema of corneal epithelium.
- Edema and opacity of corneal stroma.
- Tears and breaks in Descemet's membrane.
- Sclera is thin and appears blue.
- Anterior chamber is deep.

- Lens is flattened and displaced backwards.
- Anterior chamber is deep.
- Iris shows tremulousness.
- Ophthalmoscopy shows cupping of the disk.
- Gonioscopy shows a blocked angle.
- Tonometry shows a rise of ocular pressure.

Management

Surgical therapy

- Goniotomy controls ocular pressure in 70 to 80% of the cases.
- Combined trabeculotomy and trabeculectomy is the preferred surgery with better results.
- Once diagnosis is made, then it is better to undertake surgery soon to avoid further loss of vision and disk changes.

Medical therapy

- None of the medical therapy helps as there is a block at the angle most probably due to insertion of iris anteriorly into the trabeculum instead of the ciliary body.
- Hyperosmotic agents and acetazolamide can be used to lower the pressure till surgery is undertaken.

PRIMARY GLAUCOMA

Primary Open Angle Glaucoma

An elderly patient presents with complain of gradual loss of vision with mild headache and eye ache after near work.

Ocular examination shows dilated pupils with sluggish reaction to light reflex and low visual acuity with cupping of the disc.

Diagnosis—primary open angle glaucoma.

Primary open angle glaucoma affects adults and typically characterized by slowly progressive raised intraocular pressure above 21 mm Hg with cupping of the optic disk and specific visual field defects.

Etiology

- Primary open angle glaucoma has a polygenic inheritance. A glaucoma patient inherits a number of abnormal genes which influence the intraocular pressure, outflow facility and the cup/disk ratio.

- It affects both the sexes usually after sixth decade and slowly progressive disease with no specific psychological pattern.
- Prevalence is more in myopes, diabetics, hypertensive and thyrotoxic patients.

Pathogenesis

The angle of the anterior chamber is open, therefore, the pathology of primary open angle glaucoma lies beyond the angle that is:

Decrease in the aqueous outflow facility due to increased resistance caused by age-related thickening and sclerosis of the trabecular meshwork which are unable to drain the aqueous though the aqueous has reached the angle.

Symptoms

- *Headache and eye ache* without any obvious factor in an elderly person must arouse suspicion for glaucoma.
- *Gradual diminution of the visual acuity as* the disease is so insidious that the patient is unable to notice the gradual fall in his/her vision that occurs over years until the vision of one eye is almost lost and the other eye has also lost considerable vision.
- *Frequent change in the presbyopic correction* is due to gradual loss of accommodation owing to pressure upon the ciliary muscle and its nerve supply. *Any one requiring a frequent change of near glasses should be subjected to thorough examination for glaucoma.*
- *Defective light sense and dark adaptation:* Patient takes longer time to adapt to dim illumination.
- *Defects in visual field:* An intelligent and observant patient may notice defect in his/her field of vision.

Signs

- *Pupil is dilated with sluggish reaction to light reflex (Fig. 17.1):* In early stage, the pupil reacts normally to a light reflex.
  Later, it is semidilated and shows sluggish reaction to light reflex.

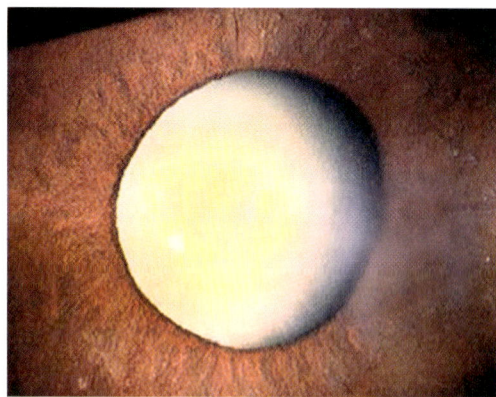

Fig. 17.1: Primary open angle glaucoma—dilated pupil

In advanced stage, the pupil is dilated and fixed showing no reaction to direct and consensual light reflex.

- *Loss of visual acuity:* Patient presents only when he has lost a considerable vision in one eye and the other eye also shows low visual acuity.
  No improvement in the visual acuity with any glasses and needs a much higher number for presbyopic correction than a normal person of his/her age.
- *Tonometry* shows raised intraocular pressure.
- *Ophthalmoscopy* shows cupping of the optic disk, change in the cup/disk ratio and hemorrhage on the disk margin
- Slit-lamp may show *Krukenberg's spindle.*
- *Defects of visual fields.*

Clinical Investigations

Digital Tonometry It is done in the same manner as testing for fluctuation in nodule or cyst in other parts of the body. Ask the patient to close both the eyes and look down. Place the bulb of two index fingers a short distance from one another above the upper border of superior tarsal plate and perform fluctuation test softly. Perform digital fluctuation first in normal eye and then compare it with the other affected eye. Repeat the test 2–3 times in both the eyes and compare. Hard feeling or no fluctuation indicates raised intraocular pressure.

It is easy and handy method for out-patient screening for glaucoma.

Schiotz tonometry

- All the normal eyes have a normal diurnal variation of 3 to 4 mm Hg in the intraocular pressure.
- *Diurnal variation* in glaucoma case may swing to 20 mm Hg or even more. Therefore, it is very essential to record the intraocular pressure at periodic interval during the day to diagnose a case for glaucoma or to assure the patient that there is no glaucoma.
- An intraocular pressure of 22 mm Hg or above should be viewed with suspicion.

Ophthalmoscopy

- Change in the cup/disk ratio
- Notching of the cup rim
- Concentric enlargement of the cup
- Splinter hemorrhage on the disk margin
- Striations and slit-like defects
- Looping of the retinal veins.

The presence of any one or more of the above mentioned findings provide an important clue for diagnosis of primary open angle glaucoma.

Cupping of the optic disk

- Cupping of the optic disk is the most important sign for glaucoma.
- Cupping of the disk occurs due to increased intraocular pressure and anoxia of the disk due to vascular sclerosis.
- Later there is glaucomatous optic atrophy.
- To begin with, the cup of the disk increases in vertical diameter giving it an oval shape extending more towards the lower temporal quadrant of the disk which results in upper arcuate scotoma.
- Cupping of the optic disk due to glaucoma must be differentiated from the *deep physiological cup* of the disk.
- *In glaucoma, the margin of the cup reaches up to the edge of the optic disk, the sides of the cup are steep and the retinal vessels appear to be broken at the margin of the disk.*
- It is essential to keep a record of the cup/disk ratio, as the ratio between the cup and

disk increases with time and it can be used to assess the progress of glaucoma.

5. *Gonioscopy:* The gonioscopy is performed with a three-mirror contact lens of Goldmann with slit-lamp. The semicircular mirror is used for examination of the angle of the anterior chamber. In primary open angle glaucoma, all the structures of the angle are seen by gonioscopy. The narrow beam of the light from the slit-lamp deflects at the transition between the anterior wall of the angle and the recess. The beam again deflects at the transition between the ciliary body and the root of the iris. In open angle, the anterior surface of the ciliary body forms the recess of the angle.

6. *Defects of the visual field:* In primary open angle glaucoma, both the central and peripheral field defects are affected. The central field defects are charted on *tangent screen* and the peripheral field on *automated perimeter.*

- *Central field defects:* The central field defects occur early due to the gradual destruction of the nerve fibers at the optic disk due to increased intraocular pressure. The central field defects are known as *nerve fiber bundle defects.*
- *Nerve fiber bundle defects* occur due to premature destruction of thick bundles of arcuate fibers which crowd on the temporal side of the disk and have an arcuate course above and below the macula.
- *Charting of central field defects is essential to assess the prognosis of glaucoma as the central vision is retained for a long time.*
- *Baring of the blind-spot:* In some cases of primary open angle glaucoma, the central field defect instead of being concentric around 30° isopter shows a curve inwards to exclude the blind spot. This defect is not pathognomonic of glaucoma. It can occur due to change in illumination and size of the pupil.
- *Seidel's sign:* There is a sickle-shaped extension of the blind spot above or below or both with concavity towards the fixation point.
- *Bjerrum's scotoma:* The scotoma is in direct continuity with blind spot. It may extend

above or below the fixation point or may form a complete ring.

- *Roenne's step:* Upper or lower sectorial defect with a horizontal edge.
- *Peripheral field defect:* In early stage of glaucoma, there is a defect in the upper or sometimes in the lower nasal field showing a characteristic sharp horizontal edge known as *Roenne's step.*

In later stage of glaucoma, there is a marked peripheral contraction of field leaving eventually a small paracentral patch in the temporal field. Central vision is lost.

Diagnosis

- An elderly patient with complain of gradual loss of vision.
- Pupil semidilated with sluggish reaction to light reflex.
- Intraocular pressure above 22 mm Hg on repeated examination during the day.
- Changes in the optic disk in form of cupping of the disk.
- Central field defect.

Differential Diagnosis

- Physiological cupping of the disk
- Coloboma of optic disk
- Anterior ischemic optic atrophy
- Chiasmal lesions.

Management

Medical therapy is the first choice. Aim to lower the pressure less than 16–18 mm Hg.

Surgery when medical therapy fails to control the intraocular pressure.

Topical medical therapy

- Timolol maleate (0.25% or 0.5%) eyedrops twice daily.
  It lowers the intraocular pressure by *reducing the aqueous secretion due to their effect on beta-receptors in the ciliary processes.* It does not affect the size of pupil, accommodation, visual acuity and tear formation. Its use is contraindicated in asthma and cardiac cases.

- *Pilocarpine (1, 2, 4%)* eyedrops two to four times daily.
  Pilocarpine reduces the intraocular pressure by opening intertrabecular spaces, thereby *increasing trabecular meshwork outflow of aqueous.* Pilocarpine may be added, if the timolol maleate fails to lower the tension to the desired level.
- *Latanoprost (0.005%)* eyedrops once daily. It is a prostaglandin by nature and lowers intraocular pressure by *increase of uveoscleral outflow of aqueous.*

Surgical therapy

- *Argon laser trabeculoplasty:* It causes shrinkage of the collagen on the inner surface of the trabecular meshwork thereby opening the intertrabecular spaces and *increases aqueous outflow.* It lowers the intraocular pressure between 8 to 10 mm Hg in about 75% of the cases.
- Most of the cases need continuation of medical therapy.
- Filtration surgery is indicated in the cases who do not respond to *argon laser trabeculoplasty.*

Filtration surgery

- Guarded partial thickness surgery—*trabeculectomy.*
- Ex-press *glaucoma filtration device.*
- Non-penetrating surgery:
  i. *Deep sclerectomy*
  ii. *Viscocanalostomy*
- Cyclodestructive surgery—cyclocryopexy, Nd: YAG laser, diode laser.

Trebeculectomy is the most common operation performed by surgeons. The success rate is about 80 to 90%.

Ex-press filtration device provides better management of intraocular pressure.

Filtration surgery is indicated in all the cases not responding to medical therapy and show progressive loss of fields with increase in the cupping or cup/disk ratio.

Primary Angle-closure Glaucoma

Primary angle-closure glaucoma is characterized by shallow anterior chamber with anteriorly placed iris-lens diaphragm resulting in narrow angle of the anterior chamber. It leads to consistent deficiency in out flow of the aqueous.

Etiology

Main factor is the closure of already existing narrow angle due to crowding of the iris at the angle, when the pupil is semidilated in the physiological states such as close work in dim light or emotional crisis.

Predisposing Factors

- *Age*: Common in fifth or sixth decade.
- *Sex:* Females are more prone (male to female ratio is 1:4).
- *Emotional personality*: People with unstable vasomotor system. Any emotional crisis results in semidilation of pupil and it causes obstruction to outflow of aqueous.
- Hypermetropic eye with shallow chamber.
- Eyes with anteriorly placed iris-lens diaphragm.
- Semidilation of pupil in dim illumination such as cloudy weather, cinema hall or near work in twilight or insufficient illumination.

Mechanism

The sequence of events that follow the semi-dilation of pupil results in rise of intraocular pressure due to *blockage in outflow of aqueous humor by angle-closure* though the drainage channels are functioning normally.

- *In an eye of normal people*, the iris lies flat with its pupillary margin gliding lightly over the anterior surface of the lens.
- *In an eye with primary angle-closure glaucoma*, there is shallow anterior chamber due to iris-lens diaphragm placed anteriorly and the iris is in close touch with the entire anterior surface of the lens resulting in *relative pupil block* for aqueous to traverse from posterior chamber to anterior chamber.
- *Out flow of aqueous* faces further block at the angle due to semidilated pupil causing crowding at the root of iris.

This results in collection of aqueous in the posterior chamber thereby pushing the relaxed iris bellies forward at the periphery resembling an *iris bombe*. The root of the iris comes close to posterior surface of cornea in the periphery of chamber tending to cut off drainage channels and the angle of anterior chamber from the rest of the anterior chamber.

The aqueous cannot reach the angle due to crowding of the iris creating a false angle. Therefore, the aqueous cannot be drained though the drainage channels are functioning normally.

Peripheral laser iridotomy or surgical iridectomy shall allow the aqueous to reach the real angle in extreme periphery beyond crowding of iris at the root of iris allowing normal drainage of aqueous through trabecular meshwork.

Laser iridotomy should be preferred over surgical iridectomy.

Prophylaxis peripheral iridotomy in the fellow eye shall free the patient from all the ill effects of all the clinical types of primary angle-closure glaucoma.

Clinical Classification of Primary Angle-closure Glaucoma

Clinical subtypes may or may not show a step-wise progression of primary angle-closure glaucoma.

1. Latent or suspect primary angle-closure glaucoma
2. Subacute or intermittent primary angle-closure glaucoma
3. Acute primary angle-closure glaucoma
4. Post congestive primary angle-closure glaucoma
5. Chronic primary angle-closure glaucoma
6. Absolute primary angle-closure glaucoma.

1. Latent or Suspect Primary Angle-closure Glaucoma

Patient presents with complain of mild discomfort, slight blurring of vision and colored rings around the light bulb occasionally after long hours of near work especially in late evening.

Slit-lamp shows shallow anterior chamber due to anteriorly placed iris-lens diaphragm. Digital tonometry indicates soft normal fluctuation. Schiotz's tonometry shows normal intraocular pressure.

Patient needs investigations such as gonioscopy, diurnal and provocative test to confirm.

Diagnosis—latent or suspect primary angle-closure glaucoma.

As this clinical phase is for a very short period, the patient usually ignores it unless it becomes more common. Patient presents with mild headache, slight blurring of vision and halos. The eye appears normal with no congestion though intraocular pressure if recorded, may be about 40 mm Hg or even more. Therefore, every adult should be screened for tonometry.

Symptoms

- Eye appears normal with no congestion
- Mild headache with slight blurring of vision.
- *Halos-colored rings:* Subjective appearance of halos around the light bulb is characteristic diagnostic symptom.

The appearance of *halos* can be demonstrated to the patient by his/her looking through a thin layer of lycopodium powder enclosed between two glass plates made up as a trial lens.

The main symptom of *halos* occurs due to edema of corneal epithelium and due to alteration in the refractive condition of the corneal lamellae. The *halos* are usually observed in late evening or night by the patient as colored rings around the light bulb or candle. The red color is the outer most and the blue color is the inner most. The only other condition which gives rise to *halos* is the stage of *incipient cortical soft cataract.*

Halos due to latent glaucoma and *halos* due to incipient cataract can be easily differentiated by *Fincham's test.*

Fincham's test: Stenopic slit is passed across the pupil in the line of vision. As the slit passes in front of the pupil, the *halos* due to glaucoma remain intact whereas the *halos* due to incipient cataract appear broken up into segments which revolve as slit is moved.

Signs Slit-lamp examination shows:
- Shallow chamber with decreased axial depth of chamber.
- Iris-lens diaphragm is placed anteriorly
- Proximity of iris to cornea in the periphery.

Gonioscopy demonstrates a narrow angle: In a case of latent primary angle-closure glaucoma, gonioscopy shows only the Schwalbe's line (glistening white line) and the anterior part of the trabecular band is visible. The crowding of the iris in the periphery conceals the lower part of the trabeculae, ciliary body and the root of the iris. There is a deflection of the beam of the light from the slit-lamp. This parallactic displacement of the light beam indicates that some part of the angle is open. In a completely closed angle, there is no parallactic displacement and light beam appears to meet at a point.

Tonometry: During the latent glaucoma phase when the patient complains of seeing colored rings, there is marked rise of the intraocular pressure to 40 mm Hg or even more.

Diurnal variation is high.

Provocative test: Dark-room test: The patient is made to sit in a dark room with his/her eyes open for half an hour. If there is a difference of more than 8 mm Hg in the intraocular pressure measured before and after the test then it is a positive test for primary angle-closure glaucoma.

Management

1. *Surgical therapy:* Prophylactic surgical therapy is the first and ideal choice.

One peripheral prophylactic laser iridotomy in both the eyes can cure the patient for rest of his life.
- It allows passage to aqueous from the posterior chamber to the angle of anterior chamber directly without passing through the pupil.
- It prevents occurrence of physiological iris bombe thereby crowding of the iris root at the angle to block it.
- It gives a complete cure.

2. *Topical medical therapy:* Until the patient is ready for operation, he/she should be advised to use pilocarpine (1, 2, 4%) eyedrops once or twice daily and an additional drop of pilocarpine whenever he/she expects to face emotional crisis of any kind and a dark environment or low illumination for a long time. Pilocarpine being a miotic keeps the pupil constricted, therefore, the angle remains open.

2. Subacute or Intermittent Primary Angle-closure Glaucoma

Patient presents with transient attacks more frequently with similar symptoms and signs as of latent or suspect primary angle-closure glaucoma.

Slit-lamp shows shallow anterior chamber with anteriorly placed iris-lens diaphragm.

Digital tonometry demonstrates normal fluctuation.

Patient needs to be investigated especially for gonioscopy, diurnal and provocative test.

Diagnosis—subacute primary angle-closure glaucoma.

In this subacute phase, the intermittent attacks of increased intraocular pressure become more regular. The normal diurnal variation in intraocular pressure is exaggerated, therefore, the ocular tension is very high usually in the late afternoon and evening. The ocular pressure falls spontaneously following rest or sleep.

Clinical features in subacute or intermittent phase of glaucoma are almost similar to the latent phase of glaucoma.

Tonometry during late afternoon or evening shows rise of the intraocular pressure.

Management of this phase is also similar to the management of latent phase.

3. Acute Primary Angle-closure Glaucoma (Fig. 17.2)

A male patient presents with intense agonizing pain with prostration covering the affected eye with hanky or turban and also supporting with palm as if the eyeball is just going to burst out.

As soon as he sits on the examination chair, he raises his both the feet on the chair and buries his head in between the knees.

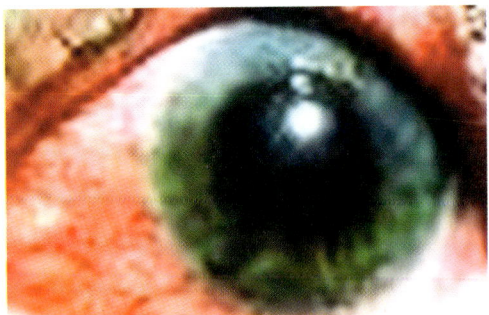
Fig. 17.2: Acute primary angle-closure glaucoma

Same patient on shifting to bed buries his head on the pillow and supports his head with both the hands in prone position, drawing his knees close to chest.

These characteristic postures are diagnostic for acute primary angle-closure glaucoma or acute uveitis.

Slit-lamp shows marked circumciliary congestion, mild haze in cornea, dilated fixed pupil.

Applanation tonometry indicates marked rise of intraocular pressure.

Diagnosis—acute primary angle-closure glaucoma.

An attack of acute phase of angle-closure glaucoma is precipitated by sudden occlusion of entire angle that remains closed for a long time due to dilation of pupil resulting in crowding of iris at the angle initiating blockage of angle and thereby causing obstruction to outflow of aqueous from normal functioning drainage channels at the real angle.

Symptoms

- *Intense pain:* The intense pain starts suddenly. It is felt in the eye and along the distribution of fifth nerve. It is due to stretching of sensory fibers of fifth nerve.
- *Headache, nausea, vomiting and prostration* may be associated with ocular pain.
- *Red eye, lacrimation and photophobia.*
- *Diminution of vision* is rapidly progressive to the extent of perception of light.

Signs

1. Lids are swollen.
2. Circumciliary congestion, lacrimation and photophobia.

3. Congestion of conjunctiva with mild chemosis.
4. Cornea appears hazy due to edema of corneal epithelium.
5. Anterior chamber is shallow.
6. Pupil is dilated, vertically oval and fixed with no reaction to consensual or direct light reflex.
7. Iris shows discoloration.
8. Schiotz's tonometry shows high intra-ocular pressure.
9. Visual acuity may be reduced to hand movements or even to perception of light only due to ischemic neuropathy.
10. Ophthalmoscopy and gonioscopy are not possible due to corneal edema and intense pain in and around the eye.
11. Fellow eye shows signs of latent phase of primary angle-closure glaucoma.

Clinical course If patient presents within short time due to acute and sudden appearance of symptoms then energetic management can abort the attack otherwise the patient enters the phase of post-congestive primary angle-closure glaucoma. It needs to be differentiated from:

- Acute conjunctivitis which presents with discharge but no pain.
- Acute anterior uveitisiridocyclitis which presents with constricted pin point pupil along with intense pain.

Management It is primarily surgical.

Start topical and systemic medical therapy to provide relief from intense pain, congestion and highly raised intraocular pressure to make the eye amenable and responsive to surgeon and surgery.

- *Medical therapy—topical and systemic:*
- Sedation and analgesics *by systemic oral or intramuscular or even intravenous route. It shall take care of general symptoms of intense ocular pain, headache, nausea, vomiting and prostration.*
- *Topical pilocarpine* 4% eyedrops to achieve miosis which helps to relieve the block of the angle by crowding of iris and breaks peripheral anterior synechia also.
- *Intravenous mannitol* (1 gm/kg body weight) as the patient may not be able to retain

medicine given orally due to nausea. Mannitol is very effective in reducing ocular tension.

- *Follow with acetazolamide* tablets 250 mg orally. Start with two tablets straight followed by one tablet every 6 hourly for 2 or 3 days.
- *Systemic and topical steroids and antibiotics* to abort the vasomotor phenomenon to reduce the conjunctival and circumciliary congestion.

2. *Surgical therapy: Slit-lamp examination and gonioscopy* on reduction in the ocular pressure and congestion of the eye is mandatory to decide the surgery needed by the patient.

- *Peripheral laser iridotomy or surgical iridectomy* is sufficient to establish the communication between posterior chamber and angle of the anterior chamber, if there are no synechia and the angle is open.
- *Trabeculectomy* a filtering surgery is the ideal choice, if the angle is blocked due to peripheral anterior synechia creating a false angle.

4. Post-congestive Primary Angle-closure Glaucoma

This phase is referred to clinical status of the eye after an attack of acute close angle glaucoma with or without any treatment.

Clinical types

- Patient may respond and achieve normal intraocular pressure.
- Patient may not respond to either medical or even surgical treatment.
- Few patients may get relief from severe symptoms without any treatment in few days as they are not able to attend eye clinic due to low socioeconomic status.
- Patient may pass into chronic congestive close angle glaucoma.

Manage this phase as acute primary angle-closure glaucoma. Aim is to provide relief from pain and annoying symptoms and save vision.

5. Chronic Primary Angle-closure Glaucoma

This phase results due to gradual synechial closure of the angle of the anterior chamber following each phase of subacute or intermittent primary angle-closure glaucoma.

This phase may also result due to combination of primary open angle glaucoma with narrow angle of anterior chamber.

Symptoms

1. Gradual loss of vision.
2. Pupil is dilated and reacts sluggishly or no reaction at all.

Signs

- Visual acuity is low.
- Pupil is dilated and reacting sluggishly or fixed.
- Tonometry shows raised intraocular pressure.
- Perimetry may show field defects—central and peripheral.
- Slit-lamp examination may show few keratic precipitates and atrophy of the iris.
- Gonioscopy shows peripheral anterior synechia or narrow angle.
- Ophthalmoscopy may show cupping of the disk.

Management

- *Lower the intraocular pressure* by timolol maleate 0.5% eyedrops twice a day and acetazolamide orally prior to surgery for few days to make the eye friendly to surgeon and surgery.
- *Trabeculectomy* a filtering surgery is the only choice of treatment to save the remaining vision.
- *Trabeculectomy* in the fellow eye, if needed as per gonioscopy and blockage at the angle.

6. Absolute Primary Angle-closure Glaucoma

Patient presents with complain of chronic pain with complete loss of vision in the affected eye and marked loss in opposite eye.

Ocular examination shows insensitive cornea, corneal haze, vertically oval dilated fixed pupil with stony hard eyeball on digital tonometry and no perception of light.

Diagnosis—absolute glaucoma.

Untreated cases of chronic primary angle-closure glaucoma pass into the phase of absolute glaucoma wherein the eye is painful and blind.

Clinical Features

1. Patient complains of pain and loss of vision in the affected eye.
2. Mild circumciliary congestion.
3. Cornea is clear but insensitive. There may be vesicles or filaments on the cornea.
4. Anterior chamber is very shallow.
5. Pupil is vertically oval, dilated and fixed.
6. Pupil appears grey.
7. Iris is atrophic.
8. Lens may be hazy.
9. Intraocular pressure is very high.
10. Ophthalmoscopy shows cupping of the disk.
11. In the end, due to degenerative changes in the ciliary processes, the ocular pressure falls and the eyeball may shrink to end as *atrophic bulbi*.

Management

- None of the medical therapy is helpful in reducing the intraocular pressure.
- Cyclocryotherapy or cyclophotocoagulation to destroy the ciliary processes thereby the tension falls and the patient gets relief from pain. It can be repeated two or three times to achieve the desired results.

SPECIFIC TYPES OF GLAUCOMA

Normal/Low Tension Glaucoma

Patient presents with all the typical findings of open angle glaucoma such as gonioscopically open angle, cupping of the disk, with or without visual field changes and associated with intraocular pressure constantly below 21 mm Hg even on repeated measurement on the same day or regularly even for weeks.

Diagnosis—normal/low tension glaucoma.

Clinical Features

- Variant of primary open angle glaucoma.
- Chronic low vascular perfusion makes the optic nerve susceptible to normal or low intraocular pressure.
- Some of these cases may show ocular lesions such as; ischemic optic neuropathy, juxtapapillary choroiditis, high myopia and temporal arteritis.

Management

- Excluding all other maladies.
- Bring down the intraocular pressure below 12 mm Hg by medical therapy or filtering surgery.
- Betaxolol 0.25% once or twice a day. It lowers the pressure and also increases optic nerve blood flow.
- *Latanoprost (0.005%)* eyedrops once daily. It is a prostaglandin by nature and lowers intraocular pressure by *increase of uveo-scleral outflow of aqueous.* It has greater ocular hypotensive effect in eyes with normal tension.
- Regular follow-up to save the vision.

Ocular Hypertension

Patient presents with intraocular pressure more than 21 mm Hg constantly without optic disk and visual field changes.

Ocular examination shows few signs of primary open angle glaucoma

Manage to lower the pressure by 20% that is, between 14–16 mm Hg with topical medical therapy.

Diagnosis—ocular hypertension.

Clinical Features

It is a variant of primary open angle glaucoma.
- There is significant diurnal variation.
- Provocative test is positive.
- No cupping or atrophy of the disk.
- No visual field defects.
- Positive family history

Management

Lower the intraocular pressure by about 20% by topical medical therapy—timolol maleate, latanoprost or pilocarpine eyedrops.

Filtering surgery not indicated until patient shows changes in the disk and visual fields.

Regular follow-up to save the vision.

Ciliary Block Glaucoma
(Malignant Glaucoma)

Patient presents with history of surgery for primary acute angle-closure glaucoma.

Slit-lamp shows flat anterior chamber with very high intraocular pressure.

Diagnosis—ciliary block glaucoma.

Clinical Features

- Ciliary block glaucoma occurs in a case of Primary angle closure glaucoma that has undergone filtering surgery.
- Anterior chamber is either flat or fails to reform and there is a rise of the intraocular pressure.

It is believed that the tips of ciliary processes rotate forward and press against the equator of the lens—*ciliolenticular block* in phakic eye or against the intraocular lens— *cilio-IOLs block* in pseudophakic eye or against the anterior hyaloids phase of vitreous—*ciliovitreal block* in aphakic eye.

Thus the aqueous is unable to enter the anterior chamber and is diverted posteriorly forming aqueous pockets in the vitreous or behind the vitreous. Due to this, the entire iris-lens diaphragm and the vitreous are pushed forward resulting in flat anterior chamber and rise in ocular pressure.

Ciliary block glaucoma (malignant glaucoma) may be phakic, pseudophakic or aphakic.

Miotics aggravate the condition further.

Management

The treatment lies in pulling back the iris-lens diaphragm backwards.
- Aggressive cycloplegic therapy which may help to pull back the lens in some cases by breaking the ciliolenticular or vitreal contact.
- Acetazolamide or mannitol to cause deturgescence of vitreous gel.
- YAG *laser hyaloidotomy.*
- Aspirate the trapped aqueous through the pars plana.

Aphakic/Pseudophakic Glaucoma

Patient presents with pain in the eye following lens extraction or IOLs implant.

Slit-lamp may show pupil block, flat chamber, peripheral anterior synechia or ingrowing of epithelium.

Diagnosis—aphakic glaucoma.

Clinical Features

Glaucoma following cataract extraction is known as aphakic glaucoma. This type of glaucoma usually occurs due to:

- Pupillary block by the vitreous protruding through the pupil thereby causing blockage of circulation of aqueous humor. Peripheral iridectomy prevents this type of glaucoma.
- Cycloplegic can relieve the pupillary block.
- Peripheral anterior synechia which follows, if the anterior chamber remains flat for a long time.
- A long standing case responds to cyclodialysis.
- Anterior chamber being lined with epithelium, when the healing of the incisional wound is delayed. The ingrowing epithelium blocks the angle and lines the iris.
- Ingrowing epithelium is best treated by application of laser light.

SECONDARY GLAUCOMA

The term 'secondary glaucoma' entertains a group of maladies in which rise of intraocular pressure is associated with some kind of primary ocular or systemic malady.

Lens-induced Glaucoma

Phacolytic Glaucoma

Patient presents with secondary open angle glaucoma in which the trabecular meshwork gets clogged by the lens particles, lens protein and macrophages laden with lens protein with rise of intraocular pressure.

Etiological factors

- Leak of protein from the intact thin capsule of hypermature cataractous lens.
- Macrophages laden with lens protein.
- Extracapsular cataract extraction.
- Traumatic rupture of lens.

Management IOLs implant

Phacoanaphylactic Uveitis with Glaucoma

Patient presents with severe reaction due to lens protein (antigen-antibody reaction) showing keratic precipitates, cellular reaction in aqueous and all other signs of anterior uveitis with rise of intraocular pressure. It follows usually after rupture of the lens due to trauma or following an extracapsular cataract surgery.

Management

- Systemically and topically steroids in high dose and taper gradually to maintenance dose for long time.
- Removal of the lens capsule or lens material left behind during first surgery.

Phacomorphic Galucoma

- *Intumescence of lens (Fig. 17.3):* Patient presents with all the symptoms and signs of acute primary angle-closure glaucoma due to swollen lens which pushes the iris forward thereby resulting in pupil and angle block. The hydration of cortical fibers during stage of intumescent cataract results in swelling of the lens. The intumescence of lens can occur by imbibing the

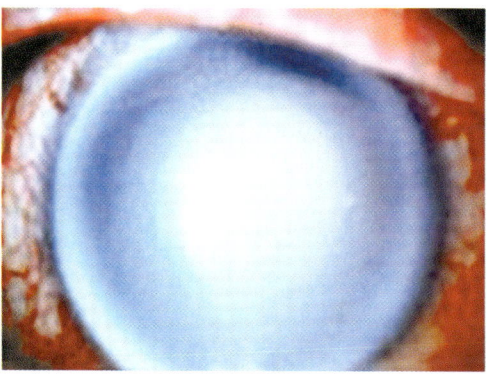

Fig. 17.3: Phacomorphic glaucoma due to intumescence of lens

aqueous following trauma resulting in rupture of lens capsule.

Manage by IOLs implant.

- *Dislocation or subluxation of lens in anterior chamber:* The dislocation or subluxation of lens can be spontaneous or traumatic.

Spontaneous dislocation of lens is commonly seen in Marfan's syndrome.

Trauma can cause hyphema and angle recession along with dislocation or subluxation of lens.

- *Spherophakia (microphakia):* Spherophakia is commonly seen in Marchesani's syndrome and in association with other ocular congenital anomalies and inborn errors of metabolism.

Lens is small and spherical thereby it causes pupil block that causes rise of intraocular pressure.

Management

- Myotic eyedrops causes rise in ocular pressure due to enhancing pupil block.
- Mydriatic relieves the ocular pressure by relieving pupil block.
- Peripheral iridectomy is the treatment of choice as aqueous can bypass the pupil block.

Hypertensive Uveitis (Fig. 17.4)

Patient presents with symptoms and signs of acute anterior uveitis with high rise of intraocular pressure due to plasmoid aqueous with anterior peripheral and posterior synechias.

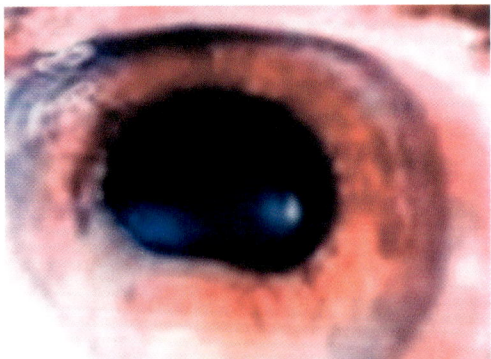

Fig. 17.4: Hypertensive uveitis

Clinical Features

Acute anterior uveitis manifests with formation of plasmoid aqueous due to increased permeability of the uveal capillaries. Due to increased viscosity of the plasmoid aqueous, its drainage is not proper, therefore, there is a rise of the intraocular pressure.

Exudates and macrophages further obstruct the trabecular drainage channels.

Later, there is the blockage of circulation of the aqueous due to peripheral anterior synechia, iris bombe, seclusio pupillae, occlusio pupillae and total posterior synechia.

Management

- An early and energetic treatment of uveitis may prevent all the causative factors which lead to rise of intraocular pressure.
- Monitor intraocular pressure and keep it under control by topical and systemic therapy.

Hemogenic Glaucoma

Presence of blood in the anterior chamber or the vitreous can raise the intraocular pressure by clogging the trabecular meshwork.

Glaucoma due to Hyphema (Red Cell Glaucoma)

- Total hyphema fills the entire anterior chamber and plugs the entire trabecular meshwork resulting in rise of intraocular pressure. Evacuate the blood from anterior chamber.
- If the hyphema is fluid in nature then nurse the patient in bed with head elevated so that the blood tends to settle down by gravity and clears the superior portion of the trabecular meshwork for drainage of the aqueous.
- If hyphema appears to be full and clotted then it is advisable to evacuate the blood by surgical procedure early as the clotted blood blocks the pupil and angle resulting in rise of the intraocular pressure.
- *Untreated hyphema associated with rise of intraocular pressure leads to blood staining of the cornea.*

Hemolytic Glaucoma

In a case with hyphema of long standing, the large mononuclear phagocytes laden with lysed hemorrhagic debris plugs the pores of trabecular meshwork causing rise in the intraocular pressure. Treat by lavage of anterior chamber.

Hemosiderotic Glaucoma

Hemosiderin released by the lysed blood cells may cause direct damage to the trabecular meshwork causing sclerosis as occurs in a case of siderosis. Treat by the lavage of the anterior chamber.

Ghost Cell Glaucoma

Old red blood cells in the vitreous migrate to the anterior chamber and plug the pores in the trabecular meshwork. These old red blood cells are not normal cells but are hollow (ghost) cells with rigid walls which do not allow them to pass through the pores in the trabeculae.

Medical therapy is effective. Few cases may need a lavage of the anterior chamber.

Pigmentary Glaucoma

Clinical Features

- Pigmentary glaucoma is characterized by the presence of Krukenberg's spindle and pigment deposition in the trabecular meshwork.
- Usually bilateral and affects young myopes and seen in diabetics.
- Slit-lamp examination shows Krukenberg's spindle.
- Gonioscopy shows the pigment accumulation along Schwalbe's line in the angle.
- Iris transillumination shows radial slit-like transillumination defects in the mid periphery.
- Treat pigmentary glaucoma like primary open angle glaucoma.

Neovascular Glaucoma

Patient presents with intense neuralgic pain in his left eye with history of very low vision but without any pain since last ten years or so.

Slit-lamp shows intense circumciliary congestion and rubeosis iridis.

Diagnosis—neovascular glaucoma.

Clinical Features

Neovascular glaucoma is usually associated with:
- Diabetic retinopathy
- Central retinal vein occlusion
- Eales' disease.

There is new vessel formation on the surface of the iris. These vessels spread and bridge the angle of anterior chamber and grow on to the corneal endothelium. It blocks the angle of anterior chamber resulting in rise of ocular pressure.

If one eye is affected then keep a watch on the other eye especially for glaucoma and occurrence of central retinal vein occlusion.

Management

Panretinal photocoagulation to prevent neovascular glaucoma.

Glaucoma Capsulare

Clinical Features

Exfoliation of the lens capsule is common among old people. On electron microscopy, the exfoliated material appears to be an amyloid like material. It appears that the pupillary movement scrapes off the material from the lens surface and this material later gets deposited in the trabecular meshwork causing rise of intraocular pressure.

Slit-lamp after full dilation of pupil may help to find signs of exfoliation. Gonioscopy reveals block of the trabeculae and early wavy pigmentary (Sampaolesi's) line in front of Schwalbe's line.

- Treat as primary open angle glaucoma.
- Medical therapy is mildly effective.
- Filtering surgery is necessary to control the glaucoma.

Steroid Glaucoma

Clinical Features

- Steroids given systemically, topically or by subconjunctival route can cause rise in the intraocular pressure.

- Patients having a long-term steroid therapy should be subjected to periodic tonometry and ophthalmoscopy to diagnose occurrence of glaucoma early.
- Glaucoma due to steroid therapy is primary open angle glaucoma.
- Ocular pressure becomes normal in a few weeks after withdrawing steroids and providing medical therapy by topical timolol maleate 0.25, 0.50% eyedrops.

Angle Recession Glaucoma

Clinical Features

- Angle recession glaucoma is due to contusion of the eyeball.
- Contusion results in the tear of the ciliary body causing angle recession.
- *Glaucoma develops after several years, therefore, it is essential to examine the patient with angle recession periodically for years.*
- Treat like primary open angle glaucoma.

GLAUCOMA ASSOCIATED WITH SYNDROMES

Posner-Schlossman Syndrome
(Glaucomatocyclitic Crisis)

Clinical Features

- Sudden and rapid rise of intraocular pressure to the level of 60 mm Hg or even more.
- Diagnosed at this stage as a case of acute angle closure glaucoma.
- Gonioscopy reveals an open angle.
- Slit-lamp shows minimal signs of inflammation in form of few keratic precipitates and mild cellular reaction in the aqueous.
- It is self-limiting.
- Steroids play a little part in its control.
- Medical therapy for primary open angle glaucoma is essential to control the ocular pressure until the disease runs its spontaneous self-limiting course.

Sturge-Weber Syndrome

Clinical Features

- Characterized by small vessel hemangioma involving structures supplied by first two branches of the trigeminal (fifth) nerve. Usually affects one side of the face.
- Rise of intraocular pressure with involvement of the upper eyelid with hemangioma.
- Treat glaucoma by goniotomy.

von Recklinghausen's Neurofibromatosis

Clinical Features

- In a typical case, the lids, orbit and temporal region are affected.
- *Swollen lid and temporal region form a characteristic picture.*
- Hypertrophied nerves can be felt by fingers through the skin of the lids as hard cords or knobs.
- Associated with infantile glaucoma, if the upper lid is involved.
- Treat by goniotomy.

Plateau Iris Syndrome

It is a condition in which the iris is inserted anteriorly on the ciliary body.
- Gonioscopy helps to diagnose it.
- Slit-lamp shows normal anterior chamber and iris plane appears flat.
- Responds well to medical therapy.

Iridocorneal Endothelial Syndrome

Clinical Features

This syndrome embraces the following three conditions:
1. Iris nevus syndrome (Cogan-Reese syndrome) is nodular or diffuse pigmented lesions of the iris.
2. Chandler's syndrome—mild iris changes with corneal edema.
3. Essential progressive iris atrophy—iris shows corectopia, atrophy and holes.

The common feature of these three anamolies is the presence of abnormal corneal endothelial cells which proliferate and form an endothelial membrane over the angle of anterior chamber.

Glaucoma manifests due to secondary synechial angle-closure due to contraction of this endothelial membrane resulting in narrow angle and peripheral anterior synechia.

Management

- Medical therapy and trabeculectomy not effective.
- Artificial filteration shunt may control the high tension.

18

Maladies of Vitreous

Vitreous

Investigations

- Ophthalmoscopy
- Slit-lamp
- B-scan ultrasonography

Specific Maladies of Vitreous

- Synchysis and syneresis
- Posterior vitreous detachment
- Persistent hyperplastic primary vitreous
- Persistent hyaloid artery

Opacities in Vitreous

- Developmental
- Muscae volitantes
- Degenerative
  - Asteroid hyalosis
  - Synchysis scintillans
  - Amyloidosis
- Inflammatory

Hereditary Hyaloidoretinopathies

- Wagner's vitreoretinal degeneration
- Goldmann-Favre's degeneration
- Hereditary juvenile retinoschisis

Intraocular Hemorrhage

- Retrovitreous hemorrhage
- Intravitreal hemorrhage
- Vitreous bands and membranes

VITREOUS

The vitreous is a clear, avascular, gelatinous gel filling the space bounded by the lens, retina and optic disk.

It consists of 99% water and 1% collagen and hyaluronic acid. It is impervious to cells and debris. Its function is to maintain the transparency and form of the eye.

The outer surface of the vitreous, the hyaloid membrane, is normally in contact with following structures—posterior lens capsule, suspensory ligaments, pars plana, retina and optic disk.

It is firmly attached to pars plana and retina behind the ora serrata. It is prone to get firmly attached to the retina at the site of degeneration of retina, scars of retina and new blood vessels.

The vitreous has all the properties of a hydrophilic gel undergoing turgescence and deturgescence. It has a tendency to become transformed into a fluid, when its protein basis becomes coagulated with age, degeneration and any kind of trauma whether mechanical or chemical.

INVESTIGATION

Ophthalmoscopy

A normal, clear, transparent and healthy vitreous gel is not visible by ophthalmoscopy or slit-lamp.

Whenever, there is a structural change in the vitreous gel due to degeneration, trauma, old age or there are foreign elements like blood, fibrovascular bands and membranes or inflammatory cells and exudates then all these are visible as black spots, floaters or bands in the red background of the fundus reflex floating freely in the fluid vitreous.

Slit-lamp

The anterior vitreous can be seen easily with the beam of the slit-lamp. The posterior and peripheral vitreous can be examined with the aid of a three-mirror contact lens. Thus, with slit-lamp and a three mirror contact lens, one can examine the whole vitreous in detail.

B-scan Ultrasonography

Ultrasonography helps to locate and identify the vitreous membranes, retinal detachment, intraocular foreign body and the state of the vitreous and structures associated with it.

SPECIFIC MALADIES OF VITREOUS

Synchysis and Syneresis

- *Patient presents with subjective symptom of seeing black floaters in front of the eye.*
- Synchysis (liquefaction) and syneresis (collapse) are two most common degenerative changes in vitreous gel.
- *Synchysis* denotes liquefaction of vitreous gel which may be total or partial.
- Synchysis senilis is an age-related phenomenon of the vitreous gel caused by alteration of its micromolecular structure.
- Synchysis of vitreous acts as a predisposing factor for posterior vitreous detachment.
- *Syneresis* denotes collapse of vitreous gel which separates its liquid from solid component of the gel.

Slit-lamp Biomicroscopy

Total synchysis: There is absence of fine fibrillar structure of the vitreous with presence of coarse aggregate floaters moving freely within vitreous cavity.

Partial synchysis: There is formation of cavity or lacuna in the posterior vitreous which appears as empty space.

Posterior Vitreous Detachment

Patient presents with complain of sudden appearance of annoying symptom of floaters and alarming symptom of flashes of light in his right eye.

Slit-lamp shows floaters in the vitreous.

Binocular indirect ophthalmoscopy shows posterior vitreous detachment.

Diagnosis—posterior vitreous detachment.

Posterior vitreous detachment (PVD) denotes separation of the cortical vitreous from the retina anywhere posterior to vitreous base. Vitreous base is a 3–4 mm wide area of attachment of vitreous to the ora serrata.

Pathogenesis

Posterior vitreous detachment (PVD) with vitreous synchysis (liquefaction) and syneresis (collapse) is an age-related phenomenon which occurs universally over the age of 65 years usually affecting the upper part of the vitreous. The liquefaction and collapse of vitreous gel can occur due to old age or any kind of trivial insult to the vitreous. In some cases, a hole develops in the thin wall of the posterior vitreous cortex which overlies the fovea. The liquid vitreous from the lacuna (cavity) of the vitreous passes through this hole into the retrohyaloid space and forcibly detaches the posterior vitreous surface from the internal limiting membrane of the retina as far as the posterior border of the vitreous base. Due to the escape of synchytic fluid, the syneresis (collapse) of the posterior vitreous follows thereby the retrohyaloid space is completely filled by the synchytic fluid. This process is known as *acute rhegmatogenous posterior vitreous detachment with collapse*. It occurs more frequently in aphakics and myopes than phakics and emmetropes.

Symptoms

Vitreous floaters Most of the patients describe the annoying symptom, as if seeing a fly or a mosquito consistently flying before the eyes.

Patient complains of seeing various types of dark spots floating or moving before the eyes.

Vitreous opacities appear to him as fine, thick, regular irregular, thread, worm or cotton wool like dark spots.

Vitreous opacities appear as moving freely with the movement of the eye and even after it is stationary.

Vitreous opacities appear as dark spot to the patient as the opacity in the vitreous can stimulate the retina by casting a shadow upon it.

Vitreous opacities can be diagnosed by Slit-lamp and direct ophthalmoscopy.

Photopsia (flashes of light) Patient complains of alarming awareness of the flash of a light, a glow, a streak of light in form of an arc in his field of vision.

Appearance of flash of light is for a very short duration never more than a fraction of a second and can be readily seen on moving the eyes in dark or in dim illumination.

This phenomenon of flash of light seen by the patient is due to cerebral awareness of vitreous stimulating the retina.

This is also commonly seen in cases that develop synersis (collapse) of vitreous and vitreous traction on vitreoretinal lesions.

Weiss or Fuchs ring: A ring-like opacity indicative of attachment of vitreous to the optic disk is pathognomonic of posterior vitreous detachment.

Management

- Sudden appearance of large number of floaters should arouse suspicion for an acute posterior vitreous detachment.
- Any patient with complaint of photopsia must be thoroughly examined to exclude vitreoretinal pathology.
- If there is no lesion of any kind, then assure the patient that it is due to degeneration of vitreous with age, therefore, nothing to worry but must report, if there is further and sudden appearance of symptoms.

Persistent Hyperplastic Primary Vitreous

Young mother with her infant presents with complain of white reflex from the right eye of her newborn baby.

Persistent hyperplastic primary vitreous is one of the serious developmental disorder of the vitreous due to *failure of regression of the primary vitreous.*

Anterior persistent hyperplastic primary vitreous is common and typically seen in microphthalmic eye. It is unilateral in about 90% of the cases. It is characterized by a retrolental mass. In course of time, the lens becomes opaque and glaucoma develops. If diagnosed early then treat by removal of lens and retrolental mass.

Posterior persisent hyperplastic primary vitreous is characterized by a white dense opaque membrane which extends from optic disk to retrolental region.

Symptoms

Leukocoria: White reflex from the eye.

Differential Diagnosis

- Retinoblastoma
- Congenital cataract
- Retinopathy of prematurity

Investigation

CT scan helps in diagnosis.

Management

Lensectomy and anterior vitrectomy.

Persistent Hyaloid Artery

Congenital remnants of the hyloid arterial system may persist in different form and location.

- *Bergmester's papilla:* It refers to the filament of glial tissue projecting in the vitreous from the optic disk.
- *Vascular loop or thread:* An obliterated vessel may be seen projecting forward in the vitreous.
- *Mittendrof dot:* A remnant of the anterior end of hyaloid artery may remain attached to the posterior lens capsule.

OPACITIES IN VITREOUS

Patient presents with annoying symptom of seeing a fly or a mosquito consistently flying before the eyes.

Slit-lamp shows fine, thick, regular, irregular, thread, worm or cotton wool-like dark spots moving freely with the movement of the eye.

Diagnosis—opacities in vitreous.

Developmental

The developmental opacities of the vitreous are located in Cloquet's canal and are remnants of the hyaloid system.

Muscae Volitantes

These are physiological opacities due to residues of primitive hyaloid vasculature. Patient perceives these as fine dots and filaments in his visual field against bright background.

Degenerative

Asteroid Hyalosis

- Asteroid hyalosis is characterized by appearance of small white dot-like bodies suspended in the vitreous gel.
- These are formed due to deposition of calcium containing lipids.
- These asteroid bodies are attached to interlacing fibers of vitreous, therefore, these bodies move only on movement of the eyeball otherwise these remain suspended in vitreous.
- These are asymptomatic, unilateral, affect elderly people and do not affect the vision.
- Easily seen even by torch light or slit-lamp usually on routine examination.

Synchysis Scintillans

- Synchysis scintillans is characterized by numerous white or yellow cholesterol crystals seen in the lower part of the vitreous.
- Due to fluid vitreous, these crystals are stirred up with every movement of the eye and settle down with every pause again in the lower part of vitreous.
- Bilateral, asymptomatic and do not affect the vision.
- Easily seen by a torch light or slit-lamp usually on routine examination.

Amyloidosis

- Fibrillar-glass wool-deposits of amyloid in the vitreous can accompany systemic heredo-familial amyloidosis.
- Other ocular manifestations include proptosis, ophthalmoplegia, anisocoria, perivasculitis and retinal hemorrhage.

Inflammatory

- Uveitis—anterior or posterior causes vitreous opacities.
- These opacities are due to pouring in of inflammatory cells and exudates in the vitreous and markedly affect the vision.
- These cells and exudates lead to the degeneration of the vitreous resulting in fluid vitreous.
- Easily seen with slit-lamp.
- Systemic and topical steroids effectively control exudation.

HEREDITARY HYALOIDORETINOPATHIES

Wegener's Vitreoretinal Degeneration

- An autosomal dominant inheritance.
- Dim vision with floaters.
- Refraction is usually myopic.
- Slit-lamp shows empty spaces.
- Ophthalmoscopy shows peripheral pigmentary degeneration and choroidal sclerosis with atrophy.
- Electroretinogram is abnormal.
- Complications—cataract and retinal detachment.

Goldmann-Favre's Degeneration

- Autosomal recessive inheritance.
- Clinical features include vitreous degeneration, retinoschisis, peripheral pigmentary degeneration and choroidal sclerosis with atrophy.
- Nyctalopia—night blindness.
- Electroretinogram is subnormal.
- Complications—cataract and retinal detachment.

Hereditary Juvenile Retinoschisis

- Transmitted as an X-linked recessive trait.
- Vitreous degeneration with retinoschisis.

- Foveal retinoschisis may resemble cystoid macular edema.

INTRAOCULAR HEMORRHAGE

Retrovitreous Hemorrhage (Fig. 18.1)

The retrovitreous hemorrhage or subhyaloid or preretinal hemorrhage is located between the retina and detached posterior hyaloid membrane. The blood remains fluid and changes its shape with change in position of the head of the patient.

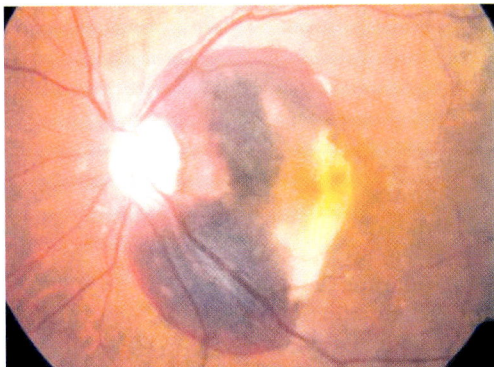

Fig. 18.1: Retrovitreous hemorrhage

In standing position, the subhyaloid blood takes up the shape of a *Boat*, i.e. there is a semicircular inferior border with a horizontal superior line with thick red cell layer on the bottom and thin yellow layer of serum on top.

It impairs the visual acuity, if the hemorrhage is located at or near the macula.

There is a rapid resolution of subhyaloid hemorrhage probably due to good retinal circulation which helps in the process of fibrinolysis, phagocytosis and hemolysis.

Intravitreal Hemorrhage

Patient presents with complain of red vision to begin with followed by marked and sudden loss of vision.

Slit-lamp shows normal anterior segment.

Ophthalmoscopy shows no red glow.

Diagnosis—intravitreal hemorrhage.

Etiology

Common causes

- Trauma, vitreous traction, retinal tear, posterior vitreous detachment, retinal vein occlusion, Eale's disease and diabetic retinopathy.
- Associated systemic diseases include: hypertension, diabetes, arteriosclerosis and anemia.

Pathogenesis

- Massive hemorrhage in the vitreous tends to diffuse anteriorly and centrally, therefore, causes a marked loss of visual acuity.
- Ophthalmoscopy shows no red reflex from the pupil.

Slit-lamp shows

- Hemorrhagic debris in the anterior vitreous and on the posterior lens capsule.
- Hemorrhage in the healthy vitreous shows finger-like projections in vitreous from the bleeding site as it moves forward along the vitreous fibers.
- Hemorrhage in a healthy vitreous clots early and takes a long time to resolve, therefore, the visual acuity is low for a long period.
- Hemorrhage in a degenerated vitreous with lacuna or cavity appears like a subhyaloid hemorrhage and has a tendency to resolve early.
- Hemorrhage in a healthy vitreous leads to its degeneration with its liquefaction and lacuna or cavity formation.

Symptoms

- Vitreous floaters and photopsia.
- Red vision to begin with followed by marked and sudden loss of vision.

Signs

- No red reflex from the pupil.
- Slit-lamp may show debris behind the lens and in the anterior vitreous.

Complications

- Hemorrhage tends to develop in a white opaque mass.
- Fibrovascular proliferation common in retinal vein occlusion and Eale's disease.
- Retinal detachment and neovascular glaucoma.

Treatment

Treat the patient by bed rest and his head elevated to minimize dispersion of blood within the vitreous gel. If the blood settles down, then upper part of fundus can be examined.

- Complete absorption of blood may occur without organization and formation of bands and membranes within 4—8 weeks.
- Look for retinal hole, tear, phlebitis or proliferative retinopathy and treat accordingly.
- Treat neovascularization with argon laser therapy.
- If there is no tendency for the blood to resolve in a week's time, then make the patient ambulatory and examine every two-week on follow-up.
- *Vitrectomy:* If blood does not resolve and patient shows good perception of light, visual acuity less than 6/60, normal electroretinogram and ultrasonography does not show detachment of retina.
- *Photocoagulation* has an important role in central retinal vein occlusion.
- Eale's disease needs medical therapy, laser therapy and even vitrectomy in a long standing case with fibrovascular proliferations.

Vitreous Bands and Membranes

Vitreous bands and membranes form after posterior vitreous detachment. These originate from hyalocytes, fibrocytes or endothelial cells of the capillaries.

Fibrovascular proliferation is seen following hemorrhage due to retinal vein occlusion, Eale's disease, and diabetic retinopathy with long standing hemorrhage not resolving.

The only treatment in early stage is by laser photocoagulation or later by vitrectomy.

19

Maladies of Retina

RETINA

Congenital Anomaly

- Coloboma of retina and choroid
- Medullated nerve fibers
- Albinism

Trauma

- Commotio retinae
- Photoretinitis (eclipse blindness)

Inflammation

- Periphlebitis retinae (Eale's disease)
- Temporal arteritis
- Subacute retinitis of Roth
- Syphilitic retinopathy
- Sarcoidosis retinopathy
- Toxoplasmosis retinopathy

Occlusive Maladies

- Central retinal artery occlusion
- Central retinal vein occlusion

Hemorrhagic and Vascular Maladies

- Exudative retinopathy of Coats
- Proliferative or neovascular retinopathy
- Retinopathy of prematurity
- Hypertensive and arteriosclerotic retinopathy
- Diabetic retinopathy
- Retinopathy in pregnancy-induced hypertension (toxemia of pregnancy)
- Idiopathic central serous choroidopathy (central serous retinopathy)

Degeneration and Dystrophy

- Retinitis pigmentosa
- Age-related macular degeneration (AMD)

- Cystoid macular edema (CME)
- Epiretinal membrane (ERM)
- Cherry-red spot at macula syndrome
- Bull's eye macular syndrome

Retinal Detachment

- Rhegmatogenous retinal detachment
- Tractional retinal detchment
- Exudative retinal detachment

Tumor

Retinoblastoma

RETINA

Retina is a part of brain. The optical system of an eye is so constituted that small images of the objects seen by the eye are brought to focus upon the outer segment of rods and cones where a complex chain of reaction begins. The ganglion cells pass the analyzed information to the brain via optic nerve. Thus, the function of the retina is to receive visual images, analyze them and pass this modified information to the brain.

The cones are used for detailed central vision and color perception. The cones are predominant at the macular, therefore, it is the macula which is concerned for central visual acuity and color vision.

The rods are present in the peripheral retina and work best in dim illumination. Thus, the peripheral retina is useful for night vision or vision in dim illumination and for visual orientation. The symptoms concerning retinal diseases are visual. Retina has no pain fibers, therefore, any inflammation of the retina does not give rise to symptom of pain or redness of the eye.

The clinical investigations for retinal maladies include visual acuity, refraction, slit-lamp, four-mirror contact lens, Schiotz's or applanation tonometry, ophthalmoscopy, visual fields, color vision, fluorescein angiography, electroretinography, electro-oculography, ultrasonography and optical coherence tomography (OCT).

CONGENITAL ANOMALY

Coloboma of Retina and Choroid

Patient presents with complain of cat's eye— white grey reflex from his pupil as observed occasionally by his relatives and friends.

Ophthalmoscopy shows typical large coloboma of retina and choroid.

Diagnosis—coloboma of retina and choroid.

Coloboma of retina and choroid occurs due to defective closure of the fetal cleft.

Ophthalmoscopic Features

- White grey color reflex of fundus.
- Glistening white sclera seen in the down and in quadrant of the fundus. Area of the coloboma may be small or large and may involve the optic disk. Coloboma is usually oval in shape with broad end towards the periphery and round narrow end towards the optic disk. Coloboma may be bridged or show several isolated defects.
- Edge of the coloboma may be sharp or fading gradually and always associated with pigmentation at the edges.
- Floor may be depressed or ectatic.
- Retinal vessels seem to dip down at the edge of the coloboma as they pass from normal fundus to the coloboma.
- Choroidal vessels are at deeper level, tortuous and broad.
- Macula is normal.

Medullated Nerve Fibers

Patient presents with complain of cat's eye—mild white reflex from the pupil as observed occasionally by his relatives and friends.

Ophthalmoscopy shows large white feathery patches all around the disk.

Diagnosis—medullated never fibers.

Normally, the myelination of optic nerve stops at lamina cribrosa. Occasionally, the process of myelination continues beyond optic disk.

Ophthalmoscopic Features

- Medullated nerve fibers are usually close to the optic disk and all around or involve a sector only.
- Large patch of medullated nerve fibers around optic disk gives rise to a *white reflex* from the pupil and exhibits *enlargement of blind spot* on visual field charting.
- Medullated nerve fibers appear as white striated patches with feathery edges usually covering the retinal vessels at some places. Sometimes these patches are far away from the optic disk and appear as isolated patches.
- One small isolated patch is likely to be mistaken for exudative spot. *The feathery look of the patch is diagnostic.*
- Medullated nerve fibers disappear in demyelinating disorders and with onset of optic atrophic due to any cause.

Albinism

Patient presents as an albinotic with albinotic eye and complains mainly of photophobia and movement of eyes.

Diagnosis—albinism.

Albinism is a hereditary condition in which there is a defective development of pigment throughout the body. This is due to an *'inborn error of metabolism'* characterized by the lack of enzyme—tyrosinase which converts *'DOPA'* into melanin.

Partial types of albinism are probably due to some functional insufficiency or defect in distribution.

Clinical Features

- Eyebrows and eyelashes are white.
- Iris appears pink due to increased transmission of light.
- Pupil appears red, as light passing through iris and sclera is reflected back.

Ophthalmoscopic Features

- Fundus appears orange red in color.
- Retinal and choroidal vessels are seen against the sclera.
- Optic disc appears as a point of confluence of vessels.

Management

Advice to use goggles and to *accept and live the life in its totality as it is* with confidence.

TRAUMA

Commotio Retinae

Patient presents with marked loss of vision following blow to the eye.

Ophthalmoscopy shows 'cherry red spot' at macula.

Diagnosis—commotio retinae/Berlin's edema.

The commotion retinae occur commonly following a blow to the eyeball.

Ophthalmoscopic Features

Malady manifests as *milky white cloudiness* involving large area of posterior pole with a prominent red spot in the center referred as *'cherry red spot'* in the foveal region.

This typical appearance is due to edema at the posterior pole giving a white appearance and the fovea in center shines as red spot.

The edema may resolve completely or is usually followed by degenerative changes at the macula in form of pigmentation or hole.

Rest and steroids have been beneficial in reducing edema and save vision and prevent degenerative changes.

Photoretinitis (Eclipse Blindness)

Patient presents soon after watching sun eclipse with alarming and annoying complain of after image of bright light covering his entire field of vision in his left eye.

Diagnosis—photoretinitis.

Photoretinitis, *eclipse retinopathy, solar retinopathy* or *eclipse blindness* refer to burn of retina at the posterior pole the *paramacular area*.

It may be unilateral or bilateral.

Etiopathogenesis

- Looking at sun eclipse with unprotected eyes.
- Exposure of the eye to the flash of the short-circuiting of a strong electric current.

In both the circumstances, practically, all the visible ultraviolet and many infrared rays pass unimpeded to the retina wherein these are absorbed by pigment epithelium. Pathological changes are due to photochemical or thermal effect resulting in a burn of retina at the posterior pole at the paramacular area.

Severity of lesion varies directly with degree of pigmentation in retina, duration of exposure and climatic environment during exposure.

Clinical Features

- *Negative after-image* of the sun which persists for long time.
- *Positive scotoma*: Dark spot in the field of vision. It usually covers the entire field of vision.
- *Metamorphopsia*: Some patients may complain of a distorted vision that is the objects appear wavy.

Ophthalmoscopy shows a pale spot at the macula with a brownish red ring round it. Later patient develops pigmentation or small grey punctate spots or even hole at the macula.

Management

- Rest to the eye in dark and cool environment.
- Systemic and topical steroids. Start with high dose and taper to maintenance dose for long time.
- Some visual defect remains and scotoma may persist permanently.
- Prophylactic use of glasses impervious to ultraviolet and infrared wavelengths is the only preventive treatment.

INFLAMMATION

Periphlebitis Retinae (Eale's Disease)

Patient presents with sudden appearance of black spots in front of the eye followed with painless and marked loss of vision.

Diagnosis—Eale's disease.

Etiopathogenesis

- Eale's disease is an idiopathic inflammation of the peripheral retinal veins and characterized by recurrent vitreous hemorrhage.
- Eale's disease is usually bilateral and affects healthy young male adult.
- Eale's is disease considered as hypersensitivity reaction to tubercular proteins.

Ophthalmoscopic Features

- *Stage of inflammation*: The retinal veins appear full and tortuous with sheathing. There is exudation under and around the vessel wall seen at places. Superficial flame shape hemorrhages near affected veins.
- *Stage of ischemia*: Later the vessels become thin and attenuated and appear like thin white cords with avascular areas and new vessel formation.
- *Stage of retinal neovascularization*: The fragile new vessels bleed in the vitreous which may be a small leak or usually massive.
- *Stage of sequelae*: Recurrent hemorrhage in the vitreous leads to development of proliferative retinopathy, tractional retinal detachment, rubeosis iridis and neovascular glaucoma.

Management

- Antitubercular therapy in selective cases.
- Steroids orally for long period in maintenance dose.
- Laser scatter photocoagulation in early stage is effective and rewarding.
- Vitrectomy in late case with sequelae.

Temporal Arteritis

Patient presents with tenderness even to mild touch or combing in his left temporal region.

Skin in that area is normal. No pulsation in the temporal artery.

Diagnosis—temporal arteritis.
    Temporal arteritis is a chronic inflammation of temporal or occipital artery. Sometimes the process may involve the ophthalmic artery and central retinal artery also.

Clinical Features

- Intense pain over the temporal region to the extent that the affected area is tender to even touch.
- *No pulsation of the affected temporal artery due to occlusion of the vessel is pathognomonic and diagnostic*
- Loss of vision in the affected eye on affection of ophthalmic or central retinal artery.
- Erythrocyte sedimentation rate (ESR) is highly raised.
- Systemic steroid is the only treatment. Start with a high dose of steroid and taper it off to a maintenance dose taking the erythrocyte sedimentation rate as an indicator.
- Biopsy of the clogged temporal artery is the only confirmatory test.

Subacute Retinitis of Roth

Patient presents for eye check up as a referred case from cardiologist.

Ophthalmoscopy shows hemorrhages with white centers and small white spots in posterior fundus.

Diagnosis—Roth's subacute retinitis.
    Subacute retinitis of 'Roth' occurs due to metastatic infection typically seen in patients suffering with subacute bacterial endocarditis.

Ophthalmoscopic Features

- Multiple superficial recurrent retinal hemorrhages of embolic origin, some of which have white centers as in the anemia and leukemia.
- *Roth's spot*: Presence of small round or oval white spots many of which are cystoids bodies mostly in the posterior segment is the characteristic and diagnostic feature of this malady.

Subacute retinitis of Roth is diagnosed accidentally on ophthalmoscopy as a routine or in a referred case.

Syphilitic Retinopathy

Patient presents with subjective symptoms of dim vision, night blindness and tubular vision.

Ophthalmoscopy shows optic atrophy with corpuscles-like pigmentation.

Diagnosis—syphilitic retinopathy.

Ophthalmoscopic Features

- *In congenital syphilitic:* Typical fundus picture known as a *'pepper-and-salt fundus'*, i.e. there are numerous white and black spots mostly in the peripheral fundus.
- *In acquired syphilitic*: Typical fundus picture shows optic atrophy with attenuated blood vessels and corpuscles like aggregated pigmentation in the periphery of the fundus. The fundus picture resembles the pigmentary retinal dystrophy.
- Concentric contraction of visual fields resulting in tubular vision.

Sarcoidosis Retinopathy

Ophthalmoscopic Features

The typical fundus picture shows optic atrophy, patches of chorioretinitis, periphlebitis, and *'candle-wax'* like deposits of exudates along the vessels due to associated posterior uveitis.

Toxoplasmosis Retinopathy

Ophthalmoscopic Features

- *In infants:* Fundus shows typical bilateral punched out scar with heavy pigmentation at the macula along with multiple chorioretinal lesions.
- *In adults:* Fundus shows typical multiple healed chorioretinal scars with heavy pigmentation.

Recurrent attack often starts at the edges of the previous scars with exudation in the vitreous.

OCCLUSIVE MALADIES

Central Retinal Artery Occlusion

Patient presents with painless and sudden marked loss of vision in right eye only few hours ago.

Ophthalmoscopy shows cherry-red spot at macula and sludging and segmentation of the blood column in both the arterioles and venules—cattle track appearance—blood column is broken and moving.

Diagnosis—central retinal artery occlusion right eye.

Etiology

Occlusion of the central retinal artery can occur due to the following factors.
- *Emboli:* Emboli are the most common cause. The important cause for emboli is an atheroma. The embolic material from the heart or carotid arteries reaches the eye directly through the ophthalmic artery which is the first branch of the internal carotid artery.
- *Vaso-obliteration:* Common cause for vaso-obliteration is arteritis which can occur in the following conditions: Giant cell arteritis, polyarteritis nodosa and systemic lupus erythematosus.
- *Raised intraocular pressure:* Raised intraocular pressure due to excessive pressure on the globe due to tight encircalage in retinal detachment surgery can lead to obstruction of the retinal circulation.

Symptoms

Sudden and painless loss of vision.

Patient feels that his vision is fading and finally goes. Vision is reduced to perception of light.

Some vision is retained in cases with presence of cilioretinal artery supplying the macula.

Signs

Pupil: Direct light reflex is absent but the consensual light reflex is present.

Ophthalmoscopic Features

- *Cherry-red spot*: The retina at the posterior pole is white and edematous in which the foveal reflex stands out as a red spot.

- *Cattle track appearance*: Sludging and segmentation of the blood column is seen in both the arterioles and venules.
- Retinal arteries are narrow and irregular.
- Retinal veins are of normal caliber.
- If the retinal circulation is not restored then the edema of the retina disappears, the arteries remains attenuated and the optic disk becomes atrophic.

Complications

- Rubeosis iridis and neovascular glaucoma in 1 to 5% of cases.
- Optic atrophy sets in, if there is no restoration of circulation.

Management

There are all the chances of restoration of circulation, if the case is treated within 48 hours of the occlusion as it is rare for a complete occlusion to occur, therefore, retina survives.

- Make the patient lie flat and nurse him also in this position as it helps to maintain circulation.
- *Lower intraocular pressure:* Massage the globe firmly and intermittently. It reduces the intraocular pressure, increases the flow of blood and may help to dislodge the emboli, if that is the factor.
- *Mannitol:* Intravenous helps to lower the intraocular pressure.
- *Giant cell arteritis:* Exclude or confirm as causative factor by measuring the erythrocyte sedimentation rate (ESR).
- *Cardiovascular system:* Thorough check-up is essential to diagnose the site of atheroma and treat accordingly.

Central Retinal Vein Occlusion
(Retinal Apoplexy, Hemorrhagic Retinitis)

Patient presents with painless and sudden marked loss of vision left eye since last evening.

Ophthalmoscopy shows marked tortuosity of veins and massive retinal hemorrhages as if the whole fundus is splashed with red ink.

Diagnosis—central retinal vein occlusion.

Etiology

The retinal vein occlusion is common in elderly in their sixth and seventh decades of life.

Systemic hypertension plays an important role for branch and central retinal vein occlusion. It is postulated that the vein is compressed by thick and arteriosclerotic artery where both have a common adventitia, i.e. just behind the lamina cribrosa and at the arteriovenous crossing in the retina.

Incidental Factors

- *Incidence of vein occlusion:* It affects both the sexes equally usually after the middle age. It affects one eye and later the other eye also gets involved. It is more common than central retinal artery occlusion.
- *Constriction of flow (pressure on vein by sclerotic retinal artery):* There is a constriction of central retinal vein by the chronic sclerotic process involving the central retinal artery just behind the lamina cribrosa and at arteriovenous crossings where the two share a common adventitia. This sets in irritative proliferation of endothelium which accelerates the process of obstruction of flow.
- *Primary venous disease:* Periphlebitis retinae affect the central or peripheral retinal veins.
- *Primary open-angle glaucoma:* Primary open-angle glaucoma and retinal vein occlusion are associated due to venous stasis induced by raised pressure in the exit veins.

1. Preocclusion of Central Retinal Vein

Ophthalmoscopic Features

- Veins are full, tortuous and engorged with retinal edema along the course.
- Venous pulsation is absent.
- Part of the disc may show swelling.
- Appearance of new formed veins at the disk with small hemorrhages.
- Hemorrhages are arranged around the terminal veins like *'berries on a twig'*.
- Few coiled venous channels may be seen.

Management

At this stage, the patient may complain of a transient obscuration of vision.

Manage by photocoagulation and control of intraocular pressure.

2. Central Retinal Vein Occlusion (Fig. 19.1)

a. Non-ischemic Occlusion or Venous Stasis Retinopathy

It is the most common clinical type of retinal vein occlusion affecting about 75% of cases. The fundus changes are mild to moderate.

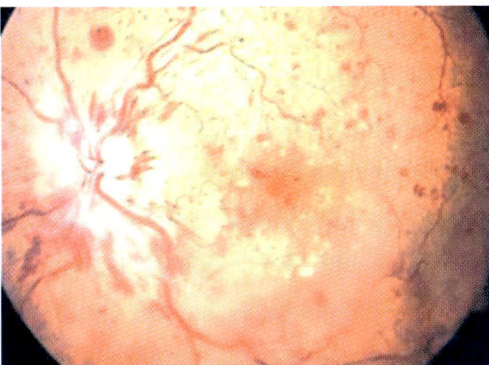

Fig. 19.1: Central retinal vein occlusion

Ophthalmoscopic Features

Early cases

- Mild venous congestion and tortuousity of veins
- Flame shape hemorrhages in periphery
- Mild papilledema and
- Mild or no macular edema.

Late cases

- Sheathing around the main vein
- Few coils at disc
- Partially absorbed hemorrhages and
- Cystoid macular edema.

Management

The malady resolves with no visual loss in about 50% of cases. The visual loss is due to cystoid macular edema. A short course of oral steroids followed by maintenance dose for 2–3 months is effective in resolving cystoid macular edema.

b. Ischemic Occlusion or Hemorrhagic Retinopathy

It refers to acute or sudden complete occlusion of the central retinal vein. Patient comes with complain of painless sudden loss of vision in the affected eye.

Ocular examination shows afferent papillary defect, visual field defect and reduced amplitude of *b*-wave of electroretinogram.

Ophthalmoscopic Features

Early cases

- Marked venous congestion and tortuousity of veins.
- Massive retinal hemorrhages in fundus as if *'splashed with red ink'*.
- Numerous cotton wool soft exudates
- Papilledema
- Macula shows edema and hemorrhages.

Late cases

- Marked sheathing around veins
- Collaterals at disk
- Neovascularization at the disc and periphery
- Macula—shows cystoids edema and pigmentary deposits.

Macula gets involved in central retinal vein and temporal retinal vein occlusion. Macula escapes in the block of inferior temporal vein branch.

3. Branch Occlusion of Retinal Vein

Superior temporal branch of central retinal vein is commonly involved.

Ophthalmoscopic Features

Fundus changes are confined to the sector supplied by superior temporal branch.
- Banking of the veins distal to arteriovenous crossing (Bonnet's sign) is often seen at the site of an impending occlusion.
- Vein distal to crossing is surrounded by a white halo due to transudation through its walls while the associated artery shows sheathing and small flame-shaped hemorrhage.
- Macula usually escapes as it is supplied by both the arteries. Yet there may be loss of central field due to hemorrhage and exudates in the central area.

c. Complications of Central Retinal Vein Occlusion

- Chronic maculopathy—edema, cyst, pigmentation, scarring, hole
- Neovascular glaucoma
- Rubeosis—iridis
- Vitreous hemorrhage and proliferative retinopathy
- Tractional retinal detachment
- Epiretinal membrane

Management

- Investigate the case fully for cardio-vascular check-up.
- Treat his hypertension.
- Measure the intraocular pressure and control it, if raised.
- Treat the cause, the inflammatory periphlebitis.
- Topical timolol maleate to control high intraocular pressure.
- There is controversy about use of anti-coagulants.
- Systemic steroid therapy in some cases is helpful especially with macular involvement.
- Intravitreal injection of triamcinolone acetonide: 4 mg/0.1 ml has been used in both types to treat macular edema and neovascularization.
- Grid laser photocoagulation for macular edema in branch occlusion.
- Panretinal photocoagulation is helpful to reestablish the circulation and saves vision and prevents neovascular glaucoma.
- Intravitreal—anti-VEGF treatment is gaining importance to treat macular edema and neovascularization.

HEMORRHAGIC AND VASCULAR MALADIES

Exudative Retinopathy of Coats

Clinical Features

- Coats' disease is the most severe form of retinal telengiectasia that typically manifests in one eye of the boys in their first decade of life.
- White reflex from the pupil, squinting eye and loss of vision.
- Needs to be differentiated from retino-blastoma.

Ophthalmoscopic Features

Large areas of intra- and subretinal yellowish exudates and hemorrhages with overlying dilated and tortuous retinal blood vessels at the posterior pole and in periphery.

Course

Some cases may show regression spontaneously.

Most of the cases show progress leading to exudative retinal detachment, retrolental mass, secondary cataract, rubeosis iridis, uveitis, secondary glaucoma, and eventually end up in phthisis bulbi.

Management

Early application of photocoagulation or cryotherapy helps to retard the progress.

Proliferative or Neovascular Retinopathy
(Fig. 19.2)

Two factors play role:
1. Massive vitreous hemorrhage
2. Neovascularization.

Etiopathogenesis

- *Massive vitreous hemorrhage,* if not resolved early has a tendency to get organized by fibrous tissue derived from the mesoblastic elements associated with the retinal vessels

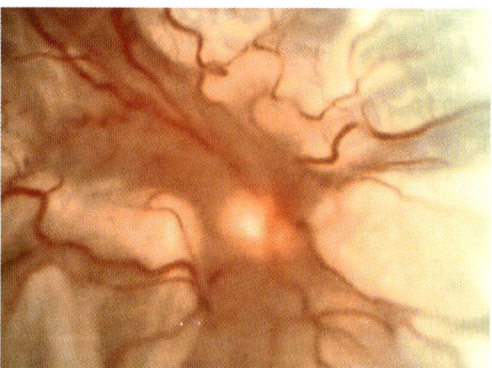

Fig. 19.2: Proliferative retinopathy

or on the optic disk. The fibrous tissue proliferates in the vitreous.

The proliferative retinopathy following vitreous hemorrhage predominates with thick fibrous tissue with few vessels.

- Neovascularization is common in diabetes and Eale's disease. These new vessels have a tendency to bleed repeatedly causing vitreous hemorrhage. Neovascularization arises from the optic nerve head and along large retinal blood vessels. These appear in the areas of capillary closure.

The proliferative retinopathy following neovascularization predominates with new vessel formation with thin membranous fibrous tissue.

Management

- Early photocoagulation to check the progress and conversion of hypoxic areas in the retina into inert scars that restrain neovascularization.
- Delay results in tractional retinal detachment, repeated hemorrhages, secondary cataract, rubeosis iridis, and neovascular glaucoma resulting in blindness—*atrophic bulbi.*

Retinopathy of Prematurity

Clinical Features

- Retinopathy of prematurity is due to formation of abnormal blood vessels over premature retina. It is prevalent in premature infant with low gestational age and low birth weight and partly related to the concentration and duration of oxygen delivered to the infant.
- This retinopathy is a leading cause of blindness in children.
- Common cause of blindness in the prenatal period.
- Potentially blinding malady, if not treated in its early stage.
- *Spontaneous resolution occurs in more than 80% of cases. All the infants who show a stage III with fibrovascular proliferation should be treated by photocoagulation.*

Hypertensive and Arteriosclerotic Retinopathy

Every person past 40 years must watch out his blood pressure as hypertension and arteriosclerotic changes affect every human being. Ophthalmoscopy helps to assess the effect on small vessels.

It shall help the person to live a long and healthy life.

1. Vascular Sclerosis

- *Tortuousity of vessels*: It is seen in small arteries near the macula which assume a cork-screw shape.
- *Attenuation of vessels:* Attenuation of vessels is first observed in small vessels. In early stage, there is a generalized attenuation. Later the changes are focal so that stretches of vessels are constricted, alternating with normal stretches. These changes are due to endothelial proliferation in intima of vessels.
- *Copper wire arteries and silver wire arteries:* This appearance is due to a change in the light reflex of vessel. The normal light streak seen on retinal vessels is due to the reflex of blood column seen through the transparent arterial wall.

  When the arterial wall becomes thickened and also reflects the light, then the light streak appears wide and burnished as copper, therefore, the appearance is known as *'copper wire arteries'.*

  When the arterial wall becomes so much thickened that it reflects all the light, then there is only light streak from the vessels, therefore, the appearance is known as *'silver wire arteries'.*
- *Sheathing of vessels*: Sheathing of vessel is known, when the sides of the arteries are visible as white lines. It occurs due to vasculitis.
- *Arteriovenous crossing changes:* Normally, a vein can be seen through an artery at the point of arteriovenous crossing. In arteriosclerosis, due to thickening of arterial wall, the translucency is lost and there is a pressure of thick artery over the underlying vein at the point of crossing.

- Normally, the crossing of vessels is oblique but in arteriosclerosis the vessels deflect and cross at right angle which is the shortest route.
- *Salu's sign* denotes deflection of vein.
- *Bonnet's sign* denotes dilation of vein distal to crossing.
- *Gunn's sign* denotes tapering of vein on either side of crossing.

It should be kept in mind that mild arteriovenous crossing changes may be seen in normal patients.

2. Intraretinal Hemorrhages

Minute leak of blood from the retinal vessels remains located or contained within the retinal tissue and assumes a characteristic shape depending on the location of the hemorrhage. The shape of the hemorrhage confirms to the anatomical configuration of the retinal layer in which they lie.

Leakage of vessels occurs due to abnormal permeability of retinal vessels which leads to *hemorrhages, retinal edema, cotton wool spot formation and hard exudates.*

Hard exudates around the fovea in the Henle's layer are distributed radially giving an appearance of a star, therefore, known as '*macular star*'.

In severe hypertension, in young adults, a swelling of the optic disk occurs in addition to all the above changes.

Flame-shaped hemorrhages occur *in the superficial nerve fiber layer, therefore, appear as striated.*

Round or dot hemorrhages occur in the deeper layers of the retina, therefore, appear as round or dot-like spots.

Intraretinal hemorrhages take a long time to resolve and usually absorb very slowly and gradually become white and rarely pigmented.

Intraretinal hemorrhages are seen in central retinal vein occlusion, central retinal branch vein occlusion, Eale's disease, papilledema, diabetic retinopathy, hypertensive retinopathy, anemia, leukemia and trauma.

Two important aspects of systemic hypertension

- Duration of hypertension
- Severity of hypertension

The vascular changes due to *duration of hypertension* are seen in *arteriosclerotic retinopathy.*

The vascular changes due to *severity of hypertension* are seen in *hypertensive retinopathy.*

3. Arteriosclerotic Retinopathy

Ophthalmoscopic features with grading

Grade I: Broadening of the arteriolar light reflex and concealment of vein at the arteriovenous crossing due to thickening of the arteriolar walls.

Grade II: Changes of grade I and associated with deflection of vein at the arteriovenous crossing—*Salu's sign.*

Grade III: Changes of grade II and associated with '*copper wire arteries*' and more changes at the arteriovenous crossing in form of dilation of vein distal to crossing—*Bonnet's sign*, tapering of vein on either side of arteriovenous crossing—*Gunn's sign* and deflection of vein at right angle to artery.

Grade IV: Changes of grade III and associated with '*silver wire arterioles*'. There may be degenerative changes at the macula and optic disk appears pale and atrophic. Some cases may present with occlusion of branch of central retinal vein.

4. Hypertensive Retinopathy

Adult patient presents himself out of his own awareness or referred by a physician for ophthalmoscopy to assess the prognosis; effect of arteriosclerosis and hypertension on the small vessels.

Ophthalmoscopic features with Keith and Wegner grading

Grade I: Mild generalized arteriolar attenuation of small branches and associated with broadening of arteriolar light reflex and concealment of vein at the arteriovenous crossing due to thickening of arteriolar walls.

Grade II: Grade I changes and associated with increased generalized arteriolar attenuation, focal arteriolar attenuation and deflection of veins at the arteriovenous crossing the *Salu's sign.*

Grade III (Fig. 19.3): Grade II changes and associated with *'copper wire arteries'*, arteriovenous crossing in form of dilation of vein distal to crossing the *Bonnet's sign*, tapering of vein on either side of arteriovenous crossing—the *Gunn's sign*, deflection of vein at right angle to artery and *flame shape hemorrhages, cotton wool (soft) and hard exudates.*

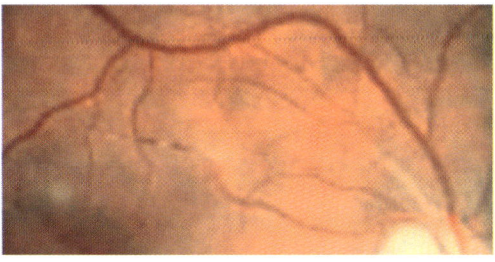

Fig. 19.3: Hypertensive retinopathy—grade III

Grade IV: Grade III changes and associated with *'silver wire arteri*oles' and *papilledema.*

Hypertensive changes are reversible up to the grade II only, therefore, it is very essential to perform ophthalmoscopy at regular intervals in a case of hypertension to save his vision.

Management

- Consultant must note down all the fundus finding in grades of hypertensive retinopathy and arteriosclerotic retinopathy so that a proper assessment can be made about the progress of hypertension and arteriosclerosis.
- Thorough cardiovascular check-up is needed at regular intervals to keep the patient free from unwanted complications of hypertension.
- Hypertension and arteriosclerosis affect almost everyone past sixth decade of life.
- A little care about health and regular check-up helps to maintain a normal blood pressure and good vision with healthy life and lifestyle for years.

Diabetic Retinopathy

Diabetic patient presents himself out of his own awareness or referred by endocrinologist, diabetologist or family physician for ophthalmoscopy to assess the prognosis; effect on vessels—micro-angiopathy; in form of microvascular occlusion and leak.

Etiology

Diabetes occurs due to lack of insulin which causes increase in blood glucose concentration, i.e. hyperglycemia. Deficiency of insulin is due to damage to B cells of pancreatic islets of Langerhans. The onset of diabetic retinopathy is related to duration of diabetes than to any other factor.

Etiopathogenesis

The diabetic retinopathy is a microangiopathy in which the retinal vessels affected are precapillary arterioles, the capillaries and venules. Diabetic retinopathy develops due to two factors namely:

1. *Microvascular occlusion* results in retinal ischemia which in turn causes retinal hypoxia which gives rise to neovascularization.
2. *Microvascular leakage* leads to hemorrhages and retinal edema.

Classification

1. Non-proliferative diabetic retinopathy
2. Proliferative diabetic retinopathy
3. Diabetic maculopathy
4. Advanced diabetic eye disease.

1. Non-proliferative Diabetic Retinopathy

It is further classified in mild, moderate, severe and very severe depending on the manifestation of ophthalmoscopic features.

Ophthalmoscopic features

- Microaneurysms *appear as small round dots usually situated on temporal side of the macula.*
- *Hemorrhages* may be either flame-shaped or round dot hemorrhages.
- *Hard exudates* (Fig. 19.4) appear as yellow waxy patches in a circinate pattern around the macula and other areas of focal leakage.
- *Cotton-wool soft exudates.*
- *Retinal veins* appear dilated, full and tortuous and show beading and looping.

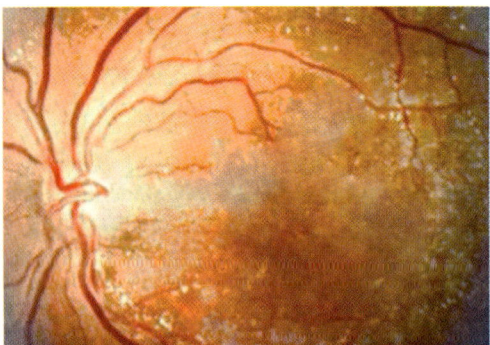

Fig. 19.4: Diabetic retinopathy—hard exudates

- *Macular edema* assumes cystoid appearance.

Management There is no cure for a diabetic retinopathy but control of certain factors helps to arrest its progress.
- Control the diabetes by diet, exercise, and antidiabetic drugs.
- Control hypertension, if associated.
- Supplement vitamins and iron to improve resistance.
- Regular check-up for blood sugar, blood cholesterol and blood urea is essential.
- Photocoagulation, if there is a macular edema.

2. Proliferative Diabetic Retinopathy

It is characterized by *neovascularization* and *hemorrhages* over the ophthalmoscopic features of very severe non-proliferative diabetic retinopathy.

Ophthalmoscopic features

- *Neovascularization* is characterized by proliferation of new vessels from the capillaries in form of neovascularization at the optic disk and temporal vascular arcades. Along with new vessel formation, there occurs condensation of connective tissue around the new vessels resulting in formation of fibrovascular epiretinal membrane.
- *Hemorrhage* follows which could be sub-hyaloid or intravitreal.

Management Panretinal 'argon laser photocoagulation'. It helps to induce involution of new vessels and prevents recurrent vitreous hemorrhage.

3. Diabetic Maculopathy

Diabetic maculopathy can be associated with non-proliferative or proliferative diabetic retinopathy. It occurs due to increased permeability of retinal capillaries. It can be *focal exudative, diffuse exudative, ischemic or mixed* maculopathy. Diabetic maculopathy is the common cause of visual loss. It is seen more in diabetics who are non-insulin dependent type.

Ophthalmoscopic feature

- Macula may show mild edema, cystic spaces and later a lamellar hole.
- Fluorescein angiography will show the areas of leakage.

Management

- Treat by argon laser avoiding the fovea.
- Intravitreal steroids to reduce macular edema have been advocated to save vision.
- Intravitreal injection of vascular endothelial growth factors (VEGFs) inhibitors is helpful in cases who do not respond to intravitreal steroids.

4. Advanced Diabetic Eye Disease

It is the ultimate result of uncontrolled diabetic retinopathy. It is associated with following complications:
- Persistent vitreous hemorrhage
- Retinal detachment
- Neovascular glaucoma
- Rubeosis iridis.

The eye ends up as a blind eye.

Retinopathy in Pregnancy-induced Hypertension

It is characterized by raised blood pressure, generalized edema, proteinuria and malady of unknown etiology.

Retinopathy occurs late practically always in the 9th month of pregnancy. There is an increase in weight due to generalized edema associated with high blood pressure. The blood pressure may range from 160/100 to 200/130 mm Hg

Ophthalmoscopic Features

* Generalized narrowing of the retinal arteries with focal constrictions.
* Flame shape-hemorrhages and cotton-wool soft exudates.
* Macular star or macular cyst.
* Retinal edema
* Exudative retinal detachment in severe cases.

Management

* Need not hurry up to terminate pregnancy until patient responds well to conservative therapy or there is danger to vision in form of maculopathy, retinal detachment or to life due to very high hypertension.
* Edema of retina is an ominous sign which indicates termination of pregnancy.
* All the features of retinopathy disappear with termination of pregnancy.

Idiopathic Central Serous Choroidopathy (Central Serous Retinopathy)

Patient presents with small dot-like positive scotoma which gradually covers up the entire field of vision.

Ophthalmoscopy shows dull foveal reflex with paramacular edema. Fluorescein angiography shows area of leak.

Diagnosis—central serous choroidopathy.
It is a common disorder of macula of unknown etiology and visually affects the males between 20 and 40 years of age.
An increase in choroidal hyperpermeability causes breach in the outer blood retina barrier. Leakage of fluid occurs at this site resulting in localized serous detachment of neuro-sensory retina at macular region.

Clinical Features

* Painless blurred vision
* Positive scotoma
* Micropsia and metamorphopsia.
* *Ophthalmoscopy* shows an oval or round elevation at the posterior pole, the macular area with a glistening reflex at the border. Foveal reflex is absent or distorted.
* *Slit-lamp with fundus lens* shows an elevation at the posterior pole with a fluid which is clear and transparent.
* *Fluorescein angiography* shows a hyper-fluorescent spot—*ink blot* at the site of leakage.
* *Prognosis* is good as 80 to 90% of cases undergo *spontaneous resolution* of subretinal fluid with return of almost normal vision.
* *Recurrence* is common.
* *Cystoid maculopathy* affects the visual acuity.
* *Manage* by photocoagulation, if edema at macula does not resolve or fluid becomes turbid.

DEGENERATION AND DYSTROPHY

Retinitis Pigmentosa (Fig. 19.5)

Patient presents with gradual loss of vision and inability to see clearly after sunset or dark background—night blindness (ratondhi).

Ophthalmoscopy shows typical bone corpuscles-like pigmentation with attenuation of vessels and pale or atrophic disk. Pigments at places are perivascular and also covering the veins.

Diagnosis—retinitis pigmentosa.
Retinitis pigmentosa is an inherited disease characterized by night blindness and constricted visual field.

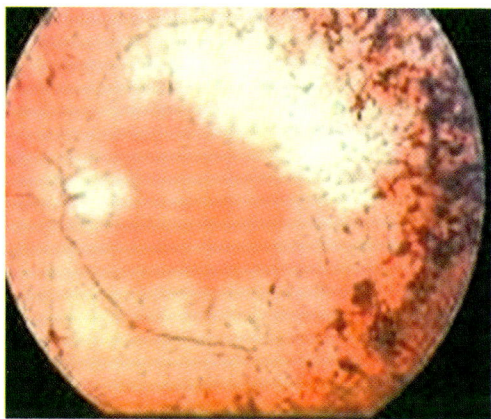

Fig. 19.5: Retinitis pigmentosa

Typical retinitis pigmentosa is a diffuse and bilateral symmetrical dystrophy of retina.

Though both the cones and rods are involved but there is a predominant damage to rods which are responsible for night vision and peripheral vision.

Ocular findings vary due to their relation with mode of inheritance. It is inherited as an *autosomal recessive, autosomal dominant or X-linked recessive* trait.

The atrophic changes in the retina begin at the equatorial region and thereafter gradually spread towards periphery.

Involvement of macula is late.

Symptoms

- *Night blindness:* Patient complains of difficulty in dim illumination. Later it becomes impossible to walk even in dim light or after sunset.
- *Dark adaptation:* Light threshold of the peripheral retina is increased.
- *Tubular vision*: Patient complains that he is not able to see anything from his side. Everything is clear in the line of vision but not on periphery.
- *Gradual loss of central vision:* With passage of time, there is loss of central vision also due to cystoid macular edema.

Ocular Features

- Myopia is most frequently associated with it.
- Posterior subcapsular cataract is seen commonly at about the age of 50 years. Its removal improves the visual acuity.
- Open angle glaucoma
- Keratoconus

Ophthalmoscopic Features

There is triad of features: (1) Bone corpuscle pigmentation, (2) attenuation of arteries and (3) pale waxy optic disk are diagnostic.

1. *Bone corpuscle pigmentation:* The typical appearance of pigment as bone corpuscle and its perivascular location is diagnostic.
2. *Attenuation of arteries:* There is marked attenuation of arteries. The pigment is seen covering the vessels at many places again a diagnostic feature.
3. *Pale waxy optic disk:* It is a late phenomenon. The optic disk appears pale and waxy—typical appearance is diagnostic feature.

Investigation

Visual fields

- *Ring scotoma:* Pigmentary degeneration starts in mid-retinal periphery. Then it extends both anteriorly and posteriorly covering a ring-shape area of the retina which gives rise to '*ring scotoma*' in the visual field which is diagnostic feature.
- *Tubular vision*: Progressive constriction of visual field ultimately leaves only a small area of central vision described by the patient as a '*tubular vision*', i.e. he feels as if seeing through a tube is diagnostic feature

Electroretinogram is subnormal or extinguished even in early stage with no fundus changes.

Dark adaptation shows elevation of both cone and rod thresholds.

Management

- There is no effective treatment for retinitis pigmentosa.
- It is treatable but not curable.
- Many measures have been adopted such as; vasodilators, placental extracts, transplantation of rectus muscles/omentum and vitamins but without any result:
  - Correct any refractive error to improve vision.
  - IOLs implant for cataract, if it is causing visual loss.
  - Low vision aids are helpful.
  - Rehabilitation as per his socioeconomic status.
  - Counseling—general, family and genetic counseling is needed.
  - *Stem cells injection* from bone marrow is under trial and showing encouraging results. Stem cells have capacity for self-renewal and differentiation into mature cell type.

Atypical Retinitis Pigmentosa

Some cases may not show typical pigmentary manifestation though fundus shows attenuation of arteries, waxy pale disc and flat ERG.

- *Retinitis pigmentosa sine pigmento:* It is characterized by all the clinical features of typical retinitis pigmentosa except the absence of pigmentary changes in the fundus.
- *Retinitis punctata albescens:* It is characterized by presence of innumerable discrete white dots scattered between posterior pole and equator without pigmentary changes. There is subsequent development of pigmentary changes, waxy pale disk and attenuation of arterioles—the characteristic features.
- *Sectorial retinitis pigmentosa:* There is involvement of only one quadrant of the fundus. The progress of the disease is very slow.
- *Pericentric retinitis pigmentosa:* The entire fundus finding is like that of a typical retinitis pigmentosa but the fundus changes are confined to central fundus sparing the periphery.

Syndromes with Retinitis Pigmentosa

- *Laurence-Moon-Bardet-Biedl syndrome:* It is an autosomal recessive genetic disorder. Its five classical features include: polydactyly or syndactyly, retinitis pigmentosa, obesity, mental retardation and hypogonadism. Some cases may also show brachycephaly, short stature, congenital heart disease, deafness and various neurological disorders. This syndrome can be confused with Alstrom-Hallgren syndrome in which there is retinitis pigmentosa, obesity, deafness and diabetes mellitus and no polydactyly, mental retardation and hypogonadism.
- *Friedreich's ataxia syndrome:* It is characterized by retinitis pigmentosa, posterior column disease, ataxia and nystagmus.
- *Kearns-Sayre syndrome:* It is characterized by retinitis pigmentosa, chronic progressive external ophthalmoplegia and heart block.
- *Refsum's syndrome (heredopathia atactica polyneuritiformis):* It is an autosomal recessive inherited syndrome. Its main features include atypical retinitis pigmentosa, peripheral neuropathy and cerebellar ataxia. Night blindness due to pigmentary retinopathy is the presenting symptom. Ophthalmoscopy shows a salt and pepper type of changes. Sudden death can occur due to acute heart failure or respiratory paralysis.
- *Cockayne's syndrome:* It is characterized by childhood dwarfism with a characteristic bird like facies, deafness, nystagmus, ataxia, progressive mental retardation and atypical pigmentary retinopathy in form of a salt-pepper fundus.
- *Usher's syndrome:* It is characterized by congenital non-progressive sensory neural deafness of varying severity with pigmentary retinopathy; thus the patient suffers from deafness and blindness. It is an autosomal recessive inherited syndrome.
- *Bassen-Kornzweig syndrome (acanthocytosis):* It manifests with atypical retinitis pigmentosa, neuromuscular disease like Friedreich's ataxia, celiac disease and malformation of erythrocytes. Disturbances of ocular motility and ptosis may also be seen.
- *Favre-Goldmann syndrome:* There is vitreoretinal degeneration with poor night vision. It shows an autosomal recessive inheritance pattern. Its features include; atypical retinitis pigmentosa, vitreous degeneration (liquefaction), retinoschisis, lens opacities and marked electroretinogram abnormalities.
- *Mucopolysaccharidoses:* This group of inborn errors of metabolism is characterized by corneal stromal infiltration, retinal pigmentary retinopathy, optic atrophy, skeletal anomalies, mental retardation and facial coarseness.

Age-related Macular Degeneration (Fig. 19.6)

An elderly patient presents with gradual loss of vision.

Ophthalmoscopy shows macular degeneration.

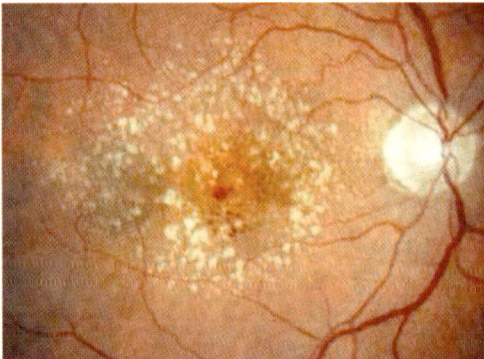

Fig. 19.6: Age-related macular degeneration

Diagnosis—age-related macular degeneration (AMD).

Age-related macular degeneration (AMD) also known as *senile macular degeneration* is a bilateral degeneration in aged past 60 years of age. This is a leading cause of blindness in developed countries. Risk factors are heredity, poor nutrition, smoking and high blood pressure. Prognosis of age-related macular degeneration is poor, therefore, it needs an early diagnosis and aggressive treatment strategy. Any permanent structural damage to the eye by other lesions should be ruled out before any treatment is commenced.

Dry AMD (Non-exudative or Atrophic or Non-neovascular)

- It affects 90% of cases.
- It causes mild to moderate gradual loss of vision.
- Patient complains of difficulty in near work due to central shadowing.
- Ophthalmoscopy shows drusens.
- Dietary supplements and antioxidants are helpful in preventing or delaying the progression.

Wet AMD (Exudative or Neovascular)

- It progresses rapidly with marked loss of vision.
- It passes through many stages and ends as disciform macular degeneration.
- Ophthalmoscopy helps in diagnosis and progress.

- Fluorescein angiography for complete categorization and subtyping of the wet AMD.
- Assess location of subfoveal hemorrhage by OCT.
- Argon green laser photocoagulation for extrafoveal choroidal neovascular membrane.
- Low fluence photodynamic therapy.
- VEGF inhibitors.

Cystoid Macular Edema (CME)

Patient presents with gradual loss of vision.

Ophthalmoscopy shows dull foveal reflex with cystoid spaces 'honeycomb appearance' at macula.

Diagnosis—cystoid macular edema (CME).

Etiological Factors

- Exact causative factor for cystoid macular edema is unknown.
- Inflammation, vitreous traction and generalized vascular diseases like hypertension, diabetes and central retinal vein occlusion have been thought of.
- Prostaglandins have been implicated.
- Seen more after an intracapsular cataract surgery.
- Implant of intraocular lens has no significant effect.
- Incidence increases with loss of vitreous.
- Incidence increases with secondary implant.

Clinical Features

Angiographic cystoid macular edema

- Angiographic cystoid macular edema develops soon after cataract extraction.
- Incidence is more with intracapsular cataract extraction.
- Fluorescein angiography shows a 'flower petal' pattern.
- Symptomless and resolves itself.

Clinical cystoid macular edema

- Clinical cystoid macular edema presents after few months to years of surgery.
- Anterior uveitis with vitritis.

- Mild irritation, redness, photophobia and dim vision.
- Fluorescein angiography shows 'flower petal' pattern with pooling of the dye.
- Ophthalmoscopy shows dull foveal reflex with cystoid spaces—'*honeycomb appearance*'.
- Most cases resolve spontaneously.
- Course of steroids or nonsteroidal anti-inflammatory drugs may help.

Epiretinal Membranes (ERM)

Patient presents with complain of gradual loss of vision and objects appear, small, large or wavy.

Ophthalmoscopy shows tortuous vessels, retinal striae, dull or loss of foveal reflex with retinal edema.

Diagnosis—epiretinal membrane.

Epiretinal membrane is an avascular, fibrocellular membrane that proliferates on the retina. It may be idiopathic as seen even in healthy eyes or secondary.

Idiopathic epiretinal membranes are associated with posterior vitreous detachment. Posterior vitreous detachment can initiate inflammation, exudation and leukocyte response. Laminocytes can form a transparent membrane which like any scar tissue creates tension on retina resulting in tortuousity of vessels, retinal striae, and loss of foveal reflex and retinal edema.

Secondary epiretinal membranes may result from ocular inflammation, retinal detachment surgery, vascular occlusions, posterior uveitis, trauma, tumors, retinal laser and cryotherapy.

Symptoms

- Epiretinal membranes are symptomatic only when macula or perimacular area is involved.
- Presenting symptoms are low vision, metamorphopsia, micropsia, macropsia, and monocular diplopia.
- Occasionally, the epiretinal membrane may detach spontaneously showing improvement in vision.

Signs

Slit-lamp is the best method to view the epiretinal membranes.
- Thin epiretinal membrane is seen as a glistening light reflex with no signs of retinal traction with normal vision.
- Transparent, translucent membrane with retinal changes such as wrinkling, vascular distortion, cystoids macular edema or pseudomacular mole with marked loss of vision.

Investigations

- Fluorescein angiography
- *Optical coherence tomography (OCT):* It helps to view vitreomacular junction and fine membranes on retina.
- *Spectral-domain optical coherence tomography (SD-OCT):* Allows three-dimensional and high resolution visualization of the dynamics of epiretinal traction through all the layers of retina up to pigment epithelium.

Management

- *No treatment for patients with mild and non-progressive symptoms.*
- *Vitrectomy:* Surgical removal of epiretinal membrane to improve visual acuity and reduce annoying symptoms of metamorphopsia, macropsia or micropsia.
- *Results are not encouraging.*

Cherry-red Spot at Macula Syndrome

Cherry-red spot at the macula is one of the most striking fundus picture seen in a rare group of following inherited metabolic diseases.
1. *Tay-Sachs disease:* This disease is also called as infantile amaurotic familial idiocy. It onsets in the first year of life and ends in death before the age of two years. A cherry-red spot is seen in about 90% of the cases.
2. *Neimann-Pick disease:* Incidence of cherry-red spot is lesser than in Tay-Sachs disease.
3. *Sandhoff disease* alike the Tay-Sachs disease.
4. *Sialidosis types 1 and 2:* Characterized by a cherry-red spot, myoclonic jerks, and pain in limbs and unsteadiness.

Pathogenesis

All these diseases are characterized by intracellular deposition of certain glycolipids and phospholipids in various tissues of the body including retina. In the retina, the lipids are stored in the ganglion cell layer giving it a white appearance on fundus examination. The fovea being free of ganglion cells so it stands out in contrast as a cherry-red spot at macula with surrounding white retina.

Bull's Eye Macular Syndrome

- In this syndrome, there is cone dystrophy.
- Patients usually present between first and third decade of their life.
- Characterized by decreased central vision, decreased vision in good illumination *'day blindness'*, defective color vision and nystagmus.

Ophthalmoscopic Features

- Typical bull eye macular lesion due to selective atrophy of retinal pigment epithelial cells.
- Vessels are attenuated with pale waxy disk and pigmentation as in retinitis pigmentosa.

RETINAL DETACHMENT

Definition

A separation of the sensory layer of the retina from the retinal pigment epithelium is known as *retinal detachment*.

Classification

1. Rhegmatogenous retinal detachment.
2. Tractional retinal detachment.
3. Exudative retinal detachment.

1. Rhegmatogenous Retinal Detachment
(Fig. 19.7)

Patient presents with complain of seeing floaters and flashes followed by black curtain in his field of vision.

Ophthalmoscopy shows retinal tear with detachment.

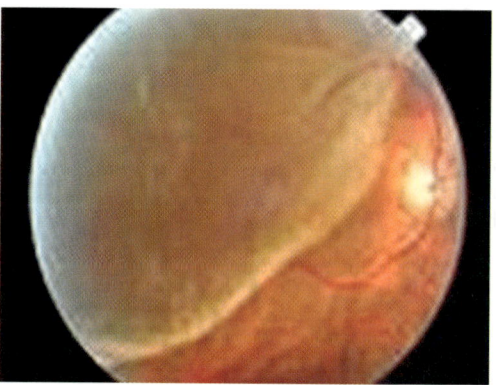

Fig. 19.7: Retinal detachment

Diagnosis—rhegmatogenous retinal detachment.

In rhegmatogenous retinal detachment, the subretinal fluid which separates the sensory layer from the retinal pigment epithelium is derived from the synchytic (liquefied) vitreous. It enters the subretinal space through a retinal hole or tear. It is mostly spontaneous but can also be due to any kind of even mild physical stress such as straining at toilet.

Predisposing Factors for Retinal Tear Leading to Detachment

Vitreoretinal Traction due to Posterior Vitreous Detachment

The synchisis (liquefaction) of vitreous gel is an age-related phenomenon caused by alteration in its micromolecular structure. In some cases, a hole develops in the posterior cortex over the foveal area. The synchytic fluid from the vitreous cavity passes through this newly created hole in the retrohyaloid space. This entry of fluid further detaches the posterior vitreous surface from the internal limiting membrane of the sensory retina. The remaining vitreous get collapses. This process is known as *acute posterior vitreous detachment*.

Due to posterior vitreous detachment, the sensory retina has lost the protective support of the healthy and stable vitreous gel; therefore, it can be now affected by any vitreoretinal traction forces. The eyes develop a retinal tear due to transmission of traction force at the strong attachment of the sensory retina at the site of peripheral retinal degenerations.

Normally, tear develops at the time of posterior vitreous detachment but it can be delayed for months. A tear caused by posterior vitreous detachment is usually symptomatic giving rise to symptoms of photopsia and floaters. The tear is usually U-shaped, mostly in upper quadrant and associated with hemorrhage.

Peripheral Retinal Degenerations

a. Lattice (palisade) degeneration: Clinical features

- Lattice degeneration of the retina is directly related to retinal detachment in about 40% of eyes and its presence in myopes is an important cause for retinal detachment in young people.
- Lattice is not an age-related phenomenon but seen commonly in young myopes above minus three dioptres.
- Lattice degeneration appears as spindle-shape sharply demarcated areas which are circumferentially oriented and located between equator and posterior border of the vitreous base. These lattice areas may form two or three rows.
- Occasionally, the lattice islands are radially oriented usually paravascularly and may extend even beyond equator.
- Lattice is usually bilateral and seen more commonly in superior temporal quadrant of fundus.
- An advanced lesion shows an arborizing network of white lines often continuous with peripheral blood vessels.
- Vitreous over the lesion is synchytic with firm attachment at borders.
- Retinal hole in the lattice remains quiet.
- Retinal tear due to lattice is usually located at its posterior border.
- Rapid progress of detachment.

b. Snail-track degeneration

- Snail-track degeneration appears as sharply demarcated bands of packed 'snowflakes'.
- Variant of lattice.
- Characteristic arborizing network of white lines seen in lattice is absent in this.

- Incidence of small holes is also less.
- Lesions are associated with phenomenon of *white with pressure*.

c. White with pressure and without pressure

- The phenomenon of *'white with pressure'* is a translucent gray appearance of the retina due to the scleral pressure induced by scleral depressor during examination of fundus with binocular indirect ophthalmoscope.
- If the retina in periphery appears translucent gray without pressure from the scleral depressor then it is known as "white without pressure". An area of peripheral retina which appears white without pressure needs strengthening with prophylactic cryotherapy.

d. Senile retinoschisis

Retinoschisis is splitting of the sensory retina into two layers: (i) an outer, and (ii) an inner layer. The split commonly occurs at the outer plexiform layer and less commonly at the level of the nerve fiber layer.

It is prevalent in young and hypermetropes. It involves both the eyes and starts at inferior and temporal quadrant.

It progresses circumferentially and involves the entire periphery of fundus. It is differentiated from retinal detachment by the immobility and transparency of the inner layers. There is an absolute field defect in the upper nasal field and it shows enlargement towards fixation point. The vision is affected with involvement of macula.

Retinal breaks occur in the inner or outer layers of retinoschisis which often leads to retinal detachment. Its progress may be arrested by photocoagulation of healthy retina ahead of retinoschisis.

Detachment is treated with scleral buckling.

e. Focal pigment proliferation or clumping

Focal pigment proliferation or clumping appears as small localized and irregular patches of pigmentation in the periphery of retina. These are usually seen with vitreoretinal traction membranes.

Clinical Features of Rhegmatogenous Retinal Detachment

Symptoms

1. *Photopsia* Photopsia is a subjective sensation of seeing a flash of light in his temporal peripheral visual field. It can be induced by eye movement and easily seen in dim illumination by the patient. It occurs due to traction at the site of vitreo retinal adhesion.

2. *Floaters* Floaters are moving vitreous opacities perceived by the patient when the opacities cast a shadow onto the retina. These are of various shapes such as small spots, large spots or rings and like a cobweb.

3. *Visual field defect* The patient complains of seeing a "black curtain" in his field of vision. The defect appears when the detachment has spread posterior to equator.

4. *Gradual loss of visual acuity* It may occur due to macular edema, vitreous hemorrhage, floaters and involvement of macula in detachment.

Signs

1. *Anterior segment* There may be signs of mild anterior uveitis in form of aqueous flare, few keratic precipitates and few anterior synechia. The intraocular pressure of the affected eye is about 5 mm Hg lower than the normal eye.

2. *Posterior segment* On ophthalmoscopy, a U-shaped retinal tear is seen usually in the upper quadrant. The detached retina is convex and slightly opaque with loss of underlying choroidal pattern. The retina is mobile on the movement of the eye. There is posterior vitreous detachment. There may be intravitreal hemorrhage.

Management

The main treatment for a retinal tear causing detachment is scleral buckling operation with explant. To this, cryopexy or photocoagulation is added depending on case.

Other surgical procedures available are drainage of subretinal fluid, and intravitreal injection of air, balanced salt solution or silicon oil.

2. Tractional Retinal Detachment

Pateint presents with complete loss of vision with old history of floaters and flashes.

Ophthalmoscopy shows bands and membranes with new vessels.

Diagnosis—tractional retinal detachment.

In this, sensory layer of retina is pulled away from retinal pigment epithelium by contraction of bands.

The most common cause for tractional retinal detachment is proliferative retinopathies in diabetes and Eale's disease following vitreous hemorrhage.

Neovascularization is one of the most important factor for traction detachment. New vessels proliferate on the optic disk and along the course of major temporal vascular arcades. The new vessels start as endothelial proliferations from veins. The mesenchyme from which new vessels are derived is also a source for fibroblasts which embraces the vessels to form a fibrovascular epiretinal membrane. This membrane becomes adherent to the posterior vitreous surface. With the detachment of posterior vitreous, the fibrovascular membrane continues to grow along its surface. Eventually, the fibrovascular membrane is pulled into the vitreous cavity resulting in detachment of retina.

Symptoms

There is the absence of photopsia and floaters. There is loss of central visual acuity and peripheral visual fields.

Signs

It may be detected on routine examination of fundus as there are almost no symptoms. On ophthalmoscopy, neither the tear nor the mobility of detached retina are seen and proliferative fibrovascular membranes are visible clearly.

Management

A pars plana vitrectomy is the only treatment of choice.

3. Exudative Retinal Detachment

Patient presents with complain of gradual loss of complete vision within last 15 days.

Ophthalmoscopy shows complete detachment.

General examination may show signs of Harada's disease.

Diagnosis—exudative retinal detachment.

There is damage to retinal pigment epithelium. It allows the fluid from choroid to gain entry and causes detachment. It is common in Harada's disease, posterior scleritis, choroidal tumors and following panretinal photocoagulation.

Symptoms

There is no symptom of photopsia as there is no vitreoretinal traction. There are symptoms of floaters mainly due to associated vitritis and uveitis. There is loss of peripheral visual fields which is fast progressive as in Harada's disease.

Signs

There are no tears in the retina. The detached retina has convexity, smooth and large balloon-like. The subretinal fluid has a tendency to shift with position of head. There is usually an associated systemic disease such as Harada's disease or rheumatoid arthritis.

Management

Treat the causative factor. The most common cause is Harada's disease and it can be treated as uveitis with steroids—topical and systemic.

TUMOR

Retinoblastoma (Fig. 19.8)

An elderly person with his grandson of about 3 years presents with propotosed and perforated eye with fungating mass.

Diagnosis—retinoblastoma.

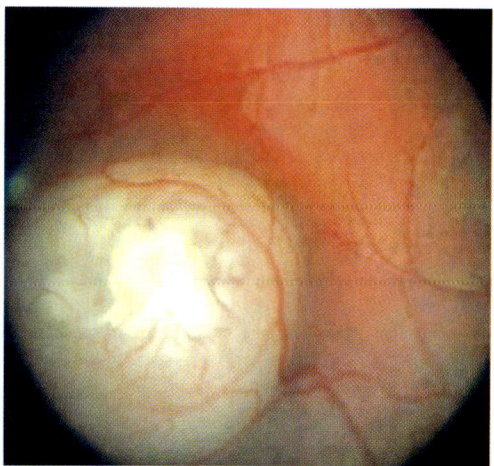

Fig. 19.8: Retinoblastoma

Incidence

- It is most common primary malignant intraocular tumor of childhood occurring 1 in 20,000 live births.
- It is bilateral in about 25 to 30% cases although one eye is affected earlier and more extensively than the other.
- There is no sexual predilection.
- In most cases, it manifests prior to the age of three.
- Tumor in each eye is independent of each other due to its multicentric origin.

Genetics and Heredity

Retinoblastoma gene identified as 14 band on the long-arm of chromosome 13 (13q14) is a *cancer suppressor or antioncogenic gene.* Inactivation of this protective gene by two mutations (*Knudson's two hit hypothesis*) is the causative factor for occurrence of retinoblastoma. Retinoblastoma may manifest as *hereditary* or *sporadic form.*

Clinical Features

The most important aspect is the clinical examination of both the eyes under full mydriasis and anesthesia to group the tumor and plan treatment accordingly.

1. Quiescent Stage

Clinical features

- *White reflex from the pupil (leukocoria or amaurosis cat's eye)* is the most common presenting symptom from the parents. The parents report that there is a white reflex from the eye or eyes of the child and these appear like a cat's eye.
- *Strabismus* is the second most common presenting symptom reported by parents. The infant develops the deviation of the eye due to loss of central vision which occurs if the tumor has involved the posterior pole affecting the macula thereby the central vision. Keeping this presenting symptom in mind, it is mandatory that a thorough examination of the fundus must be done in any case reporting with dim vision or a deviation of eye.
- *Hyphema* without any obvious cause or a history of trauma or any disease.

Clinical types with ophthalmoscopic features

1. *Endophytic retinoblastoma:* Endophytic tumors progress towards the vitreous cavity.

On ophthalmoscopy, the tumor appears as white or a pearly pink color mass with line vessels on its surface. There may be more than one mass, as the tumor has a multicentric origin. Therefore, it is essential to scale the entire fundus to avoid missing other focus of tumor. Some cases that may develop secondary calcification of tumor mass then the mass appears like a soft yellowish mass resembling the *cottage cheese.*

2. *Exophytic retinoblastoma:* Exophytic tumor grows in the subretinal space and presents an ophthalmoscopic picture of retinal detachment. Any detachment in early childhood should arouse suspicion for tumor.

Diagnosis
The age of the patient with typical presenting symptoms is enough to diagnose a case of retinoblastoma. An early diagnosis may help to treat the case with modern therapy and save the life and vision also.

Prognosis
The prognosis depends on the following points:

- *Prognosis* is favorable, if optic nerve has not been involved.
- *Prognosis* is good, if the tumor is small and located posteriorly.
- *Prognosis is very good,* if diagnosed early with a small tumor.
- *For a better prognosis:* Keep a watch on the other eye and conduct repeated examination of the fundus at regular intervals, until the child has crossed the age of 10 years at least.
- *Prognosis depends on the cellular differentiation.*
- *Well-differentiated tumor characterized by Flexner: Wintersteiner rosettes have a good prognosis.* The rosettes have a clear lumen. These need to be differentiated from *pseudorosette* in which the tumor cells cluster around blood vessels or around small areas of necrosis.
- *Highly undifferentiated tumor have a poor prognosis.*
- *Mortality rate of well-differentiated tumor is only 8% in comparison to 40% with undifferentiated tumor cells.*

Genetic counseling
It is in the interest of the patient to guide him on genetic counseling:

- Both the parents being healthy with one child affected with retinoblastoma can plan to have another child. The risk of second child getting affected is very low to about 6% only.
- Both the parents being healthy with two or more of their children being affected with retinoblastoma should not plan to have any more children. The risk increases to about 50% for the newborn.
- If any one of the parents is a survivor of hereditary retinoblastoma, then they should not plan to have a child as the risk is more than 50% of his getting a tumor.
- If both the parents are survivor of retinoblastoma then they should not plan to have any children.

2. Glaucomatous Stage (Fig. 19.9)

In later stage, child may present as a case of buphthalmos or proptosis. Intraocular pressure is high. This stage is characterized by severe pain, redness and watering.

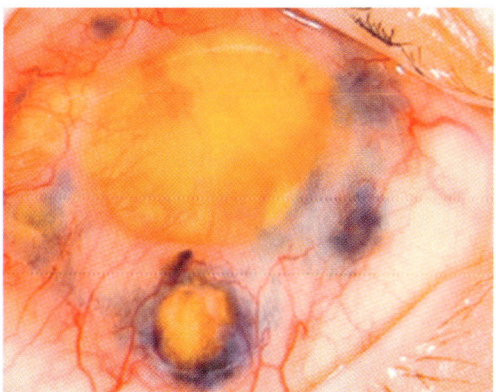

Fig. 19.9: Retinoblastoma—glaucomatous stage

3. Extraocular Extension

Globe bursts through the sclera usually at the limbus or near the optic disk. There is rapid fungative growth that involves extraocular tissue resulting in proptosis.

4. Distant Metastasis

Metastasis occurs in pre-auricular and other lymph nodes and direct extension through optic nerve. The common sites for metastases by bloodstream are skull, orbit, long bones, viscera, spinal cord and lymph nodes.

International Classification of Retinoblastoma

Group-A: Small tumor less than 3 mm.
Group-B: Large tumor more than 3 mm.
Group-C: Focal seeds of tumor subretinal and or vitreal, less than 3 mm from retinoblastoma.
Group-D: Diffuse seeds of tumor subretinal or vitreal, more than 3 mm from retinoblastoma.
Group-E: Extensive tumor occupying more than 50% of globe or associated complications.

Investigations

- Complete blood picture, ESR and hemoglobin.
- Bone free X-ray of the globe for any calcification.
- B-scan ultrasonography for presence of calcification.
- CT scan for involvement of optic nerve, orbit, pineal or central nervous system.
- Aqueous humour paracentesis for enzyme assay and cytology. An aqueous to plasma lactate dehydrogenase ratio of greater than 1.0 is suggestive.
- ELISA test to exclude toxocariasis.
- Fine needle biopsy may be required, when there is doubt about the diagnosis.
- *Metastatic workup:* Metastatic workup includes bone scan, cerebrospinal fluid analysis, bone marrow aspiration and analysis and whole body CT/MRI, when required.

Management

- Cobalt plaque irradiation is good for a small tumor.
- Photocoagulation with xenon arc is indicated in small posterior tumors not involving the optic nerve and macula.
- Cryotherapy is useful for small anterior peripheral tumors. Cryo should be repeated at least three times.
- Laser photocoagulation is useful for posterior small tumors away from macula.
- Radiotherapy with an external beam is useful for cases with medium or large tumors.
- Systemic chemotherapy is indicated in cases with metastasis.
- Enucleation with care to take a long piece of the optic nerve is the treatment of choice in advanced cases with poor vision. The involvement of the optic nerve indicates metastasis.
- Histopathology of enucleated eye is a must to assess the prognosis. Well-differentiated tumor shows rosettes. Mortality is about 8% in cases showing rosettes. Highly undifferentiated tumor has a mortality of 40%.
- Rarely spontaneous regression with shrinkage of the eyeball may occur due to necrosis followed by calcification. Role of immunological phenomenon has been thought of.

20

Maladies of Optic Nerve

Symptomatic Conditions

- Papilledema
- Optic atrophy

Inflammations

- Optic neuritis
- Arteritic anterior ischemic optic neuropathy

Toxic Optic Neuropathy or Amblyopia

- Ethyl alcohol amblyopia
- Methyl alcohol amblyopia
- Tobacco amblyopia
- Quinine amblyopia
- Ehtambutol amblyopia
- Chloroquine amblyopia
- Oral contraceptive amblyopia

Tumors

- Glioma of the optic nerve
- Meningioma of the optic nerve

Congenital Anomalies

- Drusen
- Optic disk pits

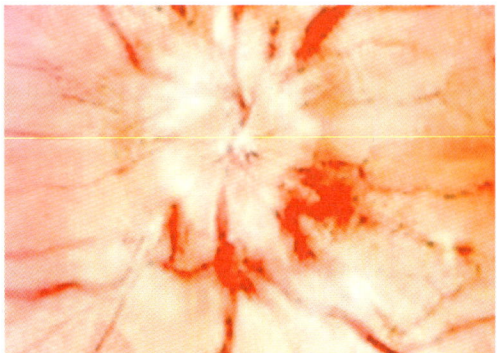

Fig. 20.1: Papilledema

It is a neurological emergency. Refer the case to neurologist for early management to reduce intracranial pressure to save the vision and life.

Papilledema is a term reserved for the passive swelling of the optic nerve head due to raised intracranial pressure which is almost always bilateral although it may be asymmetrical. Most common cause for raised intracranial pressure is space occupying lesion of brain.

Disk edema or *disk swelling* is a term that includes all the causes of active or passive edematous swelling of the optic disk.

SYMPTOMATIC CONDITIONS

Papilledema (Fig. 20.1)

Patient with raised intracranial pressure first attends ophthalmic clinic due to his presenting symptoms of headache, nausea with projectile vomiting and transient blurring of vision.

Ophthalmoscopy shows early blurring of disk margins with full vessels.

Diagnosis—papilledema.

Etiology

Intracranial space-occupying lesions such as brain tumors, abscess, tuberculoma, subdural hematoma and aneurysm are the most common causes for papilledema.

Space-occupying lesions in any position except medulla oblongata may induce papilledema.

Papilledema is most commonly associated with *tumors in posterior fossa* due to obstruction to flow of cerebrospinal fluid.

Papilledema is least with pituitary tumor.

The tumors of cerebellum, midbrain and parieto-occipital region induce early papilledema than tumors in other regions.

Fast growing lesions are associated with papilledema more frequently and acutely than the slow growing lesions.

Etiopathogenesis

Stasis of axoplasm in prelaminar region of the optic disk due to alteration in the pressure gradient across the lamina cribrosa results in the development of papilledema.

Symptoms

1. *General symptoms*
   - Headache which becomes worse by coughing or straining
   - Projectile vomiting without nausea
   - Pulsatile tinnitus
   - Consciousness may be affected
   - Diplopia—patient may complain.

2. *Ocular symptoms*
   - Transient attacks of blurred vision
   - Visual acuity remains normal for a long time.

Signs

- *Visual acuity:* The vision may remain unaffected for a long time. The vision gets affected, only when the macula is involved with hemorrhages or exudates.
- *Pupil:* Pupillary reactions are normal until optic atrophy sets in.
- *Field changes:* The earliest field change is the enlargement of the blind spot. Later there is peripheral constriction of visual field.

Ophthalmoscopic features

- *Hyperemia of the optic disk* is due to dilation of the capillaries on the optic nerve head.
- *Blurring of the optic disk margin* is first visible at the upper and lower margins then extending around the nasal side. *The temporal margin is the last to be affected.*

- *Filling of physiological cup of the optic disk is* gradual along with blurring of the peripapillary nerve fiber layer.
- *Veins are full and tortuous. Venous pulsation is absent even on pressure upon the globe.*
- *Flame-shape and round hemorrhages:* Numerous flame-shape or dot-like hemorrhages over the disk and retina. *Presence of even tiny hemorrhage over the disk must arouse the suspicion of early papilledema.*
- *Soft and hard exudates:* Numerous cotton wool spots in the posterior fundus. Later, there are hard exudates at the macula in the form of *macular star or fan-shaped* exudates on the side of the optic disk.
- *Swelling of the optic disk:* By this time, the disk is swollen. The veins appear to bend sharply over its margin.
- *Indirect binocular ophthalmoscopy: Definite parallax* may be elicited between the summit of the disk and retina.
- *Direct ophthalmoscopy:* Difference of 2–6 dioptres may be found between focusing the vessels at the summit of the disk and the vessels on the retina slightly away from the disk.
- *Post-papilledema optic atrophy:* It is the last stage in which the optic disk gets atrophied. Optic disk is pale white with blurred margins. Physiological cup is full. Veins are dilated. Exudates at the macula with atrophic changes.

Diagnosis

Nearly normal visual acuity with a typical fundus picture is more than enough to diagnose a case of papilledema.

Differential Diagnosis

There are many conditions which may give an appearance of papilledema, therefore, it is essential to differentiate it from other conditions.

- *Opaque nerve fibers* show typical appearance of feathery look of fibers with absence of other changes in the fundus.
- *Drusen of the optic nerve head:* There is the absence of physiological cup, presence of

the venous pulsation, the vessels are normal, and the disk color is normal.

- *Malignant hypertension:* Patient is young adult and comes with great loss of visual acuity. The increased blood pressure with typical fundus picture of hypertensive retinopathy shall help to differentiate it from papilledema.
- *Papillitis:* Shows marked and early loss of vision within few days. Pupillary reaction is ill-sustained. Pain on movement of the eye especially in the upward direction. Mild blurring of the disk not more than two dioptres. Typical fundus changes of papilledema are absent. Vitreous may show haze. Thus, keeping these points in mind, one can easily differentiate the papilledema from papillitis.

It is very essential to differentiate the papilledema from papillitis as any delay in the treatment of papillitis thinking it to be papilledema may cause loss of vision.

Ophthalmologist plays an important role to save the vision by early diagnosis of papilledema.

Management

It is a neurological emergency.

Refer the case to neurologist immediately with ophthalmoscopic findings to help him manage the case accordingly.

Optic Atrophy

The term 'optic atrophy' denotes degeneration of the optic nerve. It occurs as an end result of any pathological process that causes damage of axons from retinal ganglion cells to the lateral geniculate body.

Thus the optic atrophy is characterized by loss of axons. There is no regeneration of axons. The degeneration of axons is associated with proliferation of supporting and connective tissues which give rise to typical fundus picture in form of optic atrophy.

It should be kept in mind that it is not only the white color of the optic disk which is required to diagnose optic atrophy but the total composite fundus picture with associated clinical findings such as visual acuity, visual fields, pupillary reaction and changes in the retina and retinal vessels.

A person with a white optic disk may have a good central visual acuity while a person with normal disk appearance may have reduced vision. In a doubtful case, take help of all the methods of investigations including electroretinography and ultrasonography.

Clinically, it is easy to follow:

Ophthalmoscopic Classification of Optic Atrophy

1. Primary optic atrophy (Fig. 20.2)

Patient presents with gradual loss of vision since last few months.

Slit-lamp shows semidilated pupil with sluggish reaction to direct light but good reaction to consensual light.

Ophthalmoscopy shows whitish blue disk with sharp margins. Physiological cup is normal with visible lamina cribrosa. Retina and vessels are normal.

Diagnosis—primary optic atrophy.

Etiology

- Multiple sclerosis.
- Retrobulbar neuritis.
- Leber's and other hereditary optic atrophies.
- Pituitary tumors pressing directly on visual pathway.
- Toxic amblyopias.

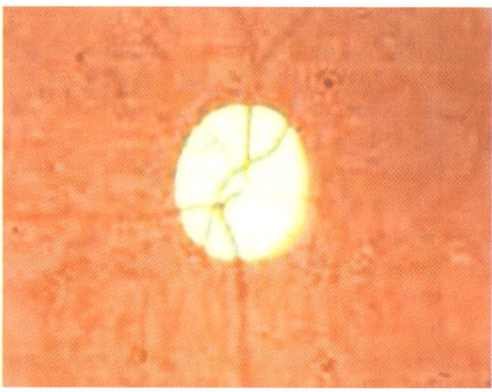

Fig. 20.2: Primary optic atrophy

Clinical features

- *Loss of vision* may be sudden or gradual.
- *Pupil* is semidilated. Direct reaction to light is sluggish or absent.
- *Visual fields* show peripheral constriction.

Ophthalmoscopic features

- Optic disk appears white with bluish hue, clear margins and decrease in its vasculature.
- Lamina cribrosa in the physiological cup is clearly visible.
- Retina and retinal vessels are normal.
- No hemorrhages and no exudates.
- Macula appears normal.

2. Postneuritic Optic Atrophy

Ophthalmoscopic features

- Optic disk appears dirty white in hue that is grayish white or pale white in color with blurred margins.
- Physiological cup is full.
- Arteries are attenuated.
- Veins are full with the perivascular sheathing seen on the disk and up to disk diameter from disk margin.
- Macula may show degenerative changes.
- Vitreous is hazy.

Postneuritic optic atrophy occurs as sequelae to long-standing papilledema or papillitis. Vision is lost early and suddenly in a case of papillitis while good vision is maintained for a long time in papilledema.

3. Consecutive Optic Atrophy

Ophthalmoscopic features

- Optic disk is yellowish and waxy in appearance.
- Margins are blurred.
- Vessels are attenuated.
- Other fundus findings shall be of the disease which is responsible for optic atrophy.

It occurs following destruction of ganglion cells due to degenerative or inflammatory lesions of the choroid and/or retina. The typical and common example is *retinitis pigmentosa.* Other common causes are diffuse chorioretinitis, central artery occlusion and pathological myopic degeneration.

4. Glaucomatous Optic Atrophy (Fig. 20.3)

Ophthalmoscopic features

- Optic disk shows deep cupping which reaches up to the margin of the disk.
- Nasal shifting of vessels which bend sharply at the margin of the optic disk.
- Parallax between the vessels on the retina and vessels at the bottom of the cup.

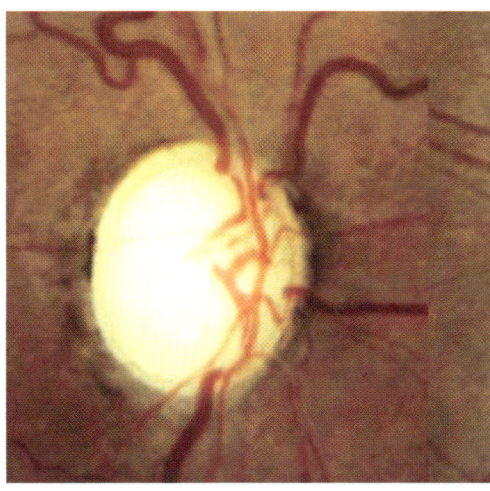

Fig. 20.3: Glaucomatous optic atrophy

It results due to high intraocular pressure in primary open-angle glaucoma.

It is to be differentiated from optic atrophy with cupping due to arteric anterior ischemic optic neuropathy in which the cup is shallow and rarely reaches up to the margin of the disk with normal intraocular pressure.

5. Vascular Optic Atrophy

Ophthalmoscopic features

- Optic disk is pale white with slight glial proliferation.
- Physiological cup is full.
- Other features are determined according to the causative vascular disease.

Vascular optic atrophy is seen in:
- Occlusion of the central retinal artery.
- Occlusion of the central retinal vein.

- Arteriosclerotic with hypertension retinopathy.
- Severe anemia.
- Arteric anterior ischemic optic neuropathy.

6. Toxic Optic Atrophy

Ophthalmoscopic features

- Optic disk is pale white or pale waxy usually with clear margins.
- Vessels are attenuated.
- Degenerative changes at the macula.
  It follows toxic neuropathies and amblyopia.

7. Ischemic Optic Atrophy

Ophthalmoscopic features

- Optic disk appears pale with blurred margins.
- Vessels are markedly attenuated.
  It occurs in giant cell arteritis and quinine amblyopia.

Management

- Treat the underlying cause. It may help to preserve some useful vision.
- Early diagnosis and energetic management shall help the patient to save some vision.

INFLAMMATION

Optic Neuritis

Patient presents with complain of veiled or misty vision, transient obscuration of vision with mild discomfort and tenderness of the eye with upward movement or even mild touch.

Slit-lamp shows an ill-sustained pupil without any doubt. Ophthalmoscopy shows mild pale disk in comparison to normal eye.

Diagnosis—retrobulbar optic neuritis.
  Optic neuritis is an inflammatory and demyelinating malady of optic nerve.

Types of Optic Neuritis

- *Retrobulbar neuritis*: Refers to involvement of the optic nerve behind the eyeball. More common in adults with multiple sclerosis.

- *Papillitis:* Refers to involvement of the optic disk in inflammatory or demyelinating disorders. More common in children.
- *Neuroretinitis*: Refers to involvement of the optic disk and macular region.

Etiology

1. *Idiopathic:* In many cases even after a thorough investigation, the cause is not established usually in cases with one attack of optic neuritis.
2. *Multiple sclerosis:* Optic neuritis is the presenting feature of multiple sclerosis in about 25% of the cases. Most of these develop multiple sclerosis within 5 years of optic neuritis. The risk of occurrence of multiple sclerosis is much increased in case with histocompatibility locus antigen (HLA-DR$_2$) positive patients with recurrences.
3. *Post-viral:* Optic neuritis follows commonly an attack of *influenza*. Post-viral optic neuritis is common in children following an attack of measles, chickenpox, mumps, whooping cough, glandular fever and even following immunization.
4. *Infection from adjacent structures:* Optic neuritis may occur following meningitis, sinusitis, extraction of septic tooth and infection in the orbit.
5. *Chronic systemic infections:* Optic neuritis has been seen in the cases of tuberculosis, sarcoidosis and syphilis.
6. *Metabolic disorder:* Optic neuritis is common among diabetics.
7. *Toxic optic neuritis*: In cases with toxic amblyopia.
8. *Miscellaneous:* Any condition which lowers the resistance of the body may help to precipitate an attack of optic neuritis such as anemia, deficiency of vitamins and protein, malnutrition, gastrointestinal disorders and collagen disorders.

Symptoms

- *Loss of visual acuity:* Most common presenting symptom is sudden and progressive loss of the central visual acuity.

- *Veiled vision*: To begin with the patient feels as if seeing through a veil and thereafter this veil gets thicker and thicker obscuring the vision even to light perception only.
- The loss of vision is due to conduction block of the optic nerve.
- *Episodic transient obscuration of vision* during exertion and exposure to heat which recovers on rest in cool environment.
- *Periocular pain:* Patient complains of pain on movement of the eye especially on upward movement of the eye *due to attachment of some fibers of superior rectus muscle to the dural sheath of the optic nerve.*
- *Headache and neuralgia:* Some patients may present with severe headache and neuralgic pain in and around the eye. These patients are unusually emotionally sensitive.
- *Dark adaptation* is reduced.
- *Color vision* is impaired.

Signs

- Reduced visual acuity.
- Decreased brightness of light
- *Pain* when asked to look upwards.
- *Tenderness* of the eye to touch on pressure.
- *Marcus-Gunn pupil* (ill-sustained pupillary reaction) is diagnostic. *It occurs due to conduction block of the impulse due to edema of the optic nerve fibers.*
- Positive central or centrocaecal scotoma.
- Impaired color vision.

Ophthalmoscopic Features

1. Ophthalmoscopic features in retrobulbar optic neuritis

- No fundus changes in the early stage.
- Later optic disk shows temporal pallor.
It is diagnosed only by symptoms and signs of which the most prominent is sudden loss of vision without any obvious fundus findings.
An ill-sustained pupillary reaction is diagnostic.

2. Ophthalmoscopic features in papillitis

- *Swelling of the optic disk:* There is swelling of the optic disk but never more than two diopters.

- *Optic disk margins* are blurred.
- *Physiological cup is full* due to edema and glial proliferation.
- *Full and tortuous veins* showing a bend at the disk margin.
- *Vitreous haze:* Due to inflammatory cells.

3. Ophthalmoscopic features in neuro-retinitis

- Features of papillitis plus extension of edema in the surrounding retina of the disk.
- Macular star.

Post-neuritic optic atrophy is the final outcome of any untreated case and presents as; disk is pale white with blurred margins, obliterated physiological cup, arteries attenuated, veins showing sheathing and some changes at the macula.

Investigation

- *Color vision* is affected even with relatively good vision.
- *Field defect:* Relative central scotoma.
- *Visually evoked response (VER)* shows reduced amplitude and delay in transmission.

Diagnosis

Optic neuritis is diagnosed on the basis of the following points:

1. Sudden and progressive loss of vision
2. Pain in the eye on upward movement
3. Ill-sustained pupillary reaction
4. Relative central scotoma
5. Defective color vision
6. Swelling of the disk is never more than two diopters.
7. Associated history of influenza or any inflammation.

Differential Diagnosis

1. *Pseudo-optic neuritis* Fundus examination in a case of hypermetropia or irregular astigmatism may show a blurred disk giving an impression of optic neuritis. All other clinical features are absent.

A change of lenses in ophthalmoscope makes the fundus picture clear.

2. *Papilledema:* In papilledema, the following points help to differentiate it from papillitis.
   - Vision is nearly normal.
   - No pain on movement of the eye upwards or any direction.
   - Pupil reacts normally.
   - Enlargement of the blind spot or the peripheral constriction of the visual fields.
   - Swelling of disk is more than two diopters and may be up to six diopters. Veins are full with hemorrhages and cotton-wool spots.

Management

Antibiotics and steroids therapy: Systemic broad-spectrum antibiotics and steroids. Taper steroids gradually to maintenance dose for long time.

Supportive therapy

- Vitamins, good diet and rest are helpful.
- Advise patient to avoid physical stress and exposure to heat and bright light for few days until the malady responds well.
- Most of the patients do recover the normal vision with residual defect in the color vision and light brightness.
- Visual prognosis is good in cases of *multiple sclerosis.*

Arteritic Anterior Ischemic Optic Neuropathy (AAION)

Patient presents with tenderness in temporal region, transient obscuration of vision and flashes of light for few seconds followed with severe and localized headache.

Ophthalmoscopy shows pale or hyperemic disk with splinter hemorrhages.

Diagnosis—arteritic anterior ischemic optic neuropathy.

Arteritic anterior ischemic optic atrophy is segmental or generalized infarction of the optic nerve. It affects elderly people usually over the age of 60 years.

Etiology

- *Giant cell arteritis—* a disease of unknown etiology.
- Common vessels affected are *superficial temporal artery, ophthalmic artery and posterior ciliary arteries.*
- Idiopathic.
- Miscellaneous factor associated with collagen vascular disorders.

Symptoms

- Transient obscuration of vision prior to onset of the malady.
- Sudden and marked loss of visual acuity.
- Patient may have a periocular pain.
- Patient may point towards a tender temporal artery.
- Headache and scalp tenderness may be present in some cases.

Ophthalmoscopic Features

There is a swelling of the disc with blurred margins.

Peripapillary splinter-shape hemorrhages.

Later the optic atrophy sets in with cupping of the disk. The cupping does not reach the margin of optic disk as in primary open-angle glaucoma.

Investigations

- Erythrocyte sedimentation rate is high.
- C-reactive protein is invariably raised.
- Elevated platelets.
- Temporal artery biopsy may give a positive report.

Management

Systemic steroid therapy Steroid is the choice in a case with giant cell arteritis as the causative factor.

Start with (2 mg/kg body weight) or 120 mg of prednisone daily and taper it to 10 mg a day in about one month's time. The daily dose of 10 mg is maintained for about 3 months.

Reduce further depending on the symptoms of the patient and erythrocyte sedimentation rate. Patient needs treatment for about 1–2 years.

Some patients may need steroid for the rest of life.

Support therapy *Good diet, vitamins, proteins.*

TOXIC OPTIC NEUROPATHY OR AMBLYOPIA

Toxic optic neuropathy embraces all the conditions of optic nerve damage due to ingestion of exogenous poisons, drugs and tobacco. The most common of these are tobacco, ethyl alcohol, methyl alcohol, quinine, ethambutol, chloroquine and oral contraceptives.

Some of these affect the ganglion cells of the retina which results in degeneration of nerve fibers while others affect the nerve fibers directly.

Alcohol (Ethyl Alcohol) Intoxication

Cute wife presents with her handsome husband with complain that my husband shows squint, when he drinks whisky even of a reputed brand. He appears normal by morning, when he wakes up.

Clinician said: All the people who get intoxicated develop not only squint but many more visual disturbances which are life-threatening for the self and family.

Diagnosis—alcohol (ethyl alcohol) intoxication.
Alcohol (ethyl alcohol) is most important class of chemical from the practical, social, family and public point of view that it is consumed by people throughout the universe irrespective of class, color, religion, race or social and educational status.

Alcohol consumption even from reputed brand too manifests visual disturbances and intoxication. Alcohol is alcohol and it does not spare any one even god man, spiritualist, king or pauper.

Alcohol intoxication causes visual disturbances such as diplopia and impairment of perception and judgment due to affection of higher visual functions, preliminary to unconsciousness.

- Alcohol intoxication is not a gradual process but it manifests quickly, when the concentration in the blood rises to a certain level that varies considerably with each individual—from 170 to 183 mg per 100 ml blood.

- Critical level is relatively constant for the same individual.
- Effects due to concentration in the blood achieved rapidly are more potent than achieved by slow drinking though the intoxication level is maintained with either rapid or slow consumption of alcohol.
- Time involved in slow drinking has a sobering influence.
- Thus each person who takes to social drinking must know his limits and should not drink more than 50% of his limit in the society to save himself and family from social disrespect and accidents particularly at night on the return journey home.

Any person who boosts about increase in his mental and physical power and shows indifference and lack of fear is diagnostic for reaching critical level for alcohol intoxication.

Alcoholic denies himself about his own observation. Family members, friends or any aware observer can notice that he is missing to pick up the eatables or drink. This occurs due to failure or markedly depressed fusional ability resulting in diplopia. This is the critical time, when that alcoholic should be tactfully moved away or even out to avoid any kind of non-sensical social accident.

Clinical Features

Symptomatic visual disturbances

- Visual acuity is lowered from 5 to 20%, an appreciable loss for late evening or night drive.
- Sensitivity to light is lowered by 30% or more.
- Threshold to brightness difference is increased by 50% or more.
- Retardation in recovery from glare.
- Depth perception is disturbed.
- Retardation in reaction time.
- Retardation in the ocular movements.
- Fusional ability is lost resulting in diplopia.
- Heterophoria breaks down causing increase in esophoria and decrease in exophoria amounting to about 2 prism dioptre.
- Failure or depressed fusional ability results in diplopia.

2. Visual Signs

- Habitual drinker develops *alcoholic peripheral neuritis.*
- Field of vision may show central scotoma.
- Incidence of tobacco amblyopia increases many folds in tobacco inhalers.
- *Protein-energy malnutrition in rich and elite professionals.*

Visual disturbances and protein (energy) malnutrition are enough to jeopardize your life, when you are at the peak of success, the *Mt Kailash.*

Self-management

- Professionals are not likely to enter the domain of intoxication.
- Professionals are possessed with strong will power.
- Professionals are successful persons, therefore, to keep alive, climb and maintain high position, they must have driver or family member to drive back.
- Professionals who are successful always make others drink rather than get drunk themselves.
- Professionals who desire to get drunk for fun—say once at least then they must get drunk at home to avoid social elite to enjoy your utterly non-ethical personality. Request your sweet heart to video graph it and show you, when you come out of your intoxication to enjoy your own utterly non-presentable disgusting act. After visualizing the self, you are likely to abandon the bottle forever.

Management

Complete abstention from alcohol and good diet helps in restoring the vision, inner vision, peace and bliss and safe, long and happy life for the self and family.

Methyl Alcohol (Wood Spirit) Amblyopia

Wood painter presents with complain of misty vision following drinking wood spirit as he had no money to buy local made alcohol.

Slit-lamp shows sluggish reaction of pupil.

Ophthalmoscopy shows pale disk.

Diagnosis—methyl alcohol amblyopia.

Methyl alcohol amblyopia takes long time-years to manifest.

Methyl alcohol amblyopia is an acute process that follows even after one time ingestion of even small quantity.

Methyl alcohol can be ingested by three routes:

1. Drinking cheap adulterated or fortified beverage is the most common way. Even a teaspoonful may result in amblyopia and an ounce can result in death. Painter is likely to drink the spirit used in painting, when his body-mind complex demands due to addiction.
2. Inhalation of fumes in industries.
3. Industrial worker may absorb it through skin.

Methyl alcohol amblyopia is commonly seen in the area where there is prohibition for alcohol. The people then drink wood alcohol or even methylated spirit. It usually occurs in an acute form and affects large number of people.

Symptoms

In acute form:
- Headache, nausea, giddiness and vomiting.
- Pain in abdomen
- Prostration, delirium, convulsions, coma and death.
- If the patient survives then there is marked loss of visual acuity.

Signs

- Pupils are dilated and fixed.
- Ophthalmoscopy shows blurring of disk margins with attenuated vessels ending as primary optic atrophy.
- *It is due to degeneration of the ganglion cells of the retina.*
- *Characteristic odor from the breath of patient is diagnostic.*

The odor is due to excretion of formaldehyde which is the breakdown product of methyl alcohol.

Management

1. *Self-management* Complete abstention from alcohol and good diet helps in restoring the vision, inner vision, peace and bliss and safe, long and happy life for the self and family.

2. *Supportive therapy*
- Gastric lavage 2–3 times a day for 3–4 days as there is evidence that the methyl alcohol in the system is continuously returning back to stomach.
- Intravenous fluids—sodium biocarbonate to neutralize acidosis by methyl alcohol.
- Prophylactic, i.e. by educating the people about the outcome of drinking wood alcohol and methylated spirit.

Tobacco Amblyopia

Clinical Features

Tobacco amblyopia occurs due to excessive use of tobacco in any of the following forms.
1. Pipe smoking
2. Tobacco chewing
3. Absorption of tobacco dust in tobacco factories
4. Smokers of strong tobacco mixture and cigars.
   - Cigarette smokers are rarely affected.
   - Tobacco amblyopia coincides with some intercurrent cause of debility and deficiency of vitamins and proteins with regular intake of alcohol enhances the toxic effect of tobacco.
   - An early complaint from the patient is about fogginess of vision more in day light rather than in dull light or evening. There is marked loss of central visual acuity causing difficulty in near work.
   - *Ophthalmoscopy*: Normal fundus or slight temporal pallor of the optic disk.
   - *Field defect diagnosis is made from characteristic centrocecal field defect involving an area between the fixation point and the blind spot*. This scotoma gradually enlarges to cover the fixation point. Thus, central vision is lost with an intact peripheral field.
   - *Loss of vision* is due to the *degeneration of the ganglion cells of the retina at the macular area*. It results in degeneration of the papillomacular bundle; therefore, there is centrocecal field defect and so loss of central visual acuity.

Management
- Prognosis is good, if it is treated early.
- Complete abstention from ingestion of tobacco in any form and also alcohol.
- Intake of diet rich in protein, vitamins and minerals.
- Course of injection of hydroxycobalamine enhances the improvement in vision.

Quinine Amblyopia

With better methods of abortion and better drugs for malaria, the quinine amblyopia has vanished.

Clinical Features
- Quinine was used in large doses as an abortifacient.
- Quinine amblyopia may occur even with a small dose of 60 mg in susceptible persons.
- Most of the patients become completely blind with deafness and tinitis.
- Only few cases may show a tubular vision.
- Pupil is dilated and immobile.
- *Ophthalmoscopy:* Optic atrophy with pale white disk and attenuated vessels.

Ethambutol Amblyopia

Clinical Features
- Ethambutol is one of the important anti-tubercular drugs given systemically by oral route.
- It has been observed that ethambutol affects the optic nerve, if the daily dose exceeds more than 15 mg/kg body weight per day. Thus it is advisable to keep the intake of drug below 15 mg/kg or reduce the dose on occurrence of neuritis.
- It has been thought that drug affects the nerve directly while the other view is that it interferes with zinc metabolism.
- *Field defect*: Bitemporal hemianopia indicating that the site of lesion is chiasma.
  - *Color vision*—impaired color vision for red and green.

- *Ophthalmoscopy* shows a swollen disk with hyperemia and splinter hemorrhages.
- All the patients on ethambutol therapy must be subjected to a regular check-up for visual fields, visual acuity, and color vision test and fundus examination.
- Diet rich in proteins and vitamins is necessary. Injection of hydroxycobalamine is very helpful.

Chloroquine Amblyopia

Clinical Features

- Chloroquine is an antimalarial drug also used in treatment of lupus erythematosus and arthritis.
- Its intake for a long period may give rise to keratopathy, myopathy, or retinopathy.
- *Ophthalmoscopy* shows pigmentary degeneration of retina which may result in loss of vision. Even mild pigmentary disturbance at macula must arouse suspicion and the drug should be withdrawn.

Oral Contraceptive Amblyopia

Clinical Features

- Oral contraceptives are usually a combination of progestogens and estrogens.
- Play an important part in production of *vascular occlusion.*
- Females with hypertension, migraine and other vascular syndromes are more susceptible for vascular occlusion.
- Its use may cause infarction of optic nerve resulting in loss of vision.

Management

- Only management is to prescribe the oral contraceptives after exclusion of any vascular disease in the patient.
- Withdraw the drug soon on observation of symptoms.

TUMORS

Glioma of the Optic Nerve (Fig. 20.4)

Patient presents with early visual loss associated with gradual, painless and unilateral axial proptosis.

Diagnosis—glioma of optic nerve.

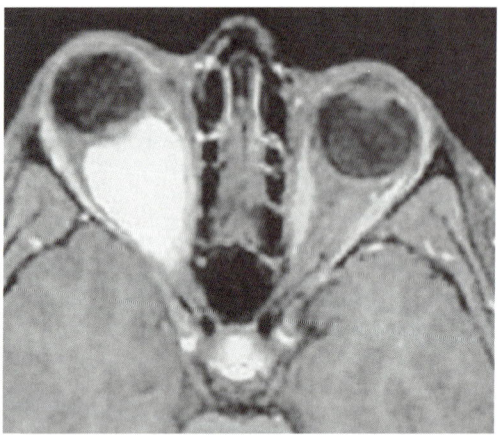

Fig. 20.4: Optic nerve glioma

Clinical Features

- Glioma is a primary ectodermal tumor of the optic nerve.
- Glial tumors are derived from the astrocytes and oligodendroglial cells of the optic nerve and can manifest either as solitary manifestation or part of neurofibromatosis.
- Glioma is a non-neoplastic and self-limiting tumor of the optic nerve with good prognosis for the life.
- Glioma is common in children manifesting before first decade of life.

Investigation

CT scan and ultrasonography show fusiform growth in relation to optic nerve and enlargement of the optic nerve.

Management

Lateral orbitotomy for removal of the glioma by preserving the eyeball is the ideal choice of surgery.

Meningioma of the Optic Nerve

Clinical Features

- Meningioma is a primary mesodermal tumor of the optic nerve sheath. These arise from the cap cells of arachnoid around the optic nerve in the orbit.
- Meningioma usually affects women in their middle age.

- Meningioma presents with early visual loss and proptosis follows later. There is restriction of ocular movements particularly in the upward direction.
- *Ophthalmoscopy* may show papilledema or optic atrophy of disk.
- *Management:* Lateral orbitotomy.

CONGENITAL ANOMALIES

Drusen

Clinical Features

- Drusen is deposits of a hyline-like calcific material within the optic disk.
- Presence of drusen may give a false appearance of papilledema. Except the full physiological cup, all the fundus findings are against papilledema.
- Presence of venous pulsation further helps to diagnose a drusen.
- Ophthalmoscopy shows drusens as waxy pearl-like irregular bodies on the surface of the optic disk. Usually, the first impression is of swollen disk.
- Fluorescein angiography shall be helpful in differentiating it from papilledema. In papilledema, there is early leakage of the dye.

Optic Disk Pits

Ophthalmoscopic Features

- Optic disk pits appear as oval or round pits on the disk.
- Optic disk pits appear darker than the surrounding disk tissue so can be easily made out with little attention to look for these.
- Optic disk pits are usually located in the inferotemporal quadrant of the disk.
- About 50% of the eyes with optic disk pits develop edema of the macula therefore, they can mimic central serous retinopathy. Photocoagulation is useful.

21

Maladies of Visual Pathways

■ I ■ I ■ I ■ I ■ I ■ I ■ I ■ I ■ I ■ I ■ I ■ I ■ I ■ I ■ I ■ I ■ I ■ I ■ I ■ I ■

Visual Pathway

Anatomy of visual pathway

Visual Field Charting

- Visual field
- Confrontation test
- Perimetry
- Manual perimetry for peripheral visual field charting
- Automated perimetry for peripheral visual field charting
- Tangent screen for central field charting

Visual Field Defects due to Visual Pathway

- Hemianopia
  Homonymous hemianopia
  Bitemporal hemianopia
  Binasal hemianopia
  Altitudinal defect
  Congruous defect
  Incongruous defect
  Sparing of macula
  Concentric contraction
  Local contraction
  Sector defect
  Quadrant defect
- Scotoma—positive, negative, relative
- Blind spot

Presenting Visual Symptom due to Lesion in Visual Pathways

- Amblyopia
- Amaurosis fugax
- Scintillating scotoma
- Night blindness (nyctalopia)
- Erythropsia (red vision)

- Cyanopsia (blue vision)
- Visual hallucinations
- Color blindness (achromatopsia)
- Word blindness
- Non-physiological visual loss

Presenting Visual Symptoms due to Lesions in Eye

- Unilateral sudden loss of vision
- Bilateral sudden loss of vision
- Bilateral transient loss of vision
- Binocular diplopia
- Uniocular diplopia
- Polyopia
- Halos
- Photopsia (flashes of light)
- Floating black spots before the eyes (vitreous floaters)
- Seeing one black spot in field of vision
- Second sight of aged
- Micropsia, macropsia and metamorphopsia
- Glare in the evening
- Day blindness

VISUAL PATHWAY (Fig. 21.1)

Anatomy of Visual Pathway

Visual pathway originates from retina consists of optic nerve, optic chiasma, optic tracts, lateral geniculate bodies, optic radiations and the visual cortex.

Visual pathway originates from nerve fiber layer of retina that consists of the axons originating from the ganglion cells. It also

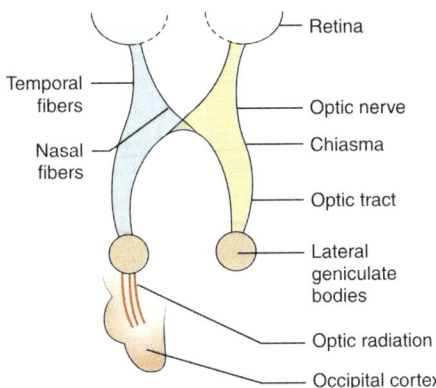

Fig. 21.1: Visual pathway

contains the afferent fibers of the pupillary light reflex.

Each optic nerve is the backward extension of the nerve fiber layer of retina. Each optic nerve extends from the optic disk to optic chiasma, where two optic nerves meet.

Optic chiasma is a flat structure 12 mm horizontally and 8 mm anteroposteriorly. It rests over the tuberculum and diaphragm sellae. Fibers originating from the nasal halves of the retina decussate at the chiasma.

Optic tracts extend outwards and backwards from the posterolateral aspect of the optic chiasma. Each optic tract consists of fibers from the temporal half of the retina of the same eye and nasal half of the opposite eye. Optic tracts terminate in lateral geniculate body of the same side.

Lateral geniculate body neurons receives the fibers of second-order neurons relayed via optic tracts.

Optic radiations extend backward from the lateral geniculate bodies to visual cortex and consist of the axons of third-order neurons of the visual pathway.

Visual cortex is located on the medial aspect of the occipital lobe, above and below the calcarine fissure and receives the fibers of the optic radiations.

THE PATHWAY

- *Fibers from the temporal half of the retina* enter the temporal part of the optic nerve,

chiasma and pass into the optic tract of the same side to terminate into the lateral geniculate body.

- *Fibers from the nasal half of the retina* enter the nasal part of optic nerve, the chiasma, and pass into the optic tract of the opposite side to terminate into the lateral geniculate body.

- *Fibers from the lateral geniculate body* enter optic radiation to end in the corresponding occipital lobes.

- *In the occipital lobes,* the part above the calcarine fissure represents the upper corresponding quadrants of both the retinas and the part below the calcarine fissure represents the lower corresponding quadrants of both the retinas.

- *Posterior part of the occipital lobe represents the macula.* Thus:

1. *Lesion of one occipital lobe or optic tract* causes blindness of the temporal half of the retina on the same side and of the nasal half of the retina on the opposite side. Projecting this outwards causes loss of vision in opposite half of binocular field—a condition called *hemianopia.*

2. *Lesion of upper occipital lobe* causes blindness of upper half of the retina on the same and opposite side. Projecting this outwards causes loss of vision in the lower half of the binocular field. It may be quadrantanopia to begin with the upper temporal quadrant of one eye and nasal quadrant of other eye or vice versa. Then it progresses in the clock or anticlockwise direction depending on the areas of cortex involved becoming *hemianopia and ultimately progresses to involve the whole field.*

VISUAL FIELD CHARTING

Visual Field

Visual field is that area of one's surrounding which is visible at one time. Visual field is limited by facial contour. Any lesion in the visual pathway produces a defect in the visual field. The defect depends on the extent of the fibers involved. There are many methods of charting the visual fields. It is essential that the visual fields are charted again on the same appliance by the same technician. The visual field charting gives information about the progress of the lesion. The visual field record the functional capacity of the visual pathway.

Confrontation Test

This method is simple and rapid to find out any gross defects in the visual field. Eye surgeon tests the visual field of the patient against his own field which is considered normal. If any defect is observed by this method, the visual field must be recorded by perimetry. This method can be used as a routine screening method for visual field.

Technique

The eye surgeon and the patient sit on a stool facing each other with the eyes at the same level adjusting the height of the stools.

Patient covers his right eye and the surgeon covers his left eye lightly with the help of their palms so that the patient is looking with his left eye in the surgeon's right eye and is asked not to deflect his eyes away from the surgeon's eye while the test is in progress.

Now the surgeon brings in stretched index finger of his right hand from the periphery keeping his hand in plane halfway between the patient and himself. Soon the surgeon observes the incoming finger himself and the patient ought to see it also. This movement is repeated in various parts of visual field, i.e. upward, downward, right and left and other meridians also covering about eight meridians.

Repeat the process with the other eye by changing hands to cover the eyes.

Perimetry

Visual field charting is purely subjective. It is essential to explain to the patient to maintain fixation at the central test object. The 5 mm white object used at the distance of 33 cm (5/330) gives the full normal peripheral field.

Extent of the normal peripheral visual field with a 5 mm white test object extends upward 50°, outward more than 90°, downward 70° and inward 60°.

Visual field varies with change in the illumination, size of the test object and the color. The field for the blue and yellow test object is roughly 10° less and that for red and green 20° less than that for the white object.

If two visual field charts of two eyes are superimposed, then there is a large central area which is common to both the eyes and this common area is the *binocular visual field*.

Size of the test object and its distance from the patient's eye are recorded by a convention similar to the mode of recording visual acuity, e.g. 5/330 both measurements in millimeters. Mention the color of the test object also.

To compare the visual field for the follow-up, use same test object and color and preferably same technician.

Equipment

Perimeter, tangent screen and test objects.

Technique

To obtain proper response and cooperation from the patients it is essential to explain— what you are going to do and what you expect from him for charting peripheral and central visual fields.

Manual Perimetry for Peripheral Visual Field Charting

The patient is seated with his chin, resting over the chin rest and adjusted to make him comfortable. The eye under examination should be in line with the fixation spot situated at the center of the arc around which the arc revolves. The other eye remains occluded. A white test object of 5 mm in size is brought in from the side at 15° intervals and the patient gives a signal by tapping the table, when he sees the test object. The readings are recorded by perforation with a sharp point incorporated in all perimeters on a chart at the back of the perimeter. Both eyes are tested in this way.

Automated Perimetry for Peripheral Field Charting

Automated perimeters (Fig. 21.2) are computer based and perform visual field test by static method. The automated perimeters automatically tests— *suprathreshold and threshold stimuli and quantify depth of field defect.*

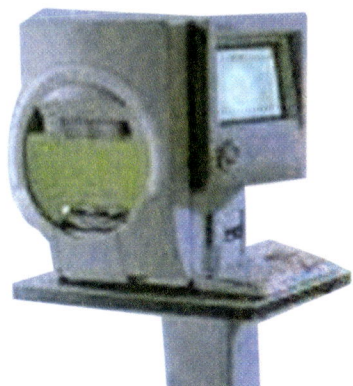

Fig. 21.2: Automated perimeter

Tangent Screen for Central Field Charting

Tangent screen of one meter is used. The patient is seated one meter from the screen comfortably fixing the eye to be examined and adjusting the chair so that the eye under examination is in line with the fixation spot in the center of screen and the other eye being covered. A white test object of 5 mm is brought in from the side at 15° intervals by a black thin test rod on which the test object is attached. The patient gives a signal on seeing the test object. The responses are carefully charted on the chart by the surgeon or he can put pins with black heads at the point on the screen where the patient gives a signal and later chart it out in one sitting.

Blind spot is charted out with this tangent screen (Fig. 21.3).

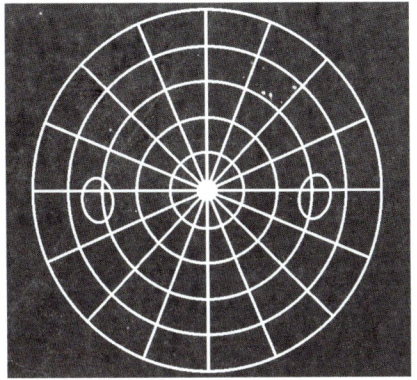

Fig. 21.3: Tangent screen

VISUAL FIELD DEFECTS DUE TO VISUAL PATHWAY

Hemianopia

Hemianopia is a condition in which there is loss of half visual field in both the eyes. Hemianopia of any kind is quickly discovered by the patient.

Patient with left hemianopia presents with difficulty in near work. Patient with bitemporal hemianopia presents with history of hitting the pedestrians unknowingly as he tends to over ride the pedestrian pathway and gets scolded.

Patient with binasal hemianopia is unable to move about as his central field is lost.

Field charting shows hemianopic field defect (Fig. 21.4).

Diagnosis— hemianopia.

Homonymous Hemianopia

In homonymous hemianopia, either right or left half of binocular visual field is lost.

Hemianopia occurs due to any lesion in the visual pathway from chiasma to the occipital lobe.

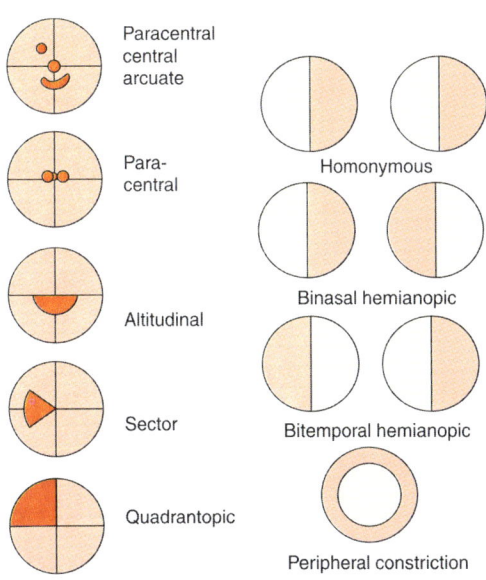

Fig. 21.4: Types of field defects

In many cases of hemianopia, the fixation area in each field escapes, particularly, if the lesion is near the occipital cortex.

- Right homonymous hemianopia—the right half of temporal field and left half of nasal field are lost.
- Left homonymous hemianopia—the left half of temporal field and right half of nasal field are lost.

Common causes

- Injury by fall on the back of the head
- Cerebral tumors
- Diseases of blood vessels.

Bitemporal Hemianopia

In bitemporal hemianopia, the temporal half of the binocular field of vision in each eye is lost.

A patient with bitemporal hemianopia is likely to over-ride the pedestrian pathway.

Common causes

- Pituitary tumors, i.e. adenoma and cranio-pharyngioma
- Suprasellar meningioma
- Chiasmal archnoiditis
- Glioma of third ventricle
- Dermoid tumors
- Injury to chiasma in fractured base of skull.

Binasal Hemianopia

In binasal hemianopia, it is the nasal half of the binocular field of vision in each eye is lost.

Patient with binasal hemianopia is unable to move about as his central field is lost.

Common causes

- Distention of the third ventricle
- Atheroma of the carotids or posterior communicating arteries.

Altitudinal Defect

It is a field defect that involves either the upper or the lower half of the visual field in one or both the eyes. The line of separation is horizontal meridian.

Congruous Defect

The field defect is said to be congruous, if it is fairly similar in both the eyes.

Incongruous Defect

The field defect is said to be incongruous, if there is marked difference in the field defects of both the eyes.

Sparing of Macula

The sparing or escape of macula in vascular lesions of occipital cortex is attributed to the fact that the occipital pole is supplied by two vessels—*the posterior and middle cerebral arteries.*

Concentric Contraction

The field gradually gets narrower.

Local Contraction

The field is narrow in a particular sector.

Sector Defect

It is bounded by two radii.

Quadrant Defect

It is bounded by a horizontal and vertical line.

Scotoma

It can be positive, negative and relative. Scotoma is an area of decreased visual sensitivity surrounded by an area of normal sensitivity.

Positive Scotoma

When patient can perceive a black spot in his field of vision, then this scotoma is said to be *positive scotoma*. This is presenting symptom in a case of central choroiditis and central serous maculopathy.

Negative Scotoma

In a case of choroiditis in later stages, the affected area which was giving a sensation of a positive scotoma becomes healed with fibrosis and does not give any sensation thus it becomes a *negative scotoma*. This area of negative scotoma is like blind spot due to optic disk with no sensation.

Relative Scotoma

Sometimes a scotoma can be charted by using a small test object. Scotoma which is not charted with a 5 mm object but can be charted with a small object of 1 or 3 mm is said to be *relative scotoma*. Scotoma charted with color test object and not with white is also said to be *relative scotoma for color*, e.g. tobacco amblyopia.

Blind Spot

Mariotte's physiological blind spot is a non-seeing area in the field of vision corresponding to the position and extent of the optic nerve head which has no elements for perception, i.e. rods and cones are absent.

On plotting the blind spot; it is a vertical oval about 7.5° by 5.5°. Its center is about 15.5° temporal to the fixation point and about 1.5° below the horizontal meridian.

Its size is affected by the distance, refractive error, and illumination.

Clinically, it increases in following conditions:
- Papilledema—due to edema around disk.
- Glaucoma—due to halo around disk.
- High myopia—due to atrophy of choroid.
- Senility—due to senile halo around disk.
- Occlusion of superior or inferior central retinal vein.
- Juxtapapillary choroiditis.
- Opaque nerve fibers.
- Coloboma of optic disk.

Blind spot larger than 7.5° by 9.5° with test object of 5/1000 is pathognomonic in absence of any visible peripapillary changes. It is useful in papilledema, glaucoma, and papillitis.

PRESENTING VISUAL SYMPTOM DUE TO LESION IN VISUAL PATHWAYS

Patient presents with typical visual symptom which is pathognomonic and diagnostic for certain lesions in the visual pathway.

Visual symptoms which have their origin due to lesion in visual pathway have been considered here.

Presenting visual symptoms compel the patient to seek opinion of an ophthalmologist. It helps both the patient and the eye physician to arrive at diagnosis and early treatment.

Amblyopia

Partial loss of visual acuity is known as amblyopia.

Unilateral Amblyopia

- Congenital
- Suppression of retinal image (amblyopia ex anopsia)
- High refractive errors
- Retrobulbar optic neuritis.

Bilateral Amblyopia

- Toxic optic neuropathy—the commonest being tobacco amblyopia.
- Hysterical amblyopia can be unilateral but it is more commonly bilateral. Some of these patients may show other symptoms such as blepharospasm, frequent blinking and lacrimation. Treat the psychogenic cause, but take care to eliminate organic factor as well.

Amaurosis Fugax

There is sudden but temporary loss of vision in one eye usually as a result of *emboli in the central retinal artery.*

The attack of this loss of vision lasts for few minutes. Patient feels that a curtain is falling from above downwards and rising from below upwards. On fundus examination, there are signs of retinal ischemia in form of edema and small hemorrhages.

If there are repeated attacks, then the patient should be subjected to a thorough cardiovascular check-up.

Other Causes

- Migraine
- Papilledema
- Giant cell arteritis
- Eclampsia
- Anemia
- Hysterical.

Scintillating Scotoma

Scintillating scotoma is a typical type of scotoma in which there is a positive scotoma in the field of vision *obscuring the sight with shimmering character.*

It is diagnostic for migraine.

- Patient feels well before the attack of migraine.
- With the onset of migraine, the scotoma appears and clouds one-half of the field of vision that gradually extends to cover the entire field.
- It may affect one eye or both the eyes.
- In some cases, the fields affected are homonymous hemianopic type.
- *Scintillating scotoma*: In the dark-clouded field-bright spots and rays of various colors are seen.
- Vision gradually clears in about 15 minutes followed by severe headache which is usually on the side of head opposite to the hemianopic field.
- Headache is often associated with nausea and vomiting.
- *Management*: Rest and sleep in a comfortable, cool and noiseless room with ergotamine tartrate, analgesic, and sedative help to alleviate the headache.

Night Blindness (Nyctalopia)

Person with night blindness is confined to his home after sunset.

- *Deficiency of vitamin A and protein*: It affects malnourished children. Oral concentrated vitamin A— three lac units followed by a good diet rich in protein cure the night blindness. Provide vitamin A supplement with proteins for long time.
- *Retinitis pigmentosa*: Night blindness is the presenting symptom. It is due to dystrophy of rods.
- Congenital night blindness
- Choroideremia
- Gyrate atrophy
- Oguchi's disease
- High myopia with retinal degeneration
- Laurence-Moon-Biedl syndrome.

Erythropsia (Red Vision)

Person with red vision is alarmed.

Erythropsia is a condition in which the objects look red in color though the visual acuity remains unaffected and there is no damage to vision in anyway.

- *Aphakia*: Erythropsia occurs after cataract extraction in an aphakic eye due to exposure to the bright light. Aphakic person should be warned about it and advise him to protect his eye from bright light.
- *Mountaineer*: Red vision is also seen by mountaineer who does not protect his eyes from glare of snow.
- *Optic neuritis*: Red vision also occurs in the patients who are in the resolution period of optic neuritis.
- *Vitreous hemorrhage* may give rise to red vision.
- *Bright light*: In a normal person, if a strong light enters his eyes through the sclera from open window on left side or while reading under a table lamp then the black print of the book may appear as red print.

Cyanopsia (Blue Vision)

Aphakia: Some of the aphakic patients may complain of seeing everything blue in color rather than red vision.

Diabetic optic atrophy: Patient with diabetic optic atrophy may complain of blue vision.

Visual Hallucinations

- Visual hallucinations of unformed images such as moving lights, circles, flashes and flickering lights are diagnostic for the *occipital lobe tumor.*
- Visual hallucinations of formed images such as people, animals, objects, etc. are diagnostic for *temporal lobe tumor.*

Color Blindness (Achromatopsia)

Acquired Color Blindness

- *Retina and choroid atrophy:* Acquired color blindness for blue color is seen in the diseases of retina and choroid in which *blue end of spectrum* is affected.
- *Nuclear sclerosis of lens:* It is also seen in cases with nuclear sclerosis of lens in which the amber pigment absorbs the blue rays. It affects the pictures of artist, therefore, labeled as *blue blindness.*

Congenital Color Blindness

Total congenital color blindness is rare and is probably caused by a central defect. It is usually associated with nystagmus and a central scotoma. In this condition, all the colors appear grey of different brightness.

Partial color blindness is discovered with especial color vision test. Person with partial color blindness learns to compensate for their deficiency in color vision by paying attention to shade and texture using his experience of day-to-day life.

It is an inherited condition and is being transmitted through the females who are unaffected.

Most cases of partial color blindness are deficient in *red and green colors.* This defect is a source of great danger in certain occupations like engine driver, sailor and any profession where it is important to differentiate colors.

Word Blindness (Dyslexia)

Word blindness is a congenital anomaly due to defects in association areas of brain. It runs in families. Due to poor performance in reading and writing, the child is brought to an ophthalmologist for check-up. The eyes are normal with normal visual acuity and normal fundus yet the child fails to recognize written or printed words. He is good in mathematics, numerical and music. Individual attention to the child helps him to overcome this defect gradually.

Non-physiological Visual Loss

- *Malingering:* Deliberate 'blind' behavior or feigning of blindness with a purpose to gain or avoid.
- *Hysteria:* Subconscious expression of signs and symptoms of defective vision without any specific purpose or aim.

It is easy to diagnose and treat a malingerer as he is likely to make one false move in his act of feigning blindness. Ophthalmic surgeon needs patience and must show trust to the patient for his act.

Hysterical patient needs psychiatric treatment for long time. Quite often persons of all the ages pretend to be blind by one or both the eyes to gain some favor from parents, friends or society. Most of these persons are either females or school-going children. Most of the females are young either newly married or married but have not conceived even after few years of marriage.

Most of the children pretend to be blind either few weeks before the examination or have been punished by parents or school teacher for not doing well in day-to-day home work.

If the patient pretends to be blind by both the eyes, then the patient is accompanied by two to four family members to help him or her to move about.

Ophthalmologist can judge the pretence about being blind by the body language as the patient enters the clinic. History of sudden loss of vision from both the eyes further confirms the diagnosis. In such a case, make the patient sit comfortably and allow one female or elderly member in the chamber to attend to the patient asking other members to wait outside in the waiting hall.

Examine the patient with torch and ask the patient to look towards you or in your eyes. *One false move by the patient of looking in your eyes further confirms the diagnosis.*

Now the patient knows that you have come to know about his/her pretence of being blind. From this moment onwards, it is the turn of the ophthalmologist to pretend that the patient is blind, only then you shall be able to cure the patient in few days. Start the treatment by instillation of antibiotic drops with the positive suggestion to the patient that the vision shall improve to finger counting to 5 feet within 15 minutes. Examine after 15 minutes showing the fingers and the patient counts the fingers.

Thereafter, prescribe supportive treatment and advise the patient to report daily with suggestion that the vision will improve daily line by line on the Snellen's chart.

In a week's time, the patient is cured. In this whole process, ophthalmologists have given his trust to the patient to keep her/his pretence of being blind to the self.

Meanwhile find out the problem from the patient and family members and suggest a solution.

School-going child pretends to be blind by one eye or reduced vision in both the eyes. It is difficult to handle such case. Ask for history of excessive homework, punishment from teacher, scolding from parents, jealousy from the brother or sister, or any factor which have disturbed the child help you to understand and treat.

Make the child sit comfortably and ask certain vague questions about school, games, hobby, films, television, etc. to divert his/her attention from his/her pretence of being blind or having a dim vision. In between, ask him/her to look at you. *One false move of looking at you in your eyes shall confirm that the child is pretending to be blind.*

In such case, put a trial frame and place minus 0.25 lens in front of both the eye with suggestion that he/she will be able to see the top line of Snellen's chart. Most of the children comply with this suggestion. You have gained his/her trust that you shall play with him/her to come out of it. Simple treatment with vitamins and eyedrops and if necessary lowest minus glasses or sun glasses should be prescribed to him/her. The child is alright in a week's time.

The most important aspect of diagnosing and treating a malingerer is to gain his/her trust and keep trust about his/her pretence of being blind. Bring the patient out of his/her game of feigning blindness very slowly in a week or two weeks time.

The following test may be used for one eye blind malingerer.

Test Devised for Malingering

1. Low concave lens of 0.25 D is placed before the blind eye and a high convex lens of 10.0 D before the normal eye. If the patient is able to read to Snellen's chart, then his/her malingering is confirmed.
2. Prism is placed base downward before the normal eye and ask the patient to look at the spot light on testing drum. If he/she can see two lights, then his/her malingering is confirmed.
3. Place a red glass before the normal eye and ask the patient to read the Snellen's color letters in red and green. If the patient can read out all the letters in red and green then his/her malingering is confirmed. Though all the above tests for one eye malingerer are useful and can be employed as required. With better knowledge of the patient about the lens and the Snellen's chart, he/she is likely to dodge the examiner.

The most convenient and easy way is to gain his/her confidence. *One false move from a malingerer to peep in your eyes is enough to confirm his being a malingerer.* Then, the only treatment left is to keep his trust and treat by giving positive suggestions of improvement everyday with your treatment.

In every case of malingering, it is very essential to exclude any disease which may be responsible for loss of vision before diagnosing him/her as a malingerer.

PRESENTING VISUAL SYMPTOM DUE TO LESIONS IN EYE

Visual symptoms which have their origin due to ocular lesion have been considered here.

Presenting visual symptom compels the patient to seek opinion of an ophthalmologist. It helps both the patient and the eye physician to arrive at diagnosis and early treatment.

Patient presents with typical visual symptom which is pathognomonic and diagnostic for certain maladies of the eye.

Unilateral Sudden Loss of Vision

1. Central retinal artery occlusion
2. Central retinal vein occlusion
3. Optic neuritis
4. Giant cell arteritis
5. Intraocular hemorrhage
6. Retinal detachment.

Bilateral Sudden Loss of Vision

1. Bilateral optic neuritis
2. Quinine amblyopia
3. Methyl alcohol amblyopia
4. Sun eclipse blindness.

Bilateral Transient Loss of Vision

Transient loss of vision is alarming to the patient. Its repeated attacks are indicative of gross cardiovascular changes.

It is observed in the following conditions:
1. Hypotension which may occur in
   - Fatigue
   - Hunger
   - Vitamin deficiency
   - Hormonal disorder
   - Arteriosclerosis
2. Fainting with vasomotor collapse
3. Heart failure
4. In some cases, even stooping and straining can cause this.

Binocular Diplopia

Diplopia is an annoying symptoms and more so if it is a binocular diplopia. It occurs in the following conditions:
1. Space occupying lesions of the orbit.
2. Fracture of the orbital floor.
3. Paresis of extraocular muscle due to nerve lesion or trauma.
4. Concomitant squint without suppression
5. Deficiency of convergence.

Case with binocular diplopia needs a thorough investigation to arrive at a diagnosis and to treat the case properly.

Uniocular Diplopia

Uniocular diplopia occurs in the following conditions:
1. Dislocation or subluxation of the lens
2. Double pupil
3. Corneal irregularity
4. Air bubble in anterior chamber
5. Projectional uniocular diplopia.

Polyopia

Polyopia is a condition in which more than two images of the object are seen by the patient. Polyopia is a presenting symptom of *incipient stage of cortical (soft) cataract*. It occurs due to development of wedge-shaped opacities in the cortex of the lens, the apex towards the center and base towards the periphery. This induces a sectorial alteration in the refractive index of the lens which causes splitting of the image resulting in polyopia.

Halos

Halo is a subjective symptom in which the patient complains of seeing colored rings around the light, therefore, it is usually observed after sunset. The colors of the ring are distributed as in the spectrum with red color the outermost and blue color the innermost. The halos can be demonstrated to the patient by asking him/her to see a bright light through a thin layer of lycopodium powder enclosed between two glass plates.

Halos are seen in the following conditions:
- *Latent, primary and subacute primary angle closure glaucoma:* Halos are due to accumulation of the fluid in the corneal epithelium thereby altering the refractive index of the corneal lamellae.
- *Incipient stage of cortical cataract:* Halos occur due to sectorial alteration in the refractive index of the lens.

These two conditions can be differentiated clinically without any doubt. Yet with Fincham's test in which a slit is passed in front of the eye then halos are seen broken in a case of cataract and continuous in a case of glaucoma.

Photopsia (Flashes of Light)

Photopsia is a condition in which the patient is aware of a flash light in form of an arc in his/her field of vision. As it is a new phenomenon, the patient is quite disturbed and presents himself/herself with this complaint.

Photopsia can appear as a flash of light, a glow, a streak of light, or light in any form in his/her field of vision usually observed in dark and on movement of the eyes. It is of a very short duration never more than a fraction of a second.

This phenomenon is due to cerebral awareness of vitreous stimulating the retina.

It is seen in the following conditions:
- Posterior vitreous detachment
- Prior to retinal detachment

- Retinitis
- Oculodigital phenomenon.

Any patient presenting with this symptom of photopsia must be thoroughly examined by indirect ophthalmoscopy and three mirror contact lens to look for *posterior vitreous detachment* which is the most common and important cause for photopsia.

Floating Black Spots before Eyes
(Vitreous Floaters)

Seeing numerous black spots floating before the eyes is a common phenomenon in aged. It is due to liquefaction of the vitreous with age. The vitreous floaters appear as dark black spots to the patient, as the opacities in the vitreous cast a shadow on the retina which is projected outside as black spots.

Sudden appearance of vitreous floaters must arouse suspicion for posterior vitreous detachment.

Thorough examination must be done. If there is no pathology, then assure the patient that it is a normal phenomenon in aged.

Floating black spots are seen:
- Liquefaction of vitreous
- Posterior vitreous detachment
- High myopia with vitreous degeneration
- Cyclitis
- Vitreous hemorrhage

Floaters can be diagnosed by direct ophthalmoscopy and slit-lamp.

Seeing One Black Spot in Field of Vision

Black spot seen by the patient occupying a constant position in his/her field of vision is annoying. Wherever he/she looks, the black spot is there.

Common Causes

1. Early nuclear cataract
2. Positive scotoma due to edema at the macula seen in:
   - Central serous retinopathy
   - Choroiditis
   - Retinitis
   - Injury.

Second Sight of Aged

Some of the patients who had been using near glasses for years start feeling that their near vision has improved considerably and are able to read the prints which were not clear without glasses. This regain of near sight is referred as *second sight of the aged*.

In reality, this regain of near sight is due to sclerosis of the lens. In sclerosis of the lens, there is an increase in the refractive index thereby the refraction tends to become myopic. Because of this change in the refractive state of the eye, the patient is able to read without glasses.

Micropsia, Macropsia and Metamorphopsia

Micropsia is condition in which the patient complains that the objects appear smaller than normal.

Macropsia is a condition in which the patient complains that the objects appear larger than normal.

Metamorphopsia is a condition in which the patient complains that the linear objects appear wavy.

Micropsia and macropsia are due to crowding or separation of the cones at the macula due to macular pathology. Metamorphopsia, the wavy appearance, is due to change in the contour of the retina at the macula due to edema.

These symptoms are seen in the following conditions:
- Central serous retinopathy
- Choroiditis
- Retinitis
- Macular edema due to any cause
- Injury causing edema at the macula

Glare in Evening

Quite often, the patient comes with a complaint that he/she is not able to stand to the glare of the headlights of vehicle.

It can occur in the following conditions:
- Early cataract
- Refractive error

- Nebular corneal scar
- Heterophoria
- Glaucoma.

Patient needs thorough eye check-up.

Day Blindness

Some patients may have a complaint that they are not able to see things clearly in the day or bright light. The vision improves at sunset or in shade. Following conditions may give rise to this symptom:

1. Central lens opacity. In this condition, the pupil contracts on exposure to bright light, thereby the vision is reduced. Use of goggles shall help the patient.
2. Central scotoma
3. Congenital.

22

Maladies of Pupillary Pathways

Pupillary Pathways

- Afferent pathway
- Efferent pathway

Pupillary Reflexes

- Near reflex—accommodation and convergence reflex
- Sensory reflex
- Pupillary light reflexes—direct, consensual and ill-sustained reflex

Action of Drugs on Intraocular Pupillary and Ciliary Muscles

- Anticholinergic drugs
- Atropine
- Homatropine
- Cyclopentolate hydrochloride
- Tropicamide

Sympathomimetic Mydriatic Drugs

Phenylephrine

Abnormal Pupillary Reactions

- Argyll Robertson pupil
- Adie's tonic pupil

PUPIL

Normally, there is only one pupil and it is placed in the center of the iris. It is circular in shape. Its size varies from 3 to 4 mm depending on the illumination. It appears geryish black. Its color reflex changes depending upon the condition of the structures located behind it. White reflex from pupil (leucocoria) is seen in cases with retinoblastoma. Pupil is like a window through that we are able to visualize this infinite world and its beauty.

PUPILLARY PATHWAYS

Afferent Pathway (Fig. 22.1)

The light reflex is initiated from the rods and cones throughout the retina.

- Afferent fibers run up along the optic nerve, partially decussate in the chiasma, and enter the optic tract in exactly the same manner as the visual fibers.
- Near the upper end of the optic tract, the fibers leave the tract and enter the pretectal region to end in the pretectal nucleus.
- New fibers from pretectal nucleus after partial decussation in midbrain travel to end in the Edinger-Westphal nucleus on each side.

Note: The afferent fibers suffer a double decussation, one at chiasma and another in midbrain which explains the mechanism of direct and consensual reaction of pupil to the light reflex.

Efferent Pathway

Fibers start from the Edinger-Westphal nucleus and pass out of the midbrain and run into the main trunk of the third nerve up to orbit.

- In the orbit, the fibers pass into the branch which supplies the inferior oblique muscle, leaving it by the short root of the ciliary ganglion.

- From the ciliary ganglion, the fibers pass as short ciliary nerves to the eye, piercing the eye along with the short ciliary arteries to ciliary body and iris.

The dilator papillae muscle is supplied by the adrenergic fibers of cervical sympathetic nerve.

- Fibers from cervical sympathetic run-up in superior cervical ganglion to carotid plexus into skull.
- Then the fibers pass into the first division of the fifth nerve following the nasal branch which they leave to enter long ciliary nerves.
- Long ciliary nerves enter the eye on each side of the optic nerve accompanying long ciliary arteries, run between choroid and sclera to enter the ciliary body and thus reach the iris.

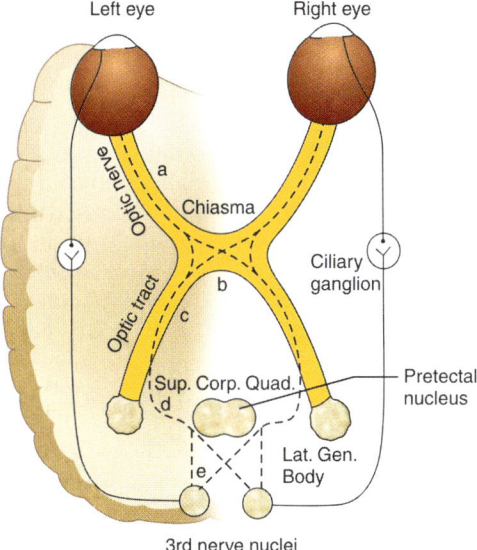

Fig. 22.1: Pathway of afferent fibers showing double decussation at chiasma and pretectal region

PUPILLARY REFLEXES

Near Reflex

Near reflex is initiated by the fibers from the medial rectus muscle which contract on convergence. The fibers from the muscle run probably by the third nerve to presumptive convergence center in tectal or pretectal region. From here, the pathway is relayed to Edinger-Westphal nucleus and then along the third nerve to the sphincter muscle of the iris, so that the pupil constricts on convergence. At the same time, the accommodation reinforces the reflex by visual impulses relayed from cortex to Edinger-Westphal nucleus.

Accommodation and Convergence Reflex (Near Reflex)

Ask the patient to look straight at the distance. While observing the pupil—ask the patient to look at the finger placed about 6 inches from the eye. As the eye converges and accommodation comes to act, the pupil constricts.

Sensory Reflex

Sensory reflex is initiated by the stimulation of any sensory nerve to the extent of causing pain, or by emotional states, and excitement. The pathway is much more complex as the dilator and constrictor both play a part in production.

Pupillary Light Reflexes

Direct Light Reflex

Ask the patient to look straight. Throw the light by a pencil-torch on the pupil of one eye and then on the other eye and note the reaction of the pupil. In a normal person, the pupil constricts briskly.

The direct light reflex is absent in the optic atrophy and following use of mydriatics.

Consensual Light Reflex

Ask the patient to look straight. Throw the light by a pencil-torch on the pupil of one eye and observe the reaction in the opposite pupil and vice versa. In a normal person, the pupil of the observed eye constricts briskly. *Its absence indicates optic atrophy of the eye in which the light was thrown.*

Ill-sustained Pupil Reflex to Light

In a normal person, when the light is thrown on the pupil, the pupil constricts, oscillates few times then comes to rest and maintains the same position on keeping the light on the eye. In an ill-sustained pupil reflex, the pupil constricts briskly and oscillates for a long time adopting a gradually dilated position on keeping the light on the eye. It indicates defective conduction of the stimulus by optic nerve.

It is seen in cases of optic neuritis, papillitis, retrobulbar neuritis, and early acute cases of macular pathology.

Ill-sustained pupil is diagnostic for defective conduction and may be the only positive finding apart from blurred vision in retrobulbar neuritis.

Absence of direct and consensual light reflex in same eye is diagnostic for chronic open angle glaucoma. Ophthalmoscopy shows glaucomatous optic atrophy.

ACTION OF DRUGS ON INTRAOCULAR PUPILLARY AND CILIARY MUSCLES

Intraocular pupillary muscles: Sphincter and dilator pupillary muscles control the size of pupil.

Intraocular ciliary muscle controls zonular laxity that is the mechanism of accommodation by the act of increased curvature of lens to visualize near objects.

- Drugs which cause dilation of pupil are *mydriatics.*
- Drugs which cause constriction of pupil are *miotics.*
- Drugs which cause paralysis of the ciliary muscle are *cycloplegics.*
- *Mydriatics* paralyze the ciliary muscle thereby abolishing the accommodation to a greater or lesser degree.
- *Miotics* stimulate the ciliary muscle thereby producing partial or complete accommodation.

Anticholinergic Drugs

These drugs cause the dilation of the pupil by abolishing the action of acetylchoiline.

Atropine

- It is the strongest mydriatic and cycloplegic drug. One drop of 1% per cent eyedrops or ointment causes dilation of pupil in about 40 minutes and marked paralysis of accommodation in about 2 hours. The effect lasts for 3 to 7 days.
- There is no antidote.
- It is known to produce local allergic reaction.

- *It reduces ciliary spasm, increases blood flow, decreases hyperemia and permeability so reduces exudation. Therefore, it is most important drug for uveitis.*

Homatropine

- It is mild cycloplegic and mydriatic. One drop of 2% eyedrops take about 40 minutes to show the effect which lasts for about 48 hears.
- One drop of Eserine 0.5% solution helps to ward off the effect earlier.

Cyclopentolate Hydrochloride

- It is available in 0.5 and 1.0% solution.
- Its effect as mydriatic and cycloplegic is rapid, mild and temporary.

Tropicamide

One drop of 0.5%, 1% eyedrop is a short-acting cycloplegic and mydriatic.

SYMPATHOMIMETIC MYDRIATIC DRUGS

Phenylephrine

- One drop of 10% solution causes full dilation of pupil in about one hour.
- Its action lasts for 5 hours.
- It causes lowering of the intraocular pressure.

ABNORMAL PUPILLARY REACTIONS

Argyll Robertson Pupil

- Reaction to near reflex is present but light reflex is absent.
- Pupil is slightly small in size.
- Both pupils are affected and dilate poorly with mydriatics.
- Its lesion is usually neurosyphilis in the region of tectum.

Adie's Tonic Pupil

- Reaction to near reflex is slow and tonic but light reflex is absent.
- Affected pupil is larger in size.
- It is usually unilateral and affects young females.
- Associated with absent knee jerk.
- Adie's pupil constricts even with weak pilocarpine (0.125%) while normal pupil is not affected.

23

Maladies of Nystagmus

Characteristics of Nystagmus

- Amplitude of nystagmus
- Frequency of nystagmus
- Types and direction of nystagmus

Ocular Nystagmus

Physiologically induced nystagmus
- End-point or deviational nystagmus
- Optokinetic nystagmus
- Physiological vestibular nystagmus

Pathologically induced nystagmus
- Amaurotic nystagmus
- Amblyopic nystagmus
- Spasmus nutans
- Occupational Miner's nystagmus
- Latent nystagmus
- Nystagmoid ocular movements

Nystagmus is defined as regular and rhythmic to and fro involuntary oscillations of the eyes. It must be differentiated from nystagmoid and myoclonic movements of the eyes.

CHARACTERISTICS OF NYSTAGMUS

Nystagmus is characterized by the following:

Amplitude of Nystagmus

Amplitude of nystagmus is said to be:
- *Fine*— if excursion is below 5°.
- *Medium*— if excursion is between 5° and 15°.
- *Course*— if excursion is over 15°.

Frequency of Nystagmus

Frequency of nystagmus can be conveniently recorded by the number of barbs on the arrow indicating the direction as *slow, medium or fast*.

Frequency is the number of oscillations per minute which can be recorded on nystagmograph.

Type and Direction of Nystagmus

Pendular Nystagmus

Eye movements are of equal velocity in each direction.

It can be horizontal, vertical, oblique or rotatory.

Jerky Nystagmus

There is a biphasic rhythm wherein slow movement in one direction is followed by a rapid saccadic return to the original position.

The direction of the jerky nystagmus is defined by direction of the fast component.

It may be right, left, up, down or rotatory.

Grades of jerky nystagmus:
- *Grade I:* Jerky nystagmus is visible only in the direction of rapid phase.
- *Grade II:* Jerky nystagmus is visible in the direction of the rapid phase and in the primary position.
- *Grade III:* Jerky nystagmus is visible in all the positions of the eyes.

OCULAR NYSTAGMUS

Ocular nystagmus is due to the defect of the central vision which does not allow fixation. There is a defect in the eye which does not allow in acquiring or maintaining fixation.

Clinical Features

1. Physiologically Induced Nystagmus

End-point or Deviational Nystagmus

- End-point or devotional nystagmus is observed in 50 to 60% of normal subjects, when the eyes are maintained in extreme lateral gaze.

- In some cases, it is seen only after a latent period of about 30 seconds.

Optokinetic Nystagmus

- Optokinetic nystagmus results, when successive objects traverse the visual field.

- Eyes follow one towards the periphery in a slow saccadic motion until the successor objects appear into the central field where on the eyes move back to primary position in a rapid movement. It is a type of jerky nystagmus.

- Clinically, it can be observed by asking the patient to gaze at a rotating drum marked with vertical stripes (Fig. 23.1).

- There is response until the patient has enough vision to see the drum.

- It is abolished in complete blindness.

- Thus it is a good test for a malingering.

- *Example:* It is seen while looking at poles outside from moving train.

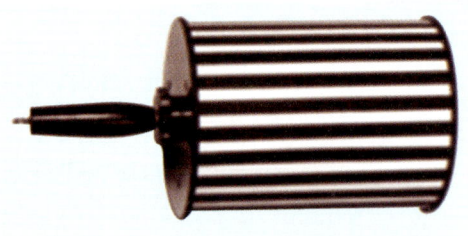

Fig. 23.1: Optokinetic drum

Physiological Vestibular Nystagmus

- It is a jerk type of nystagmus.

- It is induced by pouring cold or hot water into the ear. It is caused by altered input from the vestibular nuclei to the horizontal gaze centers. If cold water is poured into the right ear, the patient will develop a left jerk nystagmus (fast movement towards left side). Now if hot water is poured into the right ear, the patient will develop a right jerk nystagmus (fast movement towards the right side). Thus remember as— cold opposite side and warm same side.

2. Pathologically Induced Nystagmus

Amaurotic Nystagmus

Amaurotic nystagmus may occur in those who have been blind for a long time. If the infant is born blind and coordination has never developed then irregular and variable movements (searching movements, vermiform movements, or vagabond movements) are seen.

Amblyopic Nystagmus

Amblyopic nystagmus occurs due to the defect in central vision in both the eyes thereby the fixation never develops. The most common causes are albinism, achromatopsia and congenital ocular diseases of media or macula.

Spasmus Nutans

- Characterized by nystagmus, head nodding and torticollis. Head nodding and nystagmus may be present independently or together.

- Nystagmus is asymmetrical, pendular, fine and rapid.

- It is an acquired nystagmus affecting children from the age of 4 months to 1 year and resolves within a period of 4 years.

- It may be associated with squint.

- No association with any neurological problem.

Occupational Miner's Nystagmus

Miner's nystagmus is an example of occupational nystagmus. It is rapid and rotatory type of nystagmus. It is seen most commonly in coal mine workers. It occurs due to fixation problem in dim illumination.

Latent Nystagmus

Latent nystagmus can be elicited on covering up one eye. It is normally not present, when both eyes are open. It is a jerky nystagmus with rapid phase towards the uncovered eye.

Nystagmoid Ocular Movements

There are ocular movements that mimic ocular nystagmus. These are ocular flutter, opsoclonus, superior oblique myokymia and ocular bobbing. These are seen in cases of encephalitis, pontine lesions and dysfunction of brainstem.

Management

- In general treatment of nystagmus is unrewarding.
- One can only give goggles and correct the error of refraction.

24

Maladies of Squint

Ocular Investigative Evaluation

- Vision, refraction and ophthalmoscopy
- Ocular movements
- Hirschberg corneal reflex test
- Cover-uncover and alternate cover test
- Accommodation test
- Convergence test
- Prism bar vergence test
- Worth's four-light test
- Maddox rod test
- Maddox wing test
- Diplopia red-green goggle test
- Hess screen test
- After image slides
- Synoptophore

Classification of Squint

- Heterophoria—latent squint
- Heterotropia—manifest squint
- Comitant squint
- Convergent squint
- Divergent squint
- Incomitant squint
- Paralytic squint
- Restrictive squint

OCULAR INVESTIGATIVE EVALUATION

Investigative evaluation for squint is useful in an adult or an older child. These cannot be applied in a case of an infant. All the methods are not required in every case. Every case needs some investigations, while other case needs other investigations depending on the type of squint and its etiology.

Vision, Refraction and Ophthalmoscopy

These tests are mandatory in every case for evaluation. These tests may give some clue about etiological factors for squint.

Ocular Movements (Fig. 24.1)

- Test the ocular movements of each eye separately and then conjugate ocular movements.
- Test the ocular movements in the cardinal direction for each eye.
- In the lateral movement, note carefully whether the corneal margin has reached the outer canthi or not.
- Note for any nystagmoid jerks which may be normal.
- Table 24.1 depicts the different muscles in action during the change of direction of gaze of the right eye.

Hirschberg Corneal Reflex Test (Fig. 24.2)

Position of the corneal reflex gives an approximate estimation of the nature and degree of deviation of the eye.

Surgeon sitting in front of the patient throws the light on the patient's eyes and instructs him/her to look into the torch or spotlight. This will show corneal reflex.

Interpretation

Position of the corneal reflex is noted:
- If the corneal light reflex is central in the pupil, then there is no squint.

Table 24.1: Muscles in action during changing of direction of gaze

Right eye direction of gaze	*Muscles in action*
1. Right side (laterally)	Right lateral rectus and left medial rectus
2. Left side (medially)	Right medial rectus and left lateral rectus
3. Up and out	Right superior rectus and left inferior oblique
4. Down and out	Right inferior rectus and left superior oblique
5. Down and in	Right superior oblique and left inferior rectus
6. Up and in	Right inferior oblique and left superior rectus

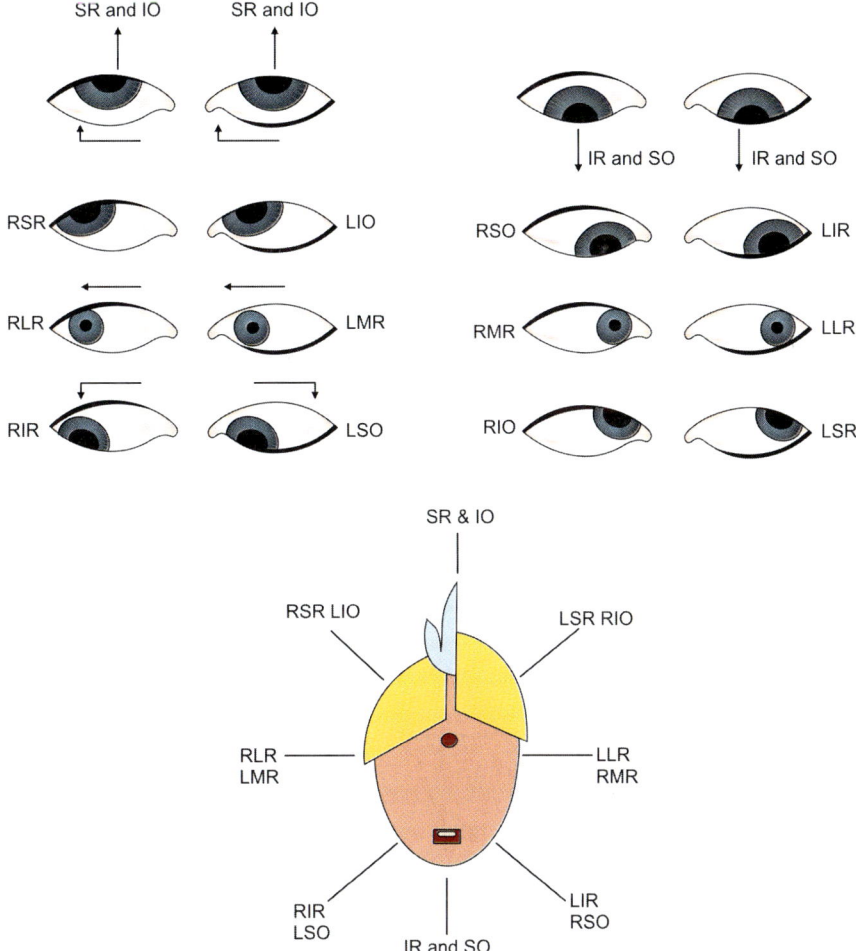

Fig. 24.1: Ocular movements

- If the corneal light reflex is just outside the pupil, then the angle of the squint is 16 degrees.

- If the corneal light reflex is midway between the pupil margin and limbus, then the squint is of 32 degrees.

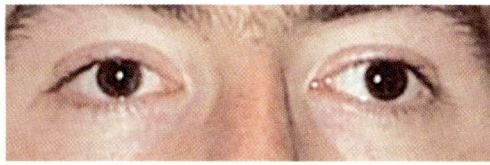

Fig. 24.2: Hirschberg corneal reflex test—left eye divergent squint

- If the corneal light reflex is at the limbus, then the squint is of 48 degrees

Corneal reflex test not only gives an approximate idea but at the same tzime is the most useful and practical method of assessing the angle of squint before and after surgery and on follow-up also.

Cover-uncover and Alternate Cover Test

Cover test is a simple, useful and reliable procedure for investigation of squint. It can be done easily in adults and children. For a very young child, use a toy with a squeaker or a light that can be flashed on and off to keep his gaze steady.

Cover test should be performed for distance and near gaze. For distance gaze, ask the patient to look at a fixation light at 6 meters. For near gaze, ask the patient to look at a spotlight at about half meter.

Surgeon while observing the movement of the eye should cover and uncover the other eye.

Repeat the process with other eye and thereafter alternately.

Interpretation

- No movement of the eye indicates *orthophoria*.
- Movement of the eye inwards indicates *esophoria*.
- Movement of the eye outwards indicates *exophoria*.
- Movement of the eye inwards or outwards may be of small degree or large degree with quick or slow recovery for fixation.
- *In concomitant squint*, the secondary deviation is equal to the primary deviation.
- *In paralytic squint*, the secondary deviation is greater than the primary deviation.
- Helps to differentiate a unilateral squint from an alternating squint.

- Movement of the eye inwards or outwards with no recovery for fixation indicates that cover test has caused a *latent squint to breakdown into a manifest squint.*
- Movement of the eye inwards or outwards with the eye wandering indicates that fixation is absent or defective due to amblyopia.

Accommodation Test

Accommodation is measured by an appliance known as *near-point rule*. Near-point rule is calibrated in centimeters and in diopters of accommodation.

Ask the patient to fix the rule at his chin and move the card in the rule towards his eye until the letters in the card are clear and distinct. He should stop immediately, when the letters become even slightly indistinct. Test each eye separately and then both together.

It gives direct reading about the *power of accommodation* present in the patient.

Convergence Test

The power of convergence is measured by an appliance known as *binocular gauge.*

- *For testing objective convergence:* Test object is placed in the groove at the far end of gauge. Patient is asked to fix the gauge at his chin and look at the test object. Move the test object towards the patient and notice the eyes for divergence.

  Measurement is taken at a point, when the one or both eyes diverge on loss of binocular fixation (Fig. 24.3).

- *For subjective convergence test:* Box with cross-shaped aperture is used which has a slide with a fine vertical line visible in the vertical limb of box. Ask the patient to fix the gauge at his chin and move the box towards the self and stop the box as soon as the vertical line appears as double.

  Point at which the line appears double is the point for measurement of convergence.

Prism Bar Vergence Test

Prism bar measures the fusional power. Ask the patient to look at a spotlight at 6 meters.

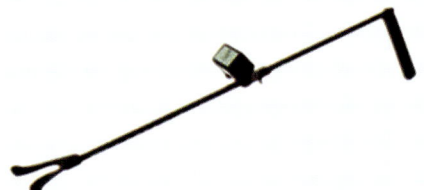

Fig. 24.3: Binocular gauge

Place the prism bar and move it for increasing strength until the spotlight appears double.

Interpretation

- Prisms placed *base-in* give the divergent fusional power.
- Prisms placed *base out* give convergent fusional power.
- The normal converging power is about 45° (25° D) and the normal divergence power is about 4° to 5°.
- Convergence below 20° is taken as a convergence insufficiency.
- Converging fusional power can be increased by exercise, if there is a convergence weakness.

Worth's Four-light Test (Fig. 24.4)

It consists of a panel containing four panes of glass arranged in a diamond fashion illuminated internally and red-green goggle.

Upper glass is of red color. Two lateral glass panes are of green color. Bottom pane is of white color.

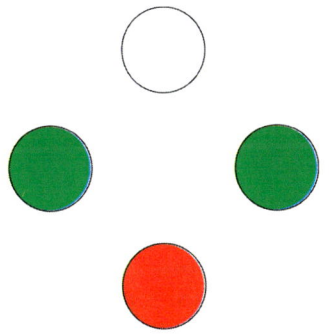

Fig. 24.4: Worth's four-light test

It is essential that the colors in the panel and goggles are complimentary.

Patient is at a distance of about 6 meters. Place red-green goggles on patient's eyes with red glass in front of the right eye and green glass in front of the left eye. Ask the patient to tell the number of light seen and the color.

Interpretation

- If the patient can see only two red lights, then it shows the suppression of the image of the left eye.
- If the patient can see only three green lights, then it shows the suppression of the image of the right eye.
- If the patient can see two red lights or three green lights alternately but never simultaneously, then there is alternating suppression.
- If the patient can see five lights two red and three green lights then there is latent or manifest squint but no suppression.

Maddox Rod Test (Fig. 24.5)

Maddox rod test ascertains the degree of heterophoria for distance.

Maddox rod is a circular piece of red glass with parallel grooves in it. It converts the image of a spotlight seen by one eye into a red streak (line) of light so that there is no stimulus for fusion of spotlight of one eye with red streak line of other eye; the two images the spotlight and red streak being different.

Streak of light is at right angles to the axis of grooves or cylinder in red glass the Maddox rod.

Make the patient sit in a semi-dark room with a spotlight at 6 meters. Place the Maddox rod horizontally before the right eye thereby converting the spotlight into vertical red streak of light.

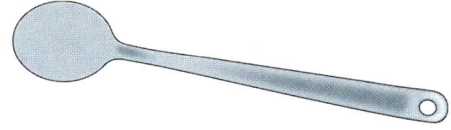

Fig. 24.5: The Maddox rod

Interpretation

- If the red vertical streak appears to pass through the spotlight, then there is horizontal orthophoria.
- If the red vertical streak appears to the left of the spotlight, then there is crossed diplopia indicating exophoria.
- If the red vertical streak appears to the right of the spotlight, then there is homonymous diplopia indicating esophoria.

Now place the Maddox rod vertically before the right eye thereby converting the spotlight into a horizontal red streak of light.

- If the red horizontal streak appears to pass through the spotlight, then there is vertical orthophoria.
- If the horizontal streak appears above the spotlight, then there is left hyperphoria.
- If the horizontal streak appears below the spotlight, then there is right hyperphoria.

Use of Prism

The degree of heterophoria can be measured by the strength of the prism placed in front of the right eye to make the streak pass through the spotlight with base-in or base-out for horizontal heterophoria and base, up or down for vertical heterophoria.

Use of Tangent Scale

The degree of heterophoria can be measured directly, if the tangent scale has been used with a spotlight at its center. The horizontal and vertical arms of the tangent scale are calibrated in degrees in bold letters which can be easily read by the patient. The number the red streak is crossing is the degree of heterophoria.

Use of Maddox Hand Frame

It provides a quick and easy method for measurement of heterophoria.

It consists of a Maddox rod placed in right side frame and 10° rotating prism in left frame. Maddox hand frame is placed before the eyes of the patient. If the red streak seen by him is not passing through the spotlight then the prism in the frame is rotated so as to make the

streak pass through the spotlight. The value of the prism is read on the scale of the frame.

Tilt in the red streak indicates cyclophoria.

Maddox Wing Test (Fig. 24.6)

Maddox wing test ascertains the degree of heterophoria for near vision. The type of heterophoria and the degree can be known and measured directly from the scale on the Maddox wing.

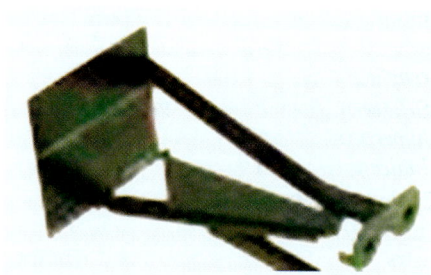

Fig. 24.6: Maddox wing test

Ask the patient to hold the Maddox wing at the handle and look through the two slit-holes in the eyepiece of the instrument.

Each eye is exposed to a certain field on the chart of the instrument due to two diaphragms which glide tangentially into each other. This provides a separate image for each eye.

With right eye, the patient is looking at the white arrow pointing vertically upwards and a red arrow pointing horizontally to the left.

With left eye, the patient is looking at the horizontal row of figures in white color and a vertical row of figures in the red color.

The figures in white and red are numericals which have been calibrated to give a direct reading of deviation in degree.

Ask the patient to keep his both the eyes open and tell white number in the horizontal row to which the white arrow is pointing at.

Interpretation

- If the white arrow is at zero, then there is no horizontal heterophoria.
- If the white arrow is pointing at any other white number, then there is heterophoria which can be either exophoria or esophoria.

Ask the patient again to look and tell the red number in vertical row to which the red arrow is pointing at.

- If the red arrow is at zero, then there is no vertical heterophoria.
- If the red arrow is pointing at any other red number, then there is hyperphoria or hypophoria.

For the convenience of the examiner:

- It should be remembered that the *even numericals in white color indicate exophoria and odd numericals in white color indicate esophoria.*
- Similarly, *even numericals in red color indicate hyperphoria, and odd numericals in red color indicate hypophoria.*

Cyclophoria can be measured by adjusting the movable shaft of the red arrow until it appears parallel with the horizontal line below the horizontal figures. Any departure from parallelism is a measure of the cyclophoria and the amount of cyclophoria can be read on the scale.

Diplopia Red-green Goggle Test (Fig. 24.7)

It is form of test in that the images in two eyes are dissociated.

This test is mainly used for the diagnosis of individual muscle palsy in cases complaining of diplopia.

The test is best performed in a semi-dark room.

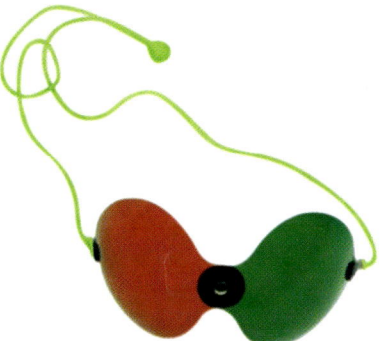

Fig. 24.7: Red-green diplopia goggles

Ask the patient to put on the diplopia goggle placing the *red glass in front of his right eye and green glass in front of his left eye.*

Ask him to look at the bar light in the examiner's hand at about one meter. Explain to him that this bar light shall be moved in all the cardinal direction of his gaze. The patient shall see two images and he should report about the *distance, level and tilt* of the two images. The examiner shall record this in diplopia chart with nine squares. The position of red image with red pencil and green image with green pencil showing the distance, level and tilt of two images as reported by the patient.

Interpretation

- The area of single vision and diplopia.
- The distance between the two images.
- The level of two images.
- One image is showing a tilt or is erect.
- There is a homonymous diplopia or crossed diplopia.

Hess Screen Test

It consists of Hess screen (Fig. 24.8), green spotlight, switch board and red-green goggle.

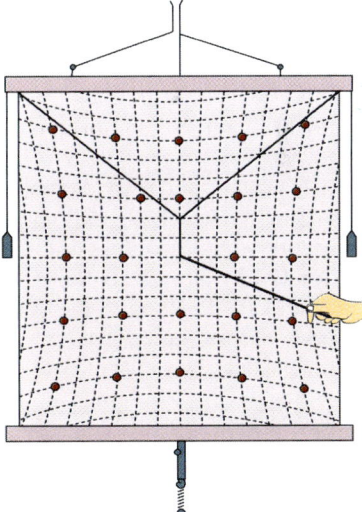

Fig. 24.8: Hess screen

Hess screen is made of wood panel of three square feet in size and painted with gray color. The screen is ruled in a grid of faint horizontal and vertical lines each separated and run parallel with a distance subtending 5° at the eye of the patient seated half meter from the screen. There is a small dot at the center of the Hess screen board. There are small circular apertures at the intersection of lines at 15° and 30° covered with pieces of red mica. There is a light source behind each aperture. The illumination of each is controlled by a control switch board. Each of the red spotlights in the screen can be switched on in turn by insertion of a plug in the corresponding switch in the control switch board.

Patient is made to sit in front of Hess screen at a distance of half meter the eyes being at the level of central point on the board. A chin rest is useful to keep him steady and maintain the level. Ask him to put on the red-green goggle; the red glass in front of the right eye and the green glass in front of the left eye.

Now the surgeon indicates each of the nine inner dots in turn by control unit. The patient is asked to shine the green spotlight in his hand over the red spot indicated by surgeon. The result is recorded on a Hess screen chart. Usually, it is the inner square which is plotted for the test.

Reverse the goggle, i.e. the red glass now in front of the left eye and green glass in front of the right eye. Repeat the test and record the result on Hess chart.

Interpretation

- Record of primary and secondary deviation.
- Hess charting at intervals provides information about progress of palsy.
- Smaller field belongs to the defective muscle and shall belong to the eye which was covered with green glass at the time the smaller field was charted out.

After Image Slides

After image slide test is the most dissociating test in which battery-powered camera flash is used to produce a vertical after image in the right eye and a horizontal after image in the left eye. *Each eye is subjected to stimulation separately. Patient is asked to draw the relative position of the two after images seen by him.*

Interpretation

- Symmetrical cross indicates normal retinal correspondence.
- Asymmetrical cross indicates abnormal retinal correspondence.
- Absence of vertical or horizontal after image indicates suppression of right or left eye, respectively.

Synoptophore (Fig. 24.9)

Synoptophore is useful to test:
- Sensory status of the eyes which includes *three grades of fusion.*
- Amplitude of fusion
- Suppression
- Retinal correspondence.

Grades of Fusion

Grade I-Simultaneous perception or macular perception (Fig. 24.10): Two dissimilar slides are used; one slide with a bird and other slide with a pot. If the patient can put the bird in the cage by seeing through the synoptophore, then he has fusion *of grade I.*

Grade II-Fusion under stress with some amplitude of fusion (Fig. 24.11): Two slides are used with

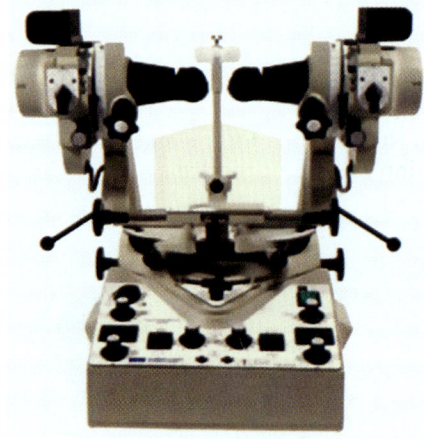

Fig. 24.9: Synoptophore

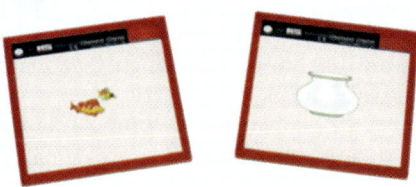

Fig. 24.10: Grade I-slides

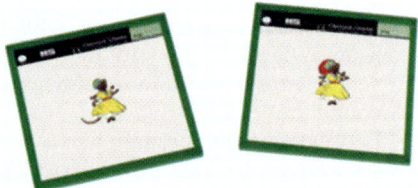

Fig. 24.11: Grade II-slides

lacking some details in each but when superimposed forms a complete picture. Popular slide with children is of a doll. In one slide, the cap is missing and in another slide the tail is missing. If the patient can fuse these two incomplete slides as one, then he has *fusion of grade II.*

Grade III-Stereopsis (Fig. 24.12): Slides must give an impression of depth. Slide of bucket gives a feeling of depth. If the patient is able to superimpose the two slides of bucket as one, then he has a good stereopsis with fusion *of grade III.*

Amplitude of Fusion

Amplitude of fusion is tested with slides meant for grade I and grade II. In this test, after superimposing the slides, the patient continues to move the arms of synoptophore

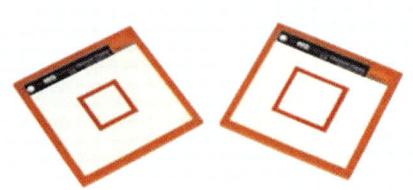

Fig. 24.12: Grade III-slides

until diplopia occurs. The point where the diplopia occurs gives the *amplitude of fusion on scale direc*tly.

The normal amplitude of fusion is about 30 diapers.

Suppression

If the patient with the slides for grade I reports that he is able to see either the bird or a pot or alternately, then he has suppression.

Retinal Correspondence

If the patient is able to superimpose the slides of grade II, then he has a normal retinal correspondence.

In case of any doubt, perform the after image test.

CLASSIFICATION OF SQUINT

Heterophoria—Latent Squint

Young mother presents with complain that she notices deviation of her son's eye especially after he finishes his homework.

Cover-uncover test reveals deviation of eyes.

Diagnosis—heterophoria— latent squint.

Heterophoria is the condition in which the eye shows deviation, when the fusion is broken. It is a condition of imperfect balance of eyes due to weak fusion, therefore, the eyes show deviation. Heterophoria can be elicited only by dissociation tests, i.e. cover-uncover test.

- Heterophoria is kept in check by subconscious effort and it is said to be a compensated heterophoria with no symptoms.
- Heterophoria requiring conscious effort to maintain fusion then it gives rise to symptoms of eye strain and eye ache.
- Decompensated heterophoria manifests as heterotropia manifest squint.

Types of Heterophoria—Latent Squint

1. *Exophoria* Exophoria is a condition of an outward (divergence) deviation of the eyes when the fusion is disturbed or broken.

Exophoria due to convergence weakness:
- Exophoria is greater for near vision than for distance vision.
- Maddox wing reading is higher than the Maddox rod reading.

Exophoria due to divergence excess:
- Exophoria is greater for distance vision than for near vision.
- Maddox rod reading is higher than the Maddox wing reading.

2. *Esophoria* Esophoria is a condition of an inward (convergence) deviation of the eyes, when the fusion is disturbed or broken.

Esophoria due to convergence excess:
- Esophoria is greater for near vision than for distance vision.
- Maddox wing reading is greater than the Maddox rod reading.

Esophoria due to divergence weakness:
- Esophoria is greater for distance vision than for near vision.
- Maddox rod reading is greater than Maddox wing reading.

3. *Hyperphoria* Hyperphoria is a condition in which the visual axis of one eye deviates upward and the visual axis of one eye deviates downward.

In clinical practice, only the term hyperphoria is used.

Right or left hyperphoria according to which eye tends to deviate upward in comparison to the other eye.

Hyperphoria may be associated with exophoria or esophoria.

4. *Cyclophoria* Cyclophoria is a condition in which there is a torsional deviation of the eye.
- If the vertical meridian of one eye shows wheel-rotation inward, then it is known as *incyclophoria.*
- If the vertical meridian of one eye shows a wheel-rotation outward, then it is known as *excyclophoria.*

Cyclophoria is usually associated with hyperphoria.

5. *Orthophoria* Orthophoria is a condition of eyes in which there is a perfect balance of eyes with no deviation even when the fusion is disturbed or broken. It is rare.

Most of the cases show some kind of mild degree of heterophoria.

Etiology

1. *Refractive state of the eyes:*
   - Esophoria develops, if there is an increased demand for accommodation as in hypermetropia and due to increased demand for convergence as in congenital myopia.
   - Exophoria develops, if there is a decreased demand of accommodation as in myopia and at a later age in presbyopia and in anisometropia with one eye hypermetropic and the other one is myopic.
2. *Factors which may cause decompensation of heterophoria:*
   - Excessive physical and mental stress
   - General fatigue or weakness or debility
   - Ocular fatigue due to excessive near work
   - Advancing age.
   - Spasm of convergence with spasm of accommodation may induce esophoria.

Symptoms

- *Headache and eye strain:* Excessive demand for accommodation and convergence usually after near work for long periods. Such cases get relief by closing one eye for few seconds or giving a break every two hours or so.
- *Blurring of print:* Patient complains that while reading there is running together of the words thereby causing blurring of the print of the book. It is annoying.
- *Difficulty in changing focus:* Patient complains of difficulty in playing fast games like badminton or table tennis as there is a need to change the focus very fast. Due to the heterophoria, the patient is not able to change his focus fast.
- *Difficulty in judging the distance:* Patient with heterophoria usually finds it a problem to

park a car. A pilot feels problem in landing and take-off.

Investigations

- Visual acuity
- Refraction
- Ophthalmoscopy
- Ocular movements
- Cover-uncover and alternate cover test
- Accommodation test
- Convergence test
- Prism bar vergence test
- Worth's four-light test
- Maddox rod test
- Maddox wing test
- Synoptophore

Diagnosis

- History of typical symptoms of heterophoria.
- Cover-uncover test shows deviation of eyes.
- Maddox rod reading shows heterophoria.
- Maddox wing reading shows heterophoria.
- Prism bar vergence test shows poor fusional reserve.
- Test for convergence shows insufficiency of convergence.
- Test for accommodation shows poor range of accommodation.

Management

- Correct even minor refractive error.
- Prescribe full hypermetropic correction.
- Exercise for increasing the fusional reserve and convergence.
- Prisms can help to relieve the symptoms.
- Surgery of the affected muscle either recession or resection as the case may be.

Supportive therapy

- Visual hygiene includes proper posture, illumination and proper distance for reading and writing.
- Break for few minutes every two hours gives break to fusional reserve and thus helps the patient to overcome his symptoms.

- Improve general health by proper diet, proper distribution of diet in whole day with addition of vitamins and general exercise.

HETEROTROPIA—MANIFEST SQUINT

1. Comitant Squint

Comitant squint is a condition in which although the eyes are misaligned yet they retain their abnormal relation to each other in all the directions of gaze. The efferent pathways are normal but the afferent pathway is defective due to poor visual acuity which again is due to either defect in the optical media of the eyes or due to breaking down of fusional reflex.

Investigative Evaluation

- History
- Visual acuity
- Refraction
- Ophthalmoscopy
- Ocular movements
- Cover-uncover and alternate cover test
- Hirschberg corneal reflex test
- Worth's four-light test
- After image test
- Synoptophore

2. Convergent Squint (Fig. 24.13)

Patient presents with one eye deviated inwards and desires treatment only for his cosmetic embarrassment among his fellow students and in society. No visual complaint of any kind.

Ocular movements are normal in all the directions of gaze.

Diagnosis—convergent squint.

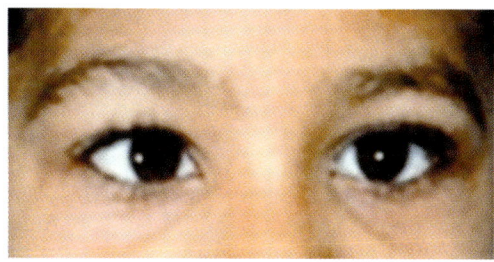

Fig. 24.13: Convergent squint

Convergent squint: Esotropia is a condition in which there is inward deviation of one eye while the other eye fixates.

Etiology

1. *High hypermetropia:* There is defective visual acuity due to high hypermetropia which demands excessive accommodation and, therefore, excessive convergence.
2. *Opacities in optical media.* Any opacity in the cornea, lens or vitreous obstructs the vision thereby the fusional reflex is not developed resulting in convergence.
3. Diseases of the eye which does not allow the fusion to develop.
4. Any acute illness or debilitating disease is the common predisposing factor for convergent squint in children.

Types of Convergent Squint

1. **Accommodational squint:** It is of four types:
   a. *Fully accommodational squint:* A case of fully accommodational squint shows no squint for distance and near with correction of his error of refraction and constant use of glasses. The squint soon appears on removal of glasses.
   b. *Accommodational with convergence excess:* These patients show no squint for distance vision with correction of refraction and constant use of glasses. But there is squint for near work even with glasses. These can be managed by prescription of additional glasses for near work.
   c. *Accommodational with divergence weakness:* Even with full correction and constant use of glasses, there is a squint for distance and esophoria for near. They respond only to surgical treatment of recession of medial rectus muscle.
   d. *Partially accommodational squint:* There is a constant convergent squint for distance and near even with full correction and constant use of glasses. The angle of squint is reduced but not fully. These cases need surgical correction with recession of medial rectus.

2. **Non-accommodational squint:** It is of three types:
   a. *Unilateral convergent squint:* It is seen early in infancy. Any acute illness may be predisposing factor. There is early suppression and amblyopia. Early surgery is the treatment of choice to achieve parallelism of the eyes and development of binocular vision.
   b. *Alternating convergent squint:* It sets early in infancy. The squint increases with the age as one uses his accommodation. In these cases, the vision is equal in both the eyes. There is free alternation of the eyes. There is no refractive error. There is a cosmetic embarrassment. Treat by surgery for cosmetic purpose. Some cases develop binocular vision, if operated early.
   c. *Secondary convergent squint:* It develops, when there is obstruction to vision due to hazy ocular media specially cornea and lens. It may follow also due to optic atrophy or anisometropia. As the convergence is strong, therefore, there is a tendency for development of the convergent squint though the eye is virtually blind with very low visual acuity. Surgical correction for cosmetic purpose is the treatment.

Management

- Correct the error of refraction and prescribe glasses for constant use.
- Surgical treatment with recession and resection of appropriate muscles of the eyes.
- In the right eye, convergent squint resect lateral rectus and recesses the medial rectus muscle.
- Some cases may need recession of the opposite medial rectus muscle.

3. Divergent Squint (Fig. 24.14)

Patient presents with one eye deviated outwards and desires treatment only for his cosmetic embarrassment among his fellow students and in society. No visual complaint of any kind.

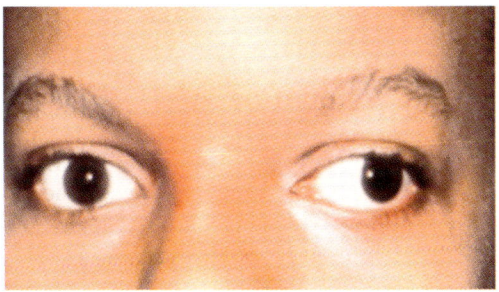

Fig. 24.14: Divergent squint

Ocular movements are normal in all the directions of gaze.

Diagnosis—divergent squint.

Divergent squint: Exotropia is a condition in which there is outward deviation of one eye while the other eye fixates.

Etiology

- *High myopia:* There is a defective visual acuity due to high myopia which demands less accommodation and therefore, less convergence. Thus there is a tendency for the eye to deviate outward.

- *No fusion:* Due to low visual acuity, there is mal-development of fusional reflex. Because of this, the eye does not take up fixation and deviates outward the normal position of rest for an eye with no fixation.

- *Opaque media:* Opacities in the optical media especially cornea and lens lead to divergence of the eye the normal position of rest.

Types of Divergent Squint

1. **Primary divergent squint:** It is of three types:
   a. *Divergence excess type:* This type of squint manifests, when the patient is looking at distance and not fixing anything particular. The patient is unaware of the squint. It is the friends or relatives who point it out about his defect in the eye. The cover-uncover test shows exophoria with good recovery for near but no recovery for distance. Later the squint becomes constant. Surgery is helpful to provide full cure from squint.
   b. *Convergence weakness type:* There is no squint for distance but there is a latent squint for near which becomes manifest in course of time. Cover-uncover test, shows exophoria for distance with good recovery but there is a manifest squint for near. On convergence test there is insufficiency of convergence. Convergence exercise may be helpful. Surgery gives full cure.
   c. *Mixed type of divergent squint:* There is squint for all the distance. This is due to divergence excess and convergence weakness. Surgery provides full cure.

2. **Secondary divergent squint:** It results due to following factors:
   - Gross visual defect leads to deviation of eye outwards.
   - Divergence occurs early, if there is a congenital defect.

Secondary divergent squint follows gross visual defect in the eye, anisometropia, aniseikonia with advancing age, high myopia and anomaly of orbit. Surgery is helpful for cosmetic purpose.

Management

- Correction of error of refraction with suitable glasses for constant use.
- Surgical treatment with resection and recession of appropriate muscles.
- *In the right eye divergent squint:* Resect the medial rectus and recess the lateral rectus muscle of the right eye.
- In some cases, a recession of the opposite lateral rectus muscle may be necessary.

Incomitant Squint

Incomitant squint is a condition in which the eyes are misaligned and do not retain their normal relative position in all the movements of the gaze. There is dissociation of ocular movements. The ocular deviation is irregular and varies in an incoordinate manner in different directions of gaze. The afferent pathway is normal and intact. It is due to defect in the efferent pathway. The efferent pathway is the motor path of the binocular reflexes. The brain is able to command but the motor apparatus is unable to function due to the lesion at the level of lower neuron, the nuclei or the nerve supplying the muscle.

1. Paralytic Squint (Fig. 24.15)

Patient presents with deviation of eye with complain of diplopia, vertigo and may show change in his head posture. Diplopia is an annoying symptom that forces the patient to attend eye clinic.

Ocular movements are dissociated.

Diagnosis—paralytic squint.

Paralytic squint is a condition in which the amount of deviation varies in different directions of gaze. It occurs due to complete or incomplete paralysis of one or more extraocular muscles.

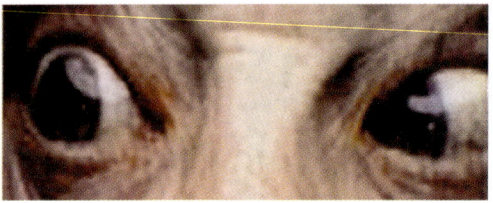

Fig. 24.15: Paralysis of 6th abducent nerve of left eye

Etiology

Most cases of paralytic squint are neurogenic. Predisposing factors for neurogenic involvement are:

- Acute and subacute infections, e.g. viral, tubercular and toxic.
- Acute demyelinating diseases.
- Metabolic diseases, e.g. diabetes, anemia, leukemia or deficiency of thiamine, nicotinic or ascorbic acid.
- Vascular lesions, e.g. hemorrhage, arteriosclerosis, aneurysm and thrombosis.
- Trauma to head, orbit and eye.
- Migraine.
- Inflammatory lesions of sinuses and orbit.
- Orbital apex syndrome.
- Sphenoidal fissure syndrome.
- Myogenic lesions, e.g. myasthenia and thyroid ophthalmopathy
- Intracranial tumors.

Symptoms

- *Diplopia:* Diplopia occurs in the cases of squint in which the binocular reflexes are well developed. It is very distressing symptom which brings the patient to the ophthalmologist early. It is likely to persist, if there is no improvement in the paralytic muscle. The adult patients do not develop suppression easily. Some patients adopt postural attitude to neutralize the deviation. It is easy for lateral diplopia but not for vertical diplopia. Patients with vertical muscle paralysis with torsional displacement of images may develop general symptoms of vertigo, nausea and vomiting with visual disturbances.

- *False orientation (confusion):* If the patient fixes with the affected eye, then there is past-pointing towards the field of action of the paralyzed muscle.

  If the patient fixes with the normal eye, then there is no past-pointing. In a recent case of paralysis of ocular muscle, this false orientation is distressing. Patient finds problem in carrying out his work requiring visual coordination. He even finds problem in his gait. In course of time, the patient fixing with the paretic eye gradually learns to adopt the new conditions.

- *Ocular vertigo with nausea:* Vertigo occurs due to these disordered subjective symptoms of diplopia and false orientation. Vertigo may produce general symptoms of nausea and vomiting. These symptoms are more pronounced in vertical paralysis and torsional defects.

- *Ocular deviation:* Its onset is sudden.

Signs

- *Abnormal deviation of the eyes:* There is an abnormal deviation of the eyes in primary position. In many cases, the deviation may be compensated by fusional reflexes and compensatory head posture. It is more common with horizontally acting muscles and particularly when the lateral rectus is involved. Thus a patient with lateral rectus paralysis may not show any deviation in the primary position but the defect is caught soon on ocular movements.

- *Restriction of ocular movement:* There is limitation of the movement of the eye in the field of action of the affected muscle during binocular movements. It is to be kept in mind that these deviations are typically seen in recent cases of palsy or complete paralysis of a muscle. *In long-standing cases, the clinical picture changes due to changes in the other muscles.*

- *Compensatory postural changes:* Change in the postural attitude occurs to overcome the inconvenience caused by distressing diplopia.

- *Face rotation:* There is rotation of the face in the direction of the field of action of the paralyzed muscle. It helps to neutralize the displacement of the diplopic image.

- *Head tilting:* There is head tilting towards the shoulder of the side of the higher image. It helps to neutralize the vertical and torsional displacement of the diplopic image. Tilting of the head lowers the image to bring it to the same level and also corrects the obliquity of the images

Investigations

All the investigative evaluation methods required can be used to evaluate a case of incomitant or paralytic squint and in addition pay more attention to the following:

- *Ocular movements:* Test ocular movements in the six diagnostic directions of gaze: (i) to the right, (ii) to the left, (iii) up and to the right, (iv) up and to the left, (v) down and to the right, and (vi) down and to the left. To these, add another two directions: (i) straight upwards, and (ii) downwards.

  Horizontal muscles can be tested with the inward and outward movements of the eyes.

  In vertical movements, each eye is moved in each direction by two muscles: (i) vertical rectus and (ii) oblique muscle.

  The diagonal movements are essential to test so that each muscle can be studied

as each muscle has a preponderant effect in that direction.

- *Cover-uncover test:* Normally, the patient fixates with his normal eye. The deviation of the affected eye is called *primary deviation* and this deviation is in the direction opposite to the primary action of the muscle.

  Cover the normal eye so that the affected eye assumes fixation. The normal eye behind the cover assumes position as brought by th e contraction of the overacting synergic muscle. This deviation of the normal eye behind the cover is called as *secondary deviation.*

  In a recent case of paresis, the secondary deviation is always greater than the primary deviation. This is due to the attempt to get the paralyzed eye into position of fixation that is an abnormal innervational effort is made to try to move the affected eye in the direction of action of the muscle. This extra-energy is involuntarily shared equally between the two eyes, therefore, there is extra-movement of the normal eye behind the cover.

  In long-standing cases due to changes in the muscles, the secondary deviation becomes equal to the primary deviation and the squint begins to assume the characteristics of concomitant strabismus.

- *Diplopia red-green goggle test:* It gives subjective analysis of the muscle involved. The direction in which there is the greatest separation of images is the direction of the action of the paralyzed muscle. It is very useful and reliable test, if only one muscle is involved. If more than one muscle is involved, then various actions must be analyzed additively.

- *Hess screen test:* It provides accurate measurement of the deviation. It helps to assess the prognosis by comparing with subsequent examination. It also allows analysis of fine details such as the presence of an over-action or contracture of the ipsilateral antagonist or the overaction of the contralateral synergist and the inhibitional palsy of the antagonist of the contralateral synergist.

Management

- Treat the causative factor. Most cases show good response to medical therapy.
- If there is no improvement and the deviation has become stabilized, then surgery can be undertaken to provide the binocular vision and cosmetic improvement.

2. Restrictive Squint

Patient usually presents with change in his head posture and difficulty in attending his daily routine work at home and office.

Restrictive squint is a condition in which the extraocular muscle is not paralyzed but its movement is mechanically restricted usually due to fibrosis.

1. Duane's Retraction Syndrome

Clinical features

- There is a marked restriction or complete abolition of the abduction (lateral) movement of one eye and rarely of both the eyes.
- There is a slight restriction of adduction (medial) movement of the affected eye.
- On attempted adduction (medial) movement of the affected eye, there is a marked retraction with up-shoot or down-shoot of the affected eye.
- On adduction (medial) movement of the eye, there is narrowing of the palpebral aperture with some degree of ptosis due to retraction of the eye.

- On attempted abduction (lateral) movement of the eye, there is widening of the palpebral aperture with some retraction of the upper lid due to minimal protraction of the eye.
- Deficiency of the convergence of the affected eye.

2. Vertical Retraction Syndrome

- Vertical retraction syndrome is a congenital condition involving only the vertical muscles.
- Limitation of movement of the affected eye on elevation or depression associated with a retraction of the globe and narrowing of the palpebral aperture.
- Hypotropia on looking upward and outward and hypertropia on looking downward and outward.

3. Superior Oblique Tendon Sheath Syndrome

- Superior oblique tendon sheath syndrome is an anomaly of cyclovertical movements.
- Clinically, the syndrome appears as a paresis of the inferior oblique muscle. In adduction, there is the absence of the elevation of the affected eye and the eye has a tendency to down-shoot.
- In primary position of the affected eye, there is either orthophoria or hypotropia. Patient may try to overcome it by tilting of head to the affected side and turning of the face slightly upwards.

Maladies of Ocular Trauma

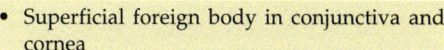

- Superficial foreign body in conjunctiva and cornea
- Contusion trauma
- Penetrating and perforating trauma
- Intraocular foreign body
- Siderosis
- Chalcosis
- Intraorbital foreign body
- Rupture of the sclera
- Chemical burn
  - Alkali burn
  - Acid burn
- Thermal burn
- Radiational trauma
  - Eclipse blindness
  - Snow blindness

OCULAR TRAUMA

Though the eyeball is well protected by the bony orbit, the nose, the lids and a cushion of fat behind the globe yet the incidence of ocular trauma is high due to industrialization, not using protective goggles, non-adoption and implementation of preventive measures for each kind of industry.

Domestic accidents can be prevented by a little awareness and care.

Strong bony orbital margin prevents many injuries of the eyeball. Lids and the eyelashes are very sensitive and the lids get closed quickly through the reflex stimuli.

Bell's phenomenon, i.e. the upward rotation of the eyeball is an additional protective reflex action which further helps to protect the globe from trauma.

New definitions as proposed by '*American Ocular Trauma Society*' for mechanical trauma are as follows:

Term *'eyeball'* has been restricted for the outer fibrous coat, the cornea and sclera.

Closed globe trauma denotes that the eyeball does not have a full thickness wound of cornea or sclera but there is an intraocular damage. It includes:

- *Contusion* results from blunt trauma.
- *Lamellar laceration* refers to partial thickness wound of eyeball may be caused by a sharp object or a blunt trauma.

Open-globe trauma denotes full thickness wound of the sclera or cornea or both. It includes:

- *Rupture* refers to full thickness rupture wound of the eyeball caused by blunt trauma. Rupture occurs due to markedly raised intraocular pressure by an *inside-out mechanism of trauma*.
- *Laceration* refers to full thickness lacerative wound of the eyeball caused by a sharp object. The laceration occurs due to an *outside-in mechanism of trauma*. It includes:
  - *Penetrating trauma:* It refers to a single laceration of eyeball caused by a sharp object. It includes *retained intraocular foreign body trauma.*
  - *Perforating trauma:* It refers to full thickness perforation with one entry and one exit point in the eyeball caused

by the same object. It includes *retained intraorbital foreign body trauma.*

Superficial Foreign Body in Conjunctiva and Cornea

Patient presents with complain of foreign body sensation each time he blinks since yesterday evening.

Slit lamp shows clear cornea. On eversion of the upper lid, the foreign body is visible lodged comfortably in the sulcus subtarsalis.

Diagnosis— superficial foreign body at sulcus subtarsalis.

Etiology

Most of the extraocular foreign bodies are small particles of coal, dust, emery, steel, glass or even small insects. Other less common objects are husk of seeds and wings of insect. As such any organic or non-organic particle floating in the atmosphere can get lodged in the conjunctival sac or the cornea while the person is moving out-doors or sometimes even when he is in-door especially during dusting or forceful air-flow from cooler fan.

With the entry of a foreign particle in the eye, there is copious watering of the eye which helps to wash out the foreign body towards the inner canthus from where it can be wiped out by the patient. It is a normal physiological phenomenon.

Often there is a tendency on the part of the patient to rub his eyes which is responsible for the foreign body to get stuck to the conjunctiva or cornea or get lodged in the sulcus subtarsalis or the fornix.

Particles of steel or emery which enter the eyeball with force get embedded straight into the cornea.

Symptoms

- Sudden discomfort in form of pain or burning in the eyes with copious watering.
- Increased reflex blinking with copious watering of the eye due to irritation of the foreign body is an effort to dislodge the foreign particle and to wash it out.

- Constant feeling of a foreign body sensation at a particular point in the lid on blinking, if the foreign body is lodged or embedded at the sulcus subtarsalis or in the cornea.

Signs

- Foreign body lodged at the sulcus subtarsalis is seen easily after eversion of the upper lid.
- Foreign body embedded in the cornea is seen clearly by slit-lamp.
- If the foreign body has been washed out, then the signs are conjunctival congestion and a feeling of foreign body sensation for few minutes or hours.

Complications

- Foreign body which has been washed out by reflex blinking and watering of the eye does not lead to any serious complication except conjunctivitis that too if the organisms have been of a virulent type.
- Foreign body lodged at the sulcus subtarsalis for a long time may cause abrasions on the cornea due to blinking that makes the foreign body rub against the cornea.
- Foreign body embedded into the cornea can cause severe conjunctivitis and ulcer which may become hypopyon ulcer.
- Nebular opacity on healing of the corneal abrasion or an ulcer.
- Foreign body of emery or steel particle often leaves a brown ring or stain of the cornea. It is a source of irritation for a long time.

Management

- Advise patient to sit quietly without rubbing his eyes or even palming his eyes to avoid the foreign body to get embedded or stuck on the conjunctiva or cornea.
- Instill topical xylocaine 2% as eyedrops and after 10 minutes perform slit-lamp examine of the conjunctiva and the cornea for a foreign body or abrasion.
- If foreign body is not visible, then wash the conjunctival sac thoroughly with normal saline.

- If foreign body is visible, then remove the foreign body after proper local anesthesia and full aseptic precautions.
- Patient can be discharged with use of topical antibiotic eyedrops four to six times a day for 5 days.
- Advise patient never to rub the eyes and if his duty is outdoors, then advise him to use goggles.

Contusion Trauma

Patient presents with history of contusion trauma by a blunt object usually a fist in minor scuffle or ball while playing.

Slit-lamp may show minor or major trauma even to the extent of rupture.

Diagnosis—contusion trauma.

Contusion trauma of the eyeball can occur due to any type of blunt object. It can produce both; the *close-globe and open-globe traumas.*

Etiology

- Blow by a fist, stone or ball hitting the eyeball.
- In rural areas or at night, the person may hit the blunt object unknowingly usually hitting a projected fixed blunt object.
- Contusion trauma to the eyeball may be a minor causing no damage to the eye or it may cause rupture of the lids and eyeball.
- Extent of the damage to the eyeball depends on the force and the angle of blunt object that hits the eyeball.
- Prognosis should be guarded as the changes in the eyeball due to contusion trauma may be delayed and slowly progressive.

Pathogenesis

In a contusion trauma, as a general rule, either the anterior segment of the eye in front of the iris-lens diaphragm or the posterior segment is preferentially affected. Due to force of the contusion trauma, the cornea is pushed inwards thereby the wave of the aqueous humor in the anterior chamber pushes the iris and lens inwards. The wave hits the retina and thereafter the compression wave rebounds and thrusts forward the iris-lens diaphragm traumatizing these structures severely.

The *compression wave* striking the cornea, iris-lens diaphragm, vitreous, retina, choroid, and the angle of the anterior chamber may cause considerable damage.

Thus, the damage due to contusion trauma depends upon the force which creates the *compression wave.*

Lesions due to Contusion Trauma

Various lesions which can be produced by a contusion trauma affecting each structure are summarized.

1. **Lids**
   - Ecchymosis—black eye due to sub-cutaneous hemorrhage.
   - Abrasions and cuts due to hitting against the orbital margin.
   - Proptosis due to orbital hemorrhage or emphysema.
2. **Conjunctiva**
   - Ecchymosis (Fig. 25.1)
   - Tear
   - Chemosis

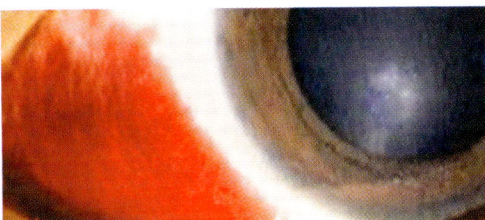

Fig. 25.1: Conjunctival ecchymosis

3. **Cornea**
   - Abrasion
   - Deep opacity of cornea due to edema
   - Partial or complete tear of the cornea
   - Tear in Descemet's membrane
   - Pigmentary deposits on endothelial surface of the cornea
   - Blood staining of the cornea.
4. **Sclera**
   - Rupture of the eyeball can occur either due to the eyeball being forced against the orbital walls or by a fall upon a projecting blunt object. The rupture

occurs at about 3 mm behind limbus and usually concentric with it.

- Conjunctiva is intact with trauma to other parts of the eye such as irido-dialysis, subconjunctival dislocation of the lens, vitreous hemorrhage and detachment of the retina.

5. **Anterior chamber**
   - Hyphema (Fig. 25.2)
   - Recession of the angle of anterior chamber.

6. **Iris, pupil and ciliary body**
   - Post-traumatic iridocyclitis
   - Traumatic miosis
   - Traumatic mydriasis

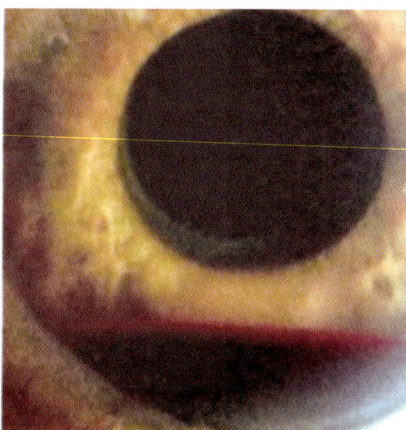

Fig. 25.2: Hyphema

- Iridodialysis, i.e. tear of iris from its ciliary attachment
- Traumatic aniridia or irideremia
- Tear of the pupillary margin
- Total inversion or retroflexion of the iris.
- Rupture of ciliary body near its anterior attachment
- Hyphema
- Recession of the angle

7. **Lens**
   - Vossius's ring on the anterior surface of lens
   - Concussion cataract
   - Subluxation of the lens
   - Dislocation of the lens

- Aphakia due to dislocation or absorption of the lens.

8. **Vitreous**
   - Liquefaction of vitreous
   - Hemorrhage in the vitreous
   - Herniation of vitreous in the anterior chamber
   - Vitreous escape
   - Posterior detachment of the vitreous

9. **Retina**
   - Hemorrhage in the retina
   - Edema of the retina
   - Tear and dialysis of retina
   - Commotioretinae (Berlin's edema)
   - Macular degeneration
   - Proliferative retinopathy
   - Detachment of retina

10. **Choroid**
    - Rupture of choroid
    - Detachment of choroid
    - Choroidal hemorrhage

11. **Optic nerve**
    - Optic atrophy
    - Avulsion of optic nerve

12. **Intraocular pressure**
    - Hypotony
    - Angle recession glaucoma
    - Ghost cell glaucoma

13. **Orbit**
    - Orbital hemorrhage or emphysema
    - Blow out fracture

Management

Refer case to trauma center and manage as required.

Penetrating and Perforating Trauma

Patient presents with history of trauma by a sharp object and complain of bleeding, pain, watering, photophobia and dim vision.

Diagnosis—penetrating or perforating trauma.
    Penetrating trauma refers to an open-globe full-thickness lacerative wound of the eyeball usually caused by sharp object.

In children
- Usual object is bow and arrow game during festive season.

- Due to sharp objects with them for their use in studies such as pen, pencil.
- Objects at home like kitchen knife, small screwdriver, etc.
- Vegetative trauma in garden or public parks with thorn, or projecting branches of the tree or bushes while playing hide and seek game.

In adults: Usually due to a stick hitting his/her eye while making small pieces of a big log of wood, or with any appliance with which he/she is working at home or workshop.

Pathogenesis

Penetrating trauma causes severe damage to the eye due to the following four factors:

1. Trauma to the ocular tissue.
2. Introduction of infection with the perforating object.
3. Post-traumatic iridocyclitis.
4. Sympathetic ophthalmitis.

Lesions and Management

1. *Tear of the conjunctiva:* It is common. A small tear with no gap can be left alone. A large tear with gap must be sutured.
2. *Corneal tear:*
   - A small linear tear of the cornea with no prolapse of iris or adhesion of the iris to the posterior surface may be left as such as it heals well, if the anterior chamber has been restored.
   - Systemic and topical broad-spectrum antibiotic therapy.
   - Topical cycloplegic in form of atropine 1% eyedrops is essential to give rest to eye and prevent anterior uveitis.
   - A large tear with prolapse of iris requires energetic surgical treatment.
3. *Trauma to lens:* There is usually a tear in the anterior or posterior capsule of the lens. The lens itself may be injured. It leads to opacification.

   If the lens has been injured severely, then IOLs implant is the first choice.

Intraocular Foreign Body

Patient presents with history of trauma while standing and watching a stone chiseler or blacksmith on its job just out of curiosity.

Slit-lamp shows point of entry with tear and hemorrhage.

Diagnosis—intraocular foreign body.

Foreign bodies which are most likely to penetrate the eyeball are minute chips of iron or steel accounting for about 90% of the intraocular foreign bodies. While chipping stone, it is the chip of chisel which enters the eyeball. Other foreign bodies which penetrate are stone, glass, lead pellets, copper percussion caps, and sometimes even small wood spicules.

Damage to the eye by penetration of an intraocular foreign body depends upon its size and velocity with which it has entered the eyeball.

Large foreign body causes considerable damage that may be beyond repair. Small foreign body gets lodged in the deeper part of the eyeball after penetrating the cornea or sclera.

An intraocular foreign body causes damage to ocular tissue by the following ways.

1. Mechanical Effect

- Foreign body after penetration of the cornea may be retained in the anterior chamber or may lie in the angle of the anterior chamber or may be caught in the iris. It can only be seen and diagnosed by slit-lamp and gonioscopy.
- Foreign body may be retained in the substance of the lens passing through the iris or pupil. If the foreign body has passed through the iris, then slit-lamp either shows a visible hole in the iris or a red reflex from the hole, if lens is clear.
- Foreign body may enter and retained in the vitreous. It can reach vitreous through various routes:
  - Through the cornea, iris and lens
  - Through the cornea, pupil and lens
  - Thorough the cornea, iris and zonule of lens

– Through the sclera, choroid and retina.

Foreign body in the vitreous remains suspended for some time until the vitreous gets liquefied due to traumatic degeneration and the foreign body may sink down. In early stage and if the foreign body is small, then probably it can be visualized ophthalmoscopically.

- Foreign body may enter the retina and retained there. In course of time, it is surrounded by exudates and later with fibrous tissue with heavy pigmentation.
- Foreign body may perforate the coats of the eyeball, double perforation and be lodged in the orbital tissue as retained intraorbital foreign body.
- If the foreign body has lodged in the posterior segment then it leads to degenerative changes in the vitreous, retina, and vision is usually lost due to formation of fibrous bands, hemorrhage and detachment of the retina.

2. Infection of the Eye

It is to be noted that metallic particles are sterile owing to heat generated on their emission and rapid transit. An infection is most certainly carried in the eye, if the particle is of stone or wood. It is essential to prevent or control infection by broad-spectrum antibiotics—systemic, topical and periocular as required.

3. Specific Reaction on Ocular Tissue

Action of intraocular foreign body varies with its chemical nature; whether the foreign body is the *non-organized material or organized material.*

Non-organized material Intraocular foreign body of non-organized material can cause the following reaction:

1. *No reaction* at all by inert substances such as glass, plastic and porcelain, gold, silver and platinum and titanium.
2. *Local irritative reaction* by lead usually occurring as shot-gun pallets become coated with carbonate and excite little

reaction forming fibrous tissue and may get encapsulated.
3. *Suppurative reaction* is excited by pure copper, zinc, nickel and mercury.
4. *Specific degenerative reaction* is produced by iron as *siderosis bulbi* and copper alloys as *chalcosis*. Iron and copper undergo electrolytic dissociation and are distributed throughout the ocular tissue causing degenerative changes.

Organized material

- Organic material tends to excite proliferative reaction characterized by formation of granulation tissue.
- Organic foreign bodies such as wood and other vegetative material produce a proliferative reaction characterized by formation of giant cells.

Other Complications

1. *Intraocular hemorrhage:* Massive hemorrhage may not absorb and leads to proliferative retinopathy and detachment of retina.
2. *Endophthalmitis* develops due to infection from foreign body. Treat by early vitrectomy and antibiotic through all the routes.
3. *Sympathetic ophthalmitis:* It is common, if the ciliary body has been damaged. Steroids are helpful to control it. Enucleate the eye, if it is completely disorganized.

Diagnosis of Intraocular Foreign Body

As an intraocular foreign body can cause irreparable damage to the ocular tissue, it is very essential to diagnose its presence as quite often the patient is unaware of it and there is very little reaction in early days.

- History may provide clue about the type of foreign body.
- Ocular examination may show the point of entry with tear and hemorrhage at the site.
- Slit-lamp and ophthalmoscopy help to locate.
- X-ray of the orbit.
- Ultrasonography.
- CT scan and MRI are the best.

Management

Surgical removal of the intraocular foreign body.

Siderosis

Siderosis occurs due to retained iron foreign body in the eye even from a small particle. In the direct siderosis, the iron is deposited in the nearby structures. In the indirect siderosis, most of the ocular tissues are involved.

Pathogenesis

The spread of the metal is due to electrolytic dissociation and dissemination throughout the eye by the intrinsic current of rest in the eye. These ions combine with the intracellular proteins resulting in degenerative changes.

Symptoms

- Gradual dim vision due to changes in the cornea, lens and retina.
- Concentric contraction of the visual fields due to degeneration of retina.
- Dim vision in dim illumination.
- Atrophic eye.

Signs

Slit-lamp

- *Cornea* shows a rusty stain; the coloration is deeper in periphery and lighter in the center.
- *Iris* also shows a rusty color reddish brown. There is a good contrast with opposite iris. Synechia has been observed indicating silent inflammatory reaction. Pupil is dilated with no reaction to light. It is probably due to atrophy of muscle fibers of the pupil-sphincter and dilator muscles.
- *Lens* shows innumerable minute brown spots in the subcapsular region. Gradually, the whole lens appears yellow tinted. In course of time, the lens becomes opaque.
- *Vitreous* is yellowish in color and shows degenerative changes.

Ophthalmoscopy

- Pigmentary degeneration of retina in the periphery.
- Optic disk shows rusty color and atrophy.

Tonometry: There is a rise of the intraocular pressure due to degenerative changes in the trabecular meshwork.

Electroretinography Electroretinogram shows diminished b-wave and later it is flat.

Management

There is no treatment for siderosis. It can be prevented by early removal of foreign body.

Chalcosis

Chalcosis occurs due to a retained foreign body of an alloy containing little pure copper. There is a slow diffusion of copper. The deposition occurs in the limiting membrane of the eye. Reaction to pure copper is a very severe suppurative type.

Chalcosis gives a typical clinical picture.

Signs

Slit-lamp

- *Kayser-Fleischer ring*: It is a golden brown ring under peripheral parts of the Descemet's membrane of cornea.
- *Sunflower cataract*: Lens shows deposition with golden green color arranged like the petals of flower.
- Aqueous humor shows many particles.
- Iris shows a greenish color.
- Vitreous may show deposits in its framework.

Ophthalmoscopy

Retina shows deposition of golden plaques which reflect as metallic sheen at the posterior pole.

Differential Diagnosis

- Hepatolenticular degeneration
- Copper poisoning.

Treatment

There is no treatment for chalcosis. It can be prevented by early removal of the foreign body.

Intraorbital Foreign Body

- An intraorbital foreign body does not excite specific reaction to it.

- Main effect is mechanical trauma and introduction of infection.
- Most metals such as iron, steel and aluminum are inert and lie quietly.
- Copper foreign body has a tendency to excite a suppurative inflammation.
- Organic foreign bodies cause granulomatous reaction.

Complications

- *Emphysema:* Orbital emphysema occurs due to fracture of the orbital wall thereby opening the air cells. It causes an acute proptosis and large swelling of lids. Emphysema can be diagnosed easily by putting mild pressure on the swollen lids. On pressure, there is a feeling of air in the lids being displaced. The air is absorbed in short time. Large emphysema may be treated by an incision to release the air.
- *Orbital hemorrhage:* It occurs due to tear of a large vein. It causes an acute proptosis and ecchymosis. A pressure bandage is enough to stop further hemorrhage. Hemorrhage takes about 3–4 weeks to absorb.
- *Orbital cellulitis:* Infection can be introduced along with the foreign body. Foreign body of wood spicule or stone is likely to set up cellulitis. Treat by broad-spectrum antibiotics and removal of foreign body.
- *Orbital granuloma:* Due to an organic foreign body.
- *Orbital neuralgia*: Trauma to infraorbital branch of the maxillary nerve.
- *Sinusitis:* Involvement of sinus causes sinusitis.
- *Cyst:* Traumatic cyst may develop following the orbital trauma.

Management

If the foreign body is of an inert material or is quiet with no reaction, then it is better to leave the foreign body in place as its removal may cause trauma to important structures which have escaped.

Remove the foreign body, if it is of wood or any organic matter. Course of broad-spectrum antibiotic is essential to prevent orbital cellulitis. An intraorbital foreign body especially near the apex can be removed by lateral orbitotomy.

Rupture of the Sclera

Patient presents with history of severe trauma covering the eye with hanky and palm as if supporting the eye.

Rupture of the sclera occurs due to a gross trauma usually due to a large blunt object being driven into the orbit between the globe and the orbital walls. Such trauma occurs commonly due to trauma by cow horn and stick. An eye having staphyloma, buphthalmos, or absolute glaucoma ruptures easily with less severe contusion trauma.

Site of indirect rupture of sclera due to trauma is almost constant. Rupture occurs concentric with limbus about 2–4 mm behind the corneoscleral junction, situated above the horizontal meridian in the upper and inner quadrant of the globe in large number of the cases.

Rupture usually extends to about 10–14 mm in length.

Clinical Features

1. Orbital hemorrhage with proptosis
2. Lids are swollen and show bruise
3. Ecchymosis (black eye) and subconjunctival hemorrhage
4. Tear in conjunctiva
5. Tear in the sclera with gap and prolapse of uveal tissue
6. Subconjunctival dislocation of lens
7. If the conjunctival tear is there, and it is large then lens and vitreous may be extruded over to cheek or lost.
8. Total hyphema.

Management

- With a severe trauma and large rupture, the prognosis is poor.

- An attempt should be made to preserve the eye and some vision as there are better facilities for operation and repair due to availability of microsurgery.
- In most cases, the ultimate result is phthisis bulbi, atrophic bulbi or rarely panophthalmitis.

Chemical Burn

There are large numbers of chemical irritants in form of solid, liquid and powder. Chemical irritants are available in chemical industries, laboratory, and even home. Thus, it is natural that chemical trauma has increased in its incidence. At the same time, the facilities for treatment has also improved. Some chemical irritants may cause a minor trauma in form of local symptoms of burning and redness while other can cause a severe damage to the eye.

Chemical agents which cause grievous trauma fall into two groups—*alkali and acid.*

1. Alkali Burn

Quite often the patient is the lab assistant or student who gets **alkali burn** *with ammonium hydroxide (liquid ammonia) while opening a tight cork of the bottle for conducting lab experiment as part of study.*

Alkali burns are caused by lime, caustic potash, caustic soda, and ammonia. The most common type of alkali burns encountered is from liquor ammonia or ammonium hydroxide.

Alkali has power to penetrate deep into the tissue, therefore, it causes more damage to the tissue in comparison to the acids.

2. Acid Burn

Quite often the patient is an employee of an automobile battery dealer who gets **acid burn** *due to spilling of sulphuric acid drop in the eye while handling the battery or acid.*

Acid burns are caused by inorganic acids like sulphuric acid, hydrochloric acid and nitric acid, the common acids in market.

Acid causes instant coagulation of all the proteins with formation of insoluble proteinates. There is coagulative necrosis which acts as a barrier for further penetration of acid deep into the tissue.

Thus, the damage caused by acid is much less in comparison to alkali. The lesion becomes sharply demarcated.

Ocular Features

- Ocular features depend upon the duration, strength and quantity of the contact of the chemical with the ocular tissue.
- Yet another factor is how fast the chemical has been neutralized by washing with water.
- Small drop or a particle excites minimal symptoms and signs in form of congestion, chemosis and burning of the eyes.
- Large quantity or a splash of chemical on the eyes is likely to cause a severe damage to the eyes.
- *Conjunctiva shows* congestion, chemosis, necrosis, discharge and later it heals with symblepharon.
- *Cornea shows* edema of the corneal epithelium, opaque cornea, necrosis of cornea and sloughing of cornea with formation of staphyloma later.

Management

- Wash the eye with plenty of water to neutralize the effect of chemical irritation to ocular tissue.
- Examine the eye thoroughly for any particle of chemical and remove it with swab or forceps.
- Excise necrotic pieces of conjunctiva, if any.
- Topical antibiotic, steroid and cycloplegic eyedrops and ointment.
- Topical eye ointment shall help prevent formation of symblepharon.
- If cornea is damaged beyond recovery, then plan for grafting. It is better to plan for grafting early as later vascularization of the cornea occurs.

Thermal Burns

Quite often, the patient is house wife or house maid who presents with thermal burn due to release of steam from pressure cooker and kettle or spilling or splash of any hot liquid or even lighted end of match stick or spark from fire work during festive season.

Domestic accidents can be prevented by a little awareness, protective glass and care.

Thermal burn can be either industrial or domestic accident in its nature. These can be caused by fire, scalds from hot liquid and steam, electric flash due to short circuiting and molten metal to name a few.

Anything which is hot in any form can give rise to a thermal burn. Clinical feature varies with the degree of the temperature and quantity of the material which has come in contact.

Fire Burns

There are blisters on the lids with charring of eyelashes and the eyebrows. In some cases, the lid margin and lower part of the conjunctiva gets involved.

Eyeball is protected due to lids.

Scalding

Scalding of the eye and face is common with domestic liquids and gases. Most common is the hot water and steam from geyser, kettle, pressure cooker or from a splash or spilling of hot liquid

Usually, the eye is protected by lids. If there is exposure of the eye to hot liquid, then there is marked conjunctival congestion with chemosis and edema of the cornea.

Electric Flash

Most common type of thermal trauma from electric current is due to an electric flash of short circuiting during work or repair of electrical line.

It causes nearly similar clinical picture to that of fire burn.

Management

Treatment of thermal burn depends on the grade of burn. If there is burn of skin of the lids, then it is better that a surgeon dealing in burns may be involved for better treatment of burn case.

Topical antibiotic, steroid and cycloplegic eyedrops and ointment as required.

Radiational Trauma

Amateur patients present with history of watching solar eclipse and skiing on snow mountains without protective goggles.

Eclipse Blindness

- Eclipse blindness occurs due to looking at the solar eclipse.
- Due to concentration of *infrared radiation* at the macula.
- Usually, bilateral but may be unilateral, if the person has looked at the solar eclipse with one eye closed.
- Complains of photopsia, chromatopsia and positive scotoma.
- Ophthalmoscopy shows changes at the macula in form of edema, fine hemorrhages and degeneration as yellow spots.
- Early systemic and topical steroids are helpful.

Snow Blindness

- Snow blindness is seen in mountaineers who are exposed to bright sunlight which is reflected from snow at high altitude in clear weather.
- Due to *ultraviolet radiation* which cause damage to the cornea.
- Immediate or early symptoms are photophobia, feeling of foreign body sensation, lacrimation, blepharospasm, burning with intense pain in the eye.
- Ocular examination shows conjunctival congestion, chemosis with edema of corneal epithelium.
- Fluorescein staining may show partial or complete staining of cornea due to desquamation of the corneal epithelial cells.
- *Management*: Topical antibiotic eyedrops and ointment with analgesics and sedatives to make the patient sleep to provide relief from intense pain. It resolves completely in 24–48 hours.

Index

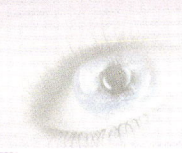